USING BASIC STATISTICS
IN THE
BEHAVIORAL SCIENCES

2nd Edition

USING BASIC STATISTICS
IN THE
BEHAVIORAL SCIENCES

Annabel Ness Evans

Concordia College (Edmonton)

Prentice-Hall Canada Inc.,
Scarborough, Ontario

Canadian Cataloguing in Publication Data
Evans, Annabel Ness
  Using basic statistics in the behavioral
sciences

2nd ed.
Includes index.
ISBN 0-13-928656-X

1. Statistics. 2. Psychology – Statistical methods.
I. Title.

QA276.12.C65 1992   001.4'22   C91-094031-2

© 1992 Prentice-Hall Canada Inc., Scarborough, Ontario

ALL RIGHTS RESERVED

No part of this book may be reproduced in any form without permission in writing from the publisher.

Prentice-Hall, Inc., Englewood Cliffs, New Jersey
Prentice-Hall International, Inc., London
Prentice-Hall of Australia, Pty., Ltd., Sydney
Prentice-Hall of India Pvt., Ltd., New Delhi
Prentice-Hall of Japan, Inc., Tokyo
Prentice-Hall of Southeast Asia (Pte.) Ltd., Singapore
Editora Prentice-Hall do Brasil Ltda., Rio de Janeiro
Prentice-Hall Hispanoamericana, S.A., Mexico

ISBN 0-13-928656-X

Acquisitions Editor: Michael Bickerstaff
Developmental Editor: Maurice Esses
Production Editors: Dick Hemingway and Maurice Esses
Production Coordinator: Anna Orodi
Design: Gail Ferreira Ng-A-Kien
Cover Design: Olena Serbyn
Figures: Greg Dorosh
Typesetting: Compeer Typographic Services Limited

1 2 3 4 5 RRD 96 95 94 93 92

Printed and bound in the U.S.A. by R.R. Donnelley and Sons Company

To Peggy Runquist

Overview

CHAPTER 1 Introduction to Statistical Concepts 1
CHAPTER 2 Organizing and Presenting Data 26
CHAPTER 3 Describing the Central Tendency of Distributions 56
CHAPTER 4 Describing the Variability of Distributions 76
CHAPTER 5 Describing the Position of Scores in Distributions 91
CHAPTER 6 Introduction to Inference: The Normal Curve 103
CHAPTER 7 Introduction to Inference: Probability 115
CHAPTER 8 Introduction to Inference: The Random Sampling Distribution 133
CHAPTER 9 Inference with the Normal Curve 156
CHAPTER 10 Inference with the t-Distribution 184
CHAPTER 11 Inference with the F-Distribution 218
CHAPTER 12 Analysis of Variance with Repeated Measures 259
CHAPTER 13 Multiple Comparison Procedures 293
CHAPTER 14 Inference with the Chi-Square Distribution 308
CHAPTER 15 Additional Non-Parametric Techniques 329
CHAPTER 16 Pearson's Correlational Technique 355
CHAPTER 17 Predictive Techniques 373
CHAPTER 18 Choosing the Appropriate Test of Significance 397
APPENDIX A Toolbox 412
APPENDIX B Statistical Tables 432
APPENDIX C Exercises for MYSTAT Software 447
Answers to Selected Exercises 462

Table of Contents

Preface   xix

Acknowledgements   xxii

CHAPTER 1   Introduction to Statistical Concepts   1
   Learning Objectives   1
   Statistics as Tools in the Research Process   2
      The Role of Statistics in Research   2
   Descriptive Statistics   2
   Inferential Statistics   3
   Correlational and Predictive Statistics   4
   Preliminary Concepts   4
      Constants versus Variables   4
      Classifying Variables   4
   Introduction to Statistical Symbolism   7
      Variables versus Constants   7
      Notation   7
   Conducting Research in the Behavioral Sciences   9
      Measurement Methods   9
      Interpreting Research Outcomes: Validity   10
      Factors Affecting Internal Validity   11
      Factors Affecting External Validity   13
      Designing the Study   14
   Using Computers in Statistics   16
   Focus on Research   19
   Summary of Terms and Concepts   21
   Exercises   22

CHAPTER 2   Organizing and Presenting Data   26
   Learning Objectives   26
   Organizing Raw Data   27
   Presenting Raw Data   28
      Presenting Data in a Table: The Frequency Distribution   29
      Presenting Data in a Graph   34

The Shape of Univariate Frequency Distributions   41
    Symmetry   41
    Kurtosis   43
Focus on Research   44
Summary of Terms and Concepts   48
Exercises   49

CHAPTER 3   Describing the Central Tendency of Distributions   56
Learning Objectives   56
Three Measures of Central Tendency   57
    Mode   57
    Median   57
    Mean   57
Calculating Measures of Central Tendency   57
    Mode   57
    Median   59
    Mean   63
Interpreting Measures of Central Tendency   64
    Mode   64
    Median   65
    Mean   65
Shape and Measures of Central Tendency   67
    Symmetrical Distributions   67
    Skewed Distributions   67
Comparing Measures of Central Tendency   68
    Sensitivity to Score Position in a Distribution   68
    Resistance to Sampling Function   69
The Mean of Combined Subgroups   69
Summary of Terms and Formulas   71
Exercises   72

CHAPTER 4   Describing the Variability of Distributions   76
Learning Objectives   76
Three Measures of Variability   77
    Range   77
    Variance   77
    Standard Deviation   77

Calculating Measures of Variability   77
   Range   77
   Variance and Standard Deviation   77
Interpreting Measures of Variability   82
   Range   82
   Variance   82
   Standard Deviation   83
The Variance and Standard Deviation of Combined Subgroups   84
Focus on Research   85
Summary of Terms and Formulas   87
Exercises   88

CHAPTER 5   Describing the Position of Scores in Distributions   91

Learning Objectives   91
Percentile and Percentile Ranks   92
   Percentiles   92
   Percentile Ranks   92
Calculating Percentiles and Percentile Ranks   93
   Percentiles   93
   Percentile Ranks   94
The Z-Score   95
Calculating Z-Scores   95
Properties of a Z-Distribution   96
   The Mean   96
   The Variance and Standard Deviation   97
   The Shape   97
Using Z to Locate Scores in a Distribution   97
Summary of Terms and Formulas   99
Exercises   100

CHAPTER 6   Introduction to Inference: The Normal Curve   103

Learning Objectives   103
Empirical vs Theoretical Frequency Distributions   103
The Normal Curve   104
   The Equation for the Standard Normal Curve   104
   Properties of the Standard Normal Curve   105

Using the Normal Curve to Solve Problems   106
    Finding Areas under the Curve   106
    Finding Z-Scores with the Curve   108
    Working with Empirical Data That Are Normally Distributed   109
Summary of Terms and Concepts   113
Exercises   113

CHAPTER 7 Introduction to Inference: Probability   115

Learning Objectives   115
Simple Probability   116
Conditional Probability   117
Probability of Compound Events   119
    Probability of A and B   119
    Probability of A or B   120
Methods of Counting   122
    Permutations   122
    Combinations   124
Binomial Probability   125
Frequency Distributions as Probability Distributions   127
Summary of Terms and Formulas   129
Exercises   130

CHAPTER 8 Introduction to Inference: The Random Sampling Distribution   133

Learning Objectives   133
Statistical Inference   134
    Descriptive vs Inferential Statistics   134
    The Random Sample   134
The Random Sampling Distribution   135
The Random Sampling Distribution of the Mean   136
    The Mean   137
    The Variance   137
    The Standard Deviation   137
    The Shape: The Central Limit Theorem   138
    Solving Problems with the Random Sampling Distribution of the Mean   139

The Random Sampling Distribution of the Difference between
  Means   142
    The Mean   143
    The Variance   143
    The Standard Deviation   144
    The Shape   145
    Solving Problems with the Random Sampling Distribution of the
      Difference   145
The Random Sampling Distribution of a Proportion   148
    The Mean   148
    The Variance   149
    The Standard Deviation   149
    The Shape   149
    Solving Problems with the Random Sampling Distribution of a
      Proportion   150
Summary of Terms and Formulas   152
Exercises   153

CHAPTER 9   Inference with the Normal Curve   156

Learning Objectives   156
Hypothesis Testing and Interval Estimation   157
Confidence Intervals Using the Normal Distribution   158
    Setting up the Confidence Interval for a Population Mean   158
    Setting up the Confidence Interval for the Difference between
      Population Means   161
    Setting up the Confidence Interval for a Population
      Proportion   162
Hypothesis Testing with the Normal Curve   163
    Types of Hypotheses   163
    The Logic and Procedure for Testing a Conceptual
      Hypothesis   164
    Testing an Hypothesis about a Population Mean   170
    Testing an Hypothesis about the Difference between Population
      Means   172
    Testing an Hypothesis about a Population Proportion   174
Consequences of Statistical Decisions   176
    Statistical Significance   176
    Type I and Type II Errors   176
    Power   177

Assumptions Underlying Inference with the Normal Curve 179
Choosing the Appropriate Test of Significance 180
Summary of Formulas 181
Exercises 181

CHAPTER 10 Inference with the t-Distribution 184

Learning Objectives 184
The t-Distribution and Unbiased Estimates 186
Relationship between the Normal and the t-Distribution 187
Degrees of Freedom when Estimating Parameters 189
When to Use the t-Distribution 191
Confidence Intervals Using the t-Distribution 192
    Setting up the Confidence Interval for a Population Mean 192
    Setting up the Confidence Interval for the Difference between Independent Population Means 193
Hypothesis Testing with the t-Distribution 195
    Testing an Hypothesis about a Population Mean 196
    Testing an Hypothesis about the Difference between Independent Population Means 197
Assumptions Underlying Inference with the t-Distribution 198
Dependent or Correlated Samples 199
    Within Subjects Designs 200
    Matched Groups Designs 201
    When to Use Dependent Groups Designs 201
    t-Test for the Difference between two Dependent Samples 203
Power Revisited 206
Choosing the Appropriate Test of Significance 207
Focus on Research 210
Summary of Formulas 211
Exercises 212

CHAPTER 11 Inference with the F-Distribution 218

Learning Objectives 218
The F-Distribution 219
    Constructing the F-Distribution 220
    Characteristics of the F-Distribution 220
Using the F-Distribution 221
    Null and Alternative Hypotheses 221

One-Way Analysis of Variance   222
    Partitioning the Variance   223
    Calculating and Interpreting the F-Ratio   229
    Running a One-Way ANOVA   229
Two-Way Analysis of Variance   232
    The Logic of Two-Way ANOVA   233
    Partitioning the Variance   237
    Calculating and Interpreting the F-Ratios   242
    Running a Two-Way ANOVA   243
Assumptions Underlying Inference with the F-Distribution   248
Inferential Error   249
Choosing the Appropriate Test of Significance   249
Focus on Research   250
Summary of Formulas   253
Exercises   254

CHAPTER 12   Analysis of Variance with Repeated Measures   259

Learning Objectives   259
One-Way ANOVA with Repeated Measures   260
    Null and Alternative Hypothesis   260
    Partitioning the Variance   260
    Calculating the F-Ratio   263
    Running a One-Way ANOVA with Repeated Measures   264
Two-Way ANOVA with Repeated Measures on One Factor   266
    Null and Alternative Hypothesis   267
    Partitioning the Variance   267
    Calculating and Interpreting the F-Ratios   272
    Running a Two-Way ANOVA with Repeated Measures   273
    Interpreting a Two-Way ANOVA with Repeated Measures   278
Assumptions Underlying ANOVA with Repeated Measures   280
Choosing the Appropriate Test of Significance   281
Focus on Research   283
Summary of Formulas   285
Exercises   287

CHAPTER 13   Multiple Comparison Procedures   293

Learning Objectives   293
Controlling the Error Rate   293

A Priori or Planned Comparisons 294
A Posteriori or *Post-Hoc* Comparisons 296
    The Scheffé Method 296
    The Tukey Method 300
Focus on Research 302
Summary of Terms and Formulas 303
Exercises 304

CHAPTER 14   Inference with the Chi-Square Distribution 308

Learning Objectives 308
The Chi-Square Distribution 309
    Constructing the Sampling Distribution of Chi-Square 310
    Characteristics of the Chi-Square Distribution 310
Using the Chi-Square Distribution 311
    The Chi-Square Test for Goodness of Fit 311
    The Chi-Square Test for Independence 315
Assumptions Underlying Inference with the Chi-Square Distribution 318
Choosing the Appropriate Test of Significance 318
Focus on Research 321
Summary of Terms and Formulas 324
Exercises 325

CHAPTER 15   Additional Non-Parametric Techniques 329

Learning Objectives 329
The Mann-Whitney U Test 330
    Null and Alternative Hypotheses 330
    The U Statistic 330
    Running the Mann-Whitney U Test 331
The Wilcoxon Signed-Ranks Test 335
    Null and Alternative Hypotheses 335
    The T Statistic 335
    Running the Wilcoxon Signed-Ranks Test 336
The Kruskal-Wallis Test 339
    Null and Alternative Hypotheses 339
    The H Statistic 340
    Running the Kruskal-Wallis Test 340

The Spearman Rank-Order Correlation Test 342
    Null and Alternative Hypotheses 342
    The rho Statistic 343
    Running the Spearman Rank-Order Correlation Test 343
Choosing the Appropriate Test of Significance 345
Focus on Research 348
Summary of Terms and Formulas 348
Exercises 350

CHAPTER 16 Pearson's Correlation Technique 355

Learning Objectives 355
Correlation as a Descriptive Technique 356
Pearson's Product-Moment Coefficient of Correlation (ρ) 357
    Calculating the Coefficient of Correlation (ρ) 357
    Factors Influencing the Correlation Coefficient 360
    Interpreting the Coefficient of Correlation 362
Correlation as an Inferential Technique 363
    Null and Alternative Hypotheses 363
    Testing the Significance of the Correlation 364
    Assumptions Underlying Inference about Correlations 365
Other Correlation Coefficients 366
Focus on Research 367
Summary of Terms and Formulas 369
Exercises 369

CHAPTER 17 Predictive Techniques 373

Learning Objectives 373
The Regression Line 374
    Criterion of Best Fit 375
    The Regression Equation 376
    Using the Regression Equation for Prediction 380
Error of Prediction: The Standard Error of Estimate 381
Interpreting the Correlation in Terms of Explained Variance 382
Regression on the Mean 384
Multiple Regression Analysis 385
    The Multiple Correlation Coefficient 385
    Using Multiple Correlation for Prediction 386
    Partial Correlation 389

Focus on Research   390
Summary of Terms and Formulas   392
Exercises   394

CHAPTER 18   Choosing the Appropriate Test of Significance   397
Learning Objectives   397
Non-Parametric versus Parametric Analysis   397
Choosing the Appropriate Parametric Test of Significance   398
Choosing the Appropriate Non-Parametric Test of Significance   402
    Testing for Identical Rank-Order Populations   402
    Testing for Differences between Obtained and Expected Frequencies   405
Exercises   408

APPENDIX A   Toolbox   412
Toolbox of Computational Formulas   412
Toolbox of Test Summaries   422

APPENDIX B   Statistical Tables   432
Table B-1.   Areas under the normal curve   432
Table B-2.   Critical values of t   434
Table B-3.   Critical values of F   435
Table B-4.   Critical values of chi-square   439
Table B-5.   Studentized range points for Tukey test   440
Table B-6.   Critical values of Mann-Whitney U   442
Table B-7.   Critical values of Wilcoxon T   444
Table B-8.   Critical values of Spearman rho   445
Table B-9.   Critical values of r   446

APPENDIX C   Exercises for MYSTAT Software   447
Exercises   447
Solutions   454

Answers to Selected Exercises   462

Index   480

Preface

Like most graduate students in psychology, I had to master graduate-level statistics in a course designed to separate the "women from the girls." It was a course we approached with a great deal of fear and trepidation. Unlike most graduate students in psychology, I thoroughly enjoyed the course and learned a great deal. I was fortunate to have as an instructor Dr. Stan Rule, who obviously appreciated the elegance of statistical procedures, and his enthusiasm for the subject matter was contagious.

I began writing this book because I could never find a text that quite suited me. Many were too quantitative, with little space given to the underlying logic of statistics. Others used such complex notation and introduced so many arithmetic and algebraic derivations that my students were unable to see through the math and get any conceptual grasp of the topic. So, I decided to write up my lecture notes and use them as my basic text. Well, as things are wont to do, that initial step escalated into a major project and this book is the result.

I have tried to keep the style of the book casual. Students are wary of statistics at the outset and I have never understood why authors of stat books promote these fears through dry, awkward, and boring prose. I think that statistics are fun and I hope that this feeling comes through in my writing. A little humor can do a lot to relax an anxious reader.

Users of the book will notice the "Canadian content" in the examples. Of course "statistics are statistics are statistics," but since I am a Canadian and my students are for the most part Canadian as well, I saw no reason to use the "number of slam dunks made by Magic Johnson" as my data base when I could use the "number of shots on goal by Glenn Anderson" instead. In a similar vein, I tried to give equal time to each gender in my examples to avoid the stereotypical emphasis on the male found in most textbooks.

I do not emphasize mechanical number crunching or rote memorization in my course, and the book reflects this orientation by avoiding unnecessary notation and jargon. I am not particularly interested in ending up with a student who can run a t-test or an analysis of variance. What I am interested in is ending up with a student who knows which is appropriate and why. With the technology available today, a trained monkey can push a button to run a particular test of significance, but not even the most sophisticated computer can examine a set of data and decide how best to analyze them in order to answer the question posed by the researcher.

The book is organized according to the format I use in my classes. I begin with descriptive techniques and follow these chapters with several designed to prepare students for inference. Inferential statistics are difficult for students to understand and I find it worthwhile to spend a lot of time laying the groundwork before I introduce inference.

The decision to place the chapters on correlation and regression near the end of the text was more or less arbitrary. Some other texts introduce these techniques early on in the course of study. I find the placement of these topics a matter of personal preference. There is no reason why these chapters could not be covered just before Chapter 9 (Inference with the Normal Curve), since they can stand alone at that point.

What's New and Different about the Second Edition of the Textbook

It was very exciting to begin work on the second edition of *Using Basic Statistics in the Behavioral Sciences*. Prentice-Hall conducted a survey of various professors across the country who had used, or were familiar with, the book. The feedback was terrific and had a strong influence on how the second edition developed. I was surprised at the number of students in disciplines other than psychology who were using my book. This became apparent to me when I received the results of the survey. The respondents included psychologists, sociologists, political scientists, biologists, and medical teachers. I realized that their special needs for their unique areas of study would require serious consideration. Clearly my insular view of statistical analysis, as a psychologist, would have to change. I learned a lot about how other disciplines approach research and data analysis. As a result, I have included new topics here, expanded chapters there, and generally tried to accommodate the suggestions of respondents and reviewers.

Each chapter of the text now opens with a list of Learning Objectives. Additional exercises have been added to each chapter, and I have attempted to include more difficult and more realistic problems. Several chapters have been expanded to include the following topics: use of computers in statistics, research design and methodology, stem and leaf diagrams, planned comparisons, multiple correlation, and regression analysis. The treatment of power has been expanded to better inform students about the importance of this concept. Several sections have been reworked at the advice of reviewers.

Beginning in Chapter 9, a new section has been added to help students decide what the appropriate analysis is for a given set of data. As new tests are introduced, this section becomes increasingly more demanding. As a result, I hope that the students' skills at selecting the appropriate test will gradually be shaped to the point where they can decide among all of the tests of significance covered in the book. These skills are further emphasized in the new Chapter 18 (Choosing the Appropriate Test of Significance). It includes the charts that formerly appeared on the inside covers.

Real research studies from a variety of journals are introduced as Focus on Research sections throughout the text in order to give students meaningful exposure to contemporary issues in psychology, sociology, political science, and other disciplines. The articles themselves are not reproduced. Rather the problem and a brief discussion of the data, the variables, and the analyses are described. I have presented only that portion of the data analysis that is relevant to the particular chapter. I did not fundamentally alter the original data, although occasionally I translated certain statistics to suit the approach adopted in the text. (For example, if the R^2 statistic from a multiple correlation analysis was reported, I gave instead the square root, R, to conform to the textbook presentation of multiple regression analysis.)

Appendix A now consists of the Toolbox (the old Chapter 18), which many users of the first edition found so handy. Appendix B consists of several statistical tables. I have added a table of Values of r to supplement the table of Critical values of Spearman rho. Appendix C provides some exercises (with solutions) that are suitable for the MYSTAT software package. The appendices are followed by Answers to Selected Exercises so that students can check for themselves whether they arrived at the correct answer for some of the exercises at the end of each chapter. The inside cover of the book now presents a List of Greek Symbols Used in Statistics.

What's New and Different about the Supplements for the Second Edition

The first edition included a *Workbook* that encouraged students to work through statistical procedures in a step-by-step fashion. I suspect that one of the reasons I prepared a workbook was because so many textbooks today provide all sorts of "bells and whistles" to accompany the basic text. One of the reviewers of the first edition commented that students shouldn't have to purchase an additional book to get enough experience in solving problems. After I bridled a bit at this, I realized that the reviewer was quite right. A statistics textbook should stand alone. Therefore, for the second edition, I have incorporated the exercises from the former *Workbook* into the text itself. I have tried to shape problem-solving skills by starting with rather elementary exercises before proceeding to more difficult problems.

For the *Instructor's Manual and Test Item File*, I have changed some questions and added some new ones. Although I didn't have an empirically based way of eliminating or refining those questions from the first edition that were unclear or poorly conceived, I did have an intuitive basis for doing so. Each question is now headed by the relevant topic in the text, the chapter learning objective, and the type of skill required to answer it (recall or application). At the end of some of the chapters, I have added some challenging problems for advanced students. This supplement also contains transparency masters for illustrating lectures. The *Test Item File* is also available separately in computerized form.

A *MYSTAT Software Package* can also be ordered from Prentice-Hall Canada Inc. As mentioned above, Appendix C of the textbook provides some appropriate exercises for it.

Acknowledgements

I took my first undergraduate statistics course from Peggy Runquist, a professor in the Psychology Department at the University of Alberta. Although she was not a statistician by training, she had a "knack" for statistics. Her approach and style greatly influenced my own when it came time for me to teach a similar course. Peggy taught me that statistics can be a lot of fun to learn and to teach. I hope this book reflects that attitude.

Bob Cahoon of the University of Alberta's Faculty of Business conducted a meticulous edit of the first edition. I believe he found every glitch that my students and I had discovered, and a few more to boot. Bob's contributions to the revision of the book for the second edition are indeed appreciated. It's nice to have friends who grant such favors.

Several people reviewed the second edition, and I thank them for the generosity of their praise and for their constructive feedback. They are Raymond S. Carteen (The University of British Columbia), Robert Gray (Carleton University), Peter G. Kepros (University of New Brunswick), Mark Sandilands (The University of Lethbridge), and Gilles L. Talbot (Champlain Regional College). A special note of thanks to Mark Sandilands who gently reminded me of the difference between "infer" and "imply" and the difference between "alternate" and "alternative."

It's hard to believe that Janis Watkin, who helped me proof the galleys for the first edition, offered to take on this onerous task again. But she did and I am grateful to her.

I am grateful to the Literary Executor of the late Sir Ronald A. Fisher, F.R.S., to Dr. Frank Yates, F.R.S., and to the Longman Group Ltd., London, for permission to reprint Tables from their book *Statistical Tables for Biological, Agricultural and Medical Research* (6th edition, 1974).

Working with the people at Prentice-Hall continues to be a rewarding experience. I would like to thank Pat Ferrier and Maurice Esses for their commitment to this project. Dick Hemingway once again assisted in the production of the book.

And as always, I thank my students, who are by far the best judges of my work.

AE
Edmonton, 1991

CHAPTER 1

Introduction to Statistical Concepts

LEARNING OBJECTIVES

After reading this chapter you should be able to:
1. Describe the role of statistics in the research process.
2. List the three goals of descriptive statistics.
3. Define sample and population.
4. Describe what inferential statistics are used for.
5. Describe what correlational statistics are used for.
6. Describe what predictive statistics are used for.
7. Describe the difference between a constant and a variable and give an example of each.
8. Describe the difference between an independent variable, a dependent variable and an organismic variable. Provide an example of each.
9. Describe the difference between a continuous variable and a discrete variable using an example.
10. Describe a nominal variable and provide an example.
11. Describe an ordinal variable and provide an example.
12. Describe an interval variable and provide an example.
13. Describe a ratio variable and provide an example.
14. Describe the three measurement methods used by researchers to collect data.
15. Describe the difference between internal and external validity.
16. List and describe each of the factors that can threaten the internal validity of a research study.
17. List and describe each of the factors that can threaten the external validity of a research study.
18. Describe five research designs typically used by behavioral scientists.
19. Describe the use of N, X, X_N, f, Σ.

Statistics as Tools in the Research Process

Statistics are tools for summarizing data, measuring relationships between sets of data, or making inferences about a large set of data by studying a subset drawn from it. This book attempts to show students in the biological, behavioral, and social sciences how to *apply* statistics to problems in their particular area of inquiry. The study of statistics per se is a mathematical discipline, much like geometry or algebra. This text, however, concentrates on how to use these techniques, provided by mathematicians, as tools to help us solve problems, in the same way that we use a slide rule or any other mathematical aid.

The Role of Statistics in Research

In research, statistics form the bridge from a question to a conclusion. Researchers begin with a question they wish to answer or some hypothesis they wish to verify. This question or hypothesis is then reworded in terms of data or evidence that might help to answer the question or verify the hypothesis. This is where statistics often come into play, helping the researcher to simplify or summarize data so that they can more easily be examined. Statistics may be used to evaluate data to determine if they adequately represent what the researcher wants to study.

The final step in research is to interpret the statistical analyses of the data and to make conclusions about the original question asked or hypothesis put forward.

Statistics, then, are tools the researcher can use to present or interpret information. There are various statistical techniques used by researchers. We will class these, for the purposes of this text, into three broad categories: *descriptive statistics*, *inferential statistics*, and *correlational/predictive statistics*.

Descriptive Statistics

Frequently, researchers need to gather large amounts of data regarding a variety of events. For example, we may wonder how well Canadian students do on high school departmental exams or how the salaries of Canadian physicians compare with those of their U.S. counterparts. When we gather information about questions such as these we are soon overwhelmed by numbers. It is very difficult to look at masses of numbers and see any trend or meaning in them. We need to summarize these numbers so that we and others can make sense out of them. Descriptive statistics serve this purpose. They allow us to *describe* a mass of numbers in terms of general trends, to tabulate data, and to present data in graphic form.

Using the tools of descriptive statistics, a mass of numbers can be presented in an organized and meaningful way, and data can be simplified so that their general trends can be seen.

Whenever our goal is to summarize, present, or organize a set of numbers for the purposes of clarification for ourselves and others, we are using the tools of **descriptive statistics.**

Inferential Statistics

Suppose that you are a psychologist interested in human memory. Let's say that you want to know how many numbers people can remember when you read off a list of 20 numbers. One way to answer this question would be to go out and test everyone and, if you did this, you would certainly have your answer. It would, however, take a lifetime or more for you to test everyone everywhere. Let's consider a less global question.

How do Catholics feel about the ordination of women? To answer this question you could send a questionnaire to every Catholic and ask, but again this would be incredibly expensive and time-consuming. A way around these dilemmas would be to find out how well *some* people remember or how *some* Catholics feel about the ordination of women, and then to generalize the findings to the whole population. For example, let's consider a water analyst who has come to test your drinking water.

She takes a **sample** from your tap, prepares a slide from that sample, examines it under a microscope and then gives you her assessment of the water. Although she has not examined all of the water, but just a small sample of it, she infers from that sample to all the water. Inference works like this. We study a small sample in some detail and then we generalize to the entire set of observations, called the **population**, from which that sample was taken.

Most psychological research is interested in people, all people. Psychological research, however, is not conducted on the population at large but rather on some portion of it. Inferential statistics provide tools for generalizing to the population at large by studying only a small sample of it. When used carefully and under appropriate conditions, researchers can use these tools to make *inferences* about populations by examining samples taken from them.

We use **inferential statistics** whenever we wish to infer things about the population at large, from information taken from a small sample of that population.

> **Population:** The entire set of observations of interest.
> **Sample:** A subset of a population.

Correlational and Predictive Statistics

Everyday we notice relationships between things. For example, we all suspect that there is a relationship between studying time and grades. We know there is a relationship between diet and good health.

Researchers often need to describe relationships between things. The statistical tools that allow us to measure the strength of various relationships are called **correlational statistics.** Correlational statistics are descriptive when they describe the relationship between two entire sets of observations; they can also be used inferentially to infer from a sample the correlation in a total population.

A correlation often used by universities is the one between high school average and university performance. These two are related in that students with high grade 12 marks tend to do well in university. This kind of established relationship can be used in **predictive statistics**. If we know that school grades and college grades are related, then we can look at a student's school grades and *predict* how he or she will do in university. Predictive statistics provide tools for making predictions about an event based on available information. How well or how accurately we can predict depends on how strong the relationship is between the two sets of observations.

When we are describing a relationship between events or when we are predicting from one event to another, we are using **correlational** or **predictive statistics**.

Preliminary Concepts

Constants versus Variables

A **constant** is just that—*constant*! A constant is a characteristic of objects, people, or events that does not vary. The temperature at which water boils (100 degrees celsius) is a constant.

A **variable** is a characteristic of objects, people, or events that can take on *different* values. It can vary in *quantity* (e.g., height of people), or in *quality* (e.g., hair color of people). Variables can be classified in different ways.

Classifying Variables

Experimental Classification

A researcher may classify variables according to the function they serve in the experiment. An **independent variable** (IV) is one which the researcher usually controls. Its values are fixed by the experimenter.

For example, if I am interested in the effects of practice on problem solving, I might choose to give lots of practice problems to one group and only a few practice problems to a different group of people. After both groups have solved the practice problems, I could measure their performance on a new set of test problems. The independent variable is amount of practice and I have selected two values of that variable to use in my experiment.

A **dependent variable** (DV) is the one controlled (we hope) by the independent variable, not by the experimenter. The performance of my subjects on the test problems is my dependent variable. It is called dependent because we assume their test performance will *depend* on the independent variable (the amount of practice they received). Usually, in psychology research, the DV is some measure of performance, e.g., score on a test, preference measure, or reaction time.

There is a special class of variables that seem like independent variables but are not directly controlled by the experimenter. Age, gender and socio-economic status, for example, are **organismic variables**. A great deal of research uses these kinds of variables. Technically they are not IV's because, although experimenters can study them, they can not manipulate them. These variables are inherent in the organism and the researcher can only select groups of subjects who already possess certain levels of these variables.

> **Independent variable:** Variable controlled by the experimenter and expected to have an effect on the behavior of the subjects.
>
> **Dependent variable:** Some measure of the behavior of subjects and expected to be influenced by the independent variable.
>
> **Organismic variable:** Characteristic of the subject and not controlled by the experimenter.

In the example discussed above, I was interested in the effects of practice on problem solving. If I were also interested in whether practice influences younger people more than older people, I might decide to compare younger people who get lots of practice with those who don't, and older people who get lots of practice with those who don't. If this were the case, amount of practice is still my independent variable. Age would be a new variable in my study and it would be an organismic variable, since I don't assign subjects to age groups. Age is inherent in the organism. All I can do is select subjects of different ages for inclusion in my study.

The dependent variable may also be influenced by an organismic variable. In the example here, I may find that test performance is not only influenced by amount of practice but also by age. Younger people may benefit more than older people by the opportunity to practice.

Mathematical Classification

Variables may also be classified in terms of the number of mathematical values they may take on within a given interval. **Continuous variables**, in theory, can take on any value within an infinite series of possible values. Weight, for example, is a continuous variable since the possible values for weight are infinite. Similarly, height is a continuous variable. In fact, the values of these continuous variables are limited only by the sensitivity of our scales or rulers, not by the variable itself.

Discrete variables can take on only a certain defined set of values. Number of children per family is a discrete variable in that certain values are not possible (e.g., 1/2 or 1 1/2). Gender is also a discrete variable; male and female are the only values possible.

> **Continuous variable:** Theoretically can take on an infinite number of values.
>
> **Discrete variable:** Can take on a finite set of values.

Measurement Classification

Variables can be classified in terms of their scale of measurement. A **nominal variable** has values that differ only qualitatively. Eye color and gender are nominal variables. For simplicity, we may assign numbers to a nominal variable (e.g., male = 1, female = 2). These numbers, however, provide no quantitative information. The numbers on the sweaters of hockey players are nominal. They are used merely for identification, not to indicate any measure of quantity. We wouldn't claim that any player numbered 99, for example, was 9 times better than one numbered 11.

Ordinal variables have values which are ordered according to quantity. Values are assigned to reflect that order. If we rated students and numbered them from best (1) to worst (90), we would have an ordinal scale. The intervals between the values, however, may not be equal. The second and third rated students are not necessarily the same distance apart as are the first and second rated students.

Interval variables have values where the intervals between them are equal. The Fahrenheit temperature scale is a good example of an interval variable. The difference between 40 degrees and 50 degrees Fahrenheit is the same as the difference between 60 and 70 degrees; that is, 10 degrees. The interval variable has an *arbitrary* zero point. Zero degrees Fahrenheit does not mean zero temperature or the absence of heat; 80 degrees is not twice as hot as 40 degrees. IQ is another interval variable. A person with an IQ of 180 is not twice as smart as someone with an IQ of 90 because a zero IQ does not mean absence of intelligence.

Ratio variables are like interval variables but with a *true* or real zero point. Height, weight and the Kelvin temperature scale are examples of ratio variables. Distance is also a ratio variable. A field goal kicker whose maximum kick is 50 metres can kick twice as far as one whose maximum is 25 metres.

> **Nominal variable:** Has values which differ in quality only.
> **Ordinal variable:** Has values ordered by quantity.
> **Interval variable:** Has values ordered by quantity with equal sized intervals between each.
> **Ratio variable:** Like interval variables with a true zero point.

Introduction to Statistical Symbolism

Statistics has its own symbolic language and every statistician adds his or her own little idiosyncracies to the language of statistics. I am no exception.

In the beginning chapters of this text, pay particular attention to the symbols and abbreviations used. This will help avoid confusion later on.

Variables versus Constants

We will be using letters at the end of the alphabet to refer to variables, for example, X, Y, Z. Letters at the beginning of the alphabet are used to refer to constants, for example, a, b, c.

Notation

The use of upper case letters at the end of the alphabet is reserved for naming collective sets or groups of scores. We refer to the X distribution or the Y distribution of numbers, for example. Sometimes X has a subscript $_i$. X_i refers to a particular score in the X distribution; X_1 is the first score in the X distribution, X_7 is the seventh score. Do not use lower case x or italicized *x* when discussing a group of scores.

N is the total number of scores in a distribution. If my psychology class has 42 students, then N = 42.

X_N is the last score in a distribution. On the final exam in my psychology class, $X_N = X_{42}$. This refers to the particular score obtained by the 42nd student.

f refers to frequency, usually the frequency of a particular score in a distribution. If 13 students got 63% on the final exam in my psychology class, then the f for 63% is 13. Do not use upper case F when referring to frequency. F has a different meaning entirely.

Σ is a summation sign. ΣX instructs you to sum or add up all the scores in the X distribution.

> **N:** The total number of observations in a population distribution.
> **X_N:** The last score in the X distribution.
> **f:** The number of times a particular score occurred in a distribution—stands for frequency.
> **Σ:** Sign for summation.

Statisticians use a particular kind of notation when they are referring to a population of scores and a different notation when they are referring to a sample drawn from a population. Descriptive statistical techniques are used to describe entire populations and so population notation should be used. An *entire* population does not mean a huge population; rather it means the population of interest. Inferential statistics are used to make inferences from a sample to a population and so sample notation should be used. Although we won't be using sample notation until the chapters on inference, many text books introduce sample notation early. The table below presents some of the standard notation used by statisticians to refer to populations and samples. We will be using these in later chapters.

Sample Versus Population Notation

Measure	Sample	Population
Size	n	N
Mean	$\overline{X}$ or $\overline{Y}$	μ_x or μ_y
Standard Deviation	S or S.D.	σ
Variance	S^2 or Var.	σ^2

Conducting Research in the Behavioral Sciences

Some research is conducted in a **laboratory** setting under highly controlled conditions. Other studies are carried out in the **field**, a natural setting outside the laboratory. Each technique presents problems to the researcher. Laboratory research, because of its contrived nature, may produce outcomes that would not occur in a more natural setting. People and animals may behave differently in a laboratory than they do in their everyday environment.

Field research attempts to study naturally occurring behavior in its usual environment. The researcher has much less control over what goes on in a field study than in a laboratory study. Which approach is used depends in part on the research question to be answered. Often more pragmatic needs limit the choices of the researcher.

Regardless of the research setting, research in the behavioral and social sciences is typically concerned with measuring behavior, animal or human. Several methods of measurement are available to the researcher. We will examine three of the more common methods of measurement.

Measurement Methods

Observation

The **observation** of behavior as it occurs is one of the primary methods of measurement used by researchers in human and animal behavior. Much of what we know about animal behavior was gathered through observation in the field. Observational methods are used in laboratory settings as well. Watching children engaging in play behavior, perhaps from behind a one-way glass, is an example of observation in the laboratory.

Self Report

Much behavior is difficult or impossible to observe directly. People's attitudes about things, for example, can't really be observed but we can ask people what their attitudes are. To measure human sexual behavior, Kinsey used self report rather than observation, which was the method chosen by Masters and Johnson. **Self report** is the method most often chosen by researchers interested in attitudes, beliefs, personality, feelings, etc. Because subjects are reporting on their own subjective inner states, and because it is often difficult to corroborate self report data, we must be careful when we interpret the results of research using this method of measurement.

Survey research gathers self report data with a questionnaire: a standard set of questions given to a large number of people. Opinion poll research is an example of this. The researcher selects a large sample of people, measures their opinions on various issues, and generalizes to the population at large.

There is always some probability of a sampling error that would bias the outcome, and survey researchers must make every attempt to construct samples that are representative of the population.

Some studies collect self report data through a one-on-one interview, often with a structured set of questions. The advantage of an interview is that the researcher can vary the questions depending on answers to previous questions. This provides the flexibility that a mail-out questionnaire lacks.

Standardized Tests

There are many psychological, educational, and sociological tests that have been standardized on a large population and can be used to assess an individual compared to those standards or norms. This method of measurement is typical in educational settings where test performance is used to predict future performance after some sort of educational experience or training. Standardized tests are also commonly used in psychotherapeutic settings to help with diagnoses of psychological pathology.

It's important to recognize that a single administration of a standardized test to an individual is not normally enough information for accurate prediction or diagnosis. **Standardized tests** must be corroborated by other measurements.

Interpreting Research Outcomes: Validity

Applying a statistical procedure to a set of numbers is the easy step in the research process. Deciding which procedure is appropriate for the particular data in hand requires expertise in both research design and statistics. But perhaps even more crucial is the interpretation of the statistical outcome and this issue we will address here. Good researchers are careful to design their studies so that the results can be accurately interpreted. It is necessary to carefully control the research situation so that the results can be attributed to the variables manipulated by the researcher rather than to some other reason. In other words, alternative explanations for the outcome must be ruled out. This is achieved by good research design. If the researcher fails to anticipate what the controlling variables are in a study, then her interpretation of which variables are responsible for the outcome may be faulty. The researcher may well believe that the outcome was a result of a particular variable and may be unaware of other variables operating that affected the data. When this occurs, we say the study lacks validity. Studies can also lack validity when the results do not generalize to other situations or to other subjects. A statistically significant outcome from a study does not guarantee that the finding has any importance in the real world.

We say that a research study is valid if (1) the outcome was dependent upon the variables specifically studied and (2) the findings generalize to other situations and subjects. The former is called **internal validity** and the latter is called **external validity**.

Factors Affecting Internal Validity

An internally valid study is one where the outcomes of importance are a result of the variables manipulated by the researcher. For example, a nursing supervisor who concludes from a study she conducted that casual clothes, rather than uniforms, worn by her nurses promote a feeling of well-being in her aged patients, must be sure that the change in dress was the responsible variable, rather than something else. Suppose that her nurses were more relaxed in casual clothes than when in uniform and the patients responded favorably. It could be important for the supervisor to realize that the change in attitude on the part of the nursing staff was the critical variable rather than the change in dress. When designing studies researchers must keep in mind several factors that can influence the internal validity of their work.

Proactive History

Many research studies compare performance of different groups of subjects who have been treated differently in some way. Perhaps one group got a special kind of training and the other group got a different type or no training at all. The object is to show that the training was the influencing factor on performance. It is important that the different groups were initially equivalent before the training was given. If the groups were not equivalent then differences following training may be due not to the training but to the inherent differences in the groups themselves. **Proactive history** then, refers to all the differences subjects bring with them into the investigation.

Imagine that the Scouting Association conducted a study to determine if scout training influenced social responsibility in young boys. Suppose they found that scouts were more socially responsible than non-scout boys. Their conclusion that scouting experience was responsible for this difference could well be faulty. Boys who join scouts may well be different to begin with than boys who do not. If the groups (scouts and non-scouts) were indeed initially different, it would be inappropriate to conclude that scout training had an effect on social responsibility.

The most common procedure for controlling the effects of proactive history is random selection of subjects and random assignment to groups.

Retroactive History

Certain events can occur during the time that the research study is conducted that may influence the behavior of the subjects involved. Suppose that a sociologist sends out a questionnaire to compare the attitudes of Torontonians and Vancouverites on the issue of capital punishment. Further suppose that during this period of time, a particularly gruesome killing in Vancouver had stimulated a great deal of media attention. The results of the study might show that Vancouverites have different opinions about capital punishment than do Torontonians. If the researcher was unaware of the events in Vancouver, his interpretation of the results of his study might be faulty. Indeed had he conducted the study at a different time he might have found quite a different outcome. One of the reasons why many researchers use animal rather than human subjects is that it is so much easier to control differences in history with animals.

Retroactive history is of particular concern to researchers conducting long term investigations.

Maturation

Developmental differences in subjects during the course of a research study can affect internal validity. As you might imagine, this is of particular concern in long-term research with children. A finding that children do better at solving math problems after receiving 6 weeks of special training must be carefully evaluated since the maturation of the children may be responsible wholly or in part for the finding rather than the special training itself. The use of an appropriate control group is the best way to deal with the influences of **maturation**.

Testing

Testing plays an important role in many research studies. A pre-test is often used to measure performance level before some special training is given. A post-test follows training to determine if the training had an effect. Sometimes the initial pre-test itself can affect performance and this obscures the role of the training on the post-test scores. For the study to be internally valid the researcher must find ways to ensure that the training, not the pre-test, was responsible for the performance differences following training.

Attrition (Experimental Mortality)

Attrition means the differential loss of subjects from certain groups in a research study. Subjects may be lost for a variety of reasons. If this loss is particularly great for one group, then internal validity may be reduced. A researcher interested in the effects of behavioral intervention with alcoholics might choose to compare two groups—a "problem drinking" group with a "chronic alcoholic" group. Subjects are trained in behavioral principles in order to help them control their drinking over a period of six months. Suppose that several members of the "chronic alcoholic" group dropped out of the study for health reasons. This is an example where the internal validity of the study is threatened because we might expect that the results would have been different had the drop-outs been able to continue in the study.

Investigator Bias

Experimenter or **investigator bias** is an issue of great concern in research today. The expectations of even the most conscientious experimenter may unintentionally influence the results of the study. One way to control for such a bias is through a double-blind control procedure where neither the individual collecting the data nor the subject participating in the study is aware of the hypotheses or expected outcomes.

Factors Affecting External Validity

An externally valid study is one where the findings have generality to subjects and situations other than the specific ones studied. Discovering that a third year anthropology student behaves in a specific way in a highly contrived laboratory context is not all that helpful if this behavior does not occur for most people in most settings. This is where we may ask the question "Is the finding really 'significant' in the real world?" Researchers must consider several factors that can influence external validity when they plan their studies.

Sampling Bias

In research we often study a **sampling** of subjects with the objective of generalizing from the sample to the population from which the sample was drawn. Such generalizations have validity only if the sample from which the generalization is made is indeed representative of the population being generalized to. One way of increasing the likelihood that the sample is representative of the population is to randomly select the subjects to be included in the sample. Unfortunately, much of the time random selection is not possible. Psychological research, for example, is often conducted on samples of university students. If university students are different in important ways from the general population, then research outcomes from such studies may not have validity in the real world.

The problems researchers face when designing studies are many. To increase the likelihood of internal validity one often has to relax concerns about external validity and vice versa. The research design itself provides the best opportunity for increasing validity.

The Hawthorne Effect

Subjects who participate in an investigation may behave differently simply because they are singled out for special treatment. The specific treatment may not be responsible for the outcome but rather the awareness on the part of subjects that they are participating in a study. This phenomenon is known as the **Hawthorne effect**.

One way to avoid this effect is to use deceptive techniques so that subjects are not aware they are participating. Obviously this is not always possible or desirable, but researchers do attempt to limit the information available to subjects about the nature of the study.

Designing the Study

The choice of a research design is made for a variety of reasons, some of which are pragmatic. Most of us would be delighted to be able to always design research where threats to internal and external validity are eliminated. Unfortunately this is not always possible. Available resources, the nature of the research question, and other variables can limit our choices about design. As long as we are aware of the problems with various designs we can temper our conclusions about our findings accordingly. A poor design does not necessarily mean poor research. Accurate and fair interpretation of the results is the critical feature of good research.

Experimental Designs

Earlier in this chapter we discussed the experimental classification of variables by the role they play in an experiment. In an experiment the investigator systematically manipulates an independent variable(s) and measures some aspect of behavior (the dependent variable) to see if the IV influenced behavior. Typically subjects are randomly assigned to an experimental group, which receives the IV, or to a control group, which does not receive the IV. Assuming the two groups were initially equivalent, the experimenter can compare their performance. If differences occur it can be concluded that they were *caused* by the IV manipulation. This type of research design, called **experimental design**, is the cornerstone of psychological research and is the only design where cause and effect can unequivocally be determined.

The researcher choosing to conduct an experiment has many decisions to make. She must decide what independent variable she wishes to investigate and what dependent variable she will measure, and she must consider the potential influence of factors other than the independent variable that might affect performance. In other words, if variables other than the ones chosen for study, often called *extraneous variables*, influence performance, then her interpretation of the effect of the IV is made much more difficult. Imagine a researcher interested in the effects of alcohol on reaction time in a simulated driving test. She might be wise to consider factors such as previous experience with alcohol and driving competency when she decides how to assign subjects to groups. Researchers using people as subjects must continually guard against the influence of extraneous variables such as differences in motivation, attention, and ability when they design their experiments. These problems help us understand why controlled laboratory experiments and animal subjects are often preferred by some researchers.

Many research questions, however, do not lend themselves to an experimental design. Medical research, in particular, often is limited by ethical issues that make true experimentation impossible. Suppose you were interested in the effects of computer radiation on fetal weight gain in pregnant women. This is a research problem that would best be studied with a correlational design.

Correlational Designs

Correlational designs attempt to measure the relationship between two or more variables. Subjects are not randomly assigned to an IV or control group; rather they already have either been exposed or not been exposed to the IV. A researcher who studies a sample of pregnant women who work on computers every day as part of their jobs and another sample of pregnant women who do not use computers is using a correlational design. He would compare the weights of the newborns born to the computer-using women with the weights of the children born to the control group to see if a relationship exists. Suppose the weights of the computer-group babies are lower. The researcher might not be able to prove conclusively that the lower weights were caused by computer radiation. But if he had carefully controlled other possible variables that might produce the difference, he could be fairly confident that a causal relationship exists.

Because correlational designs do not unequivocally determine cause and effect, and because ethical considerations limit the use of the experiment in human subjects, many health related questions are studied with animal populations. Generalizing from animals to humans, however, requires caution.

Case Study Designs

The case study is the design of choice for many investigators of personality and mental illness. Freud, for example, used this technique to gather the data he used to develop his theory of personality and psychopathology. You might be interested to know that Freud's theory of personality and personality development was based on case study research of adults in psychotherapy. He rarely studied "normal" adults or children. He based his ideas about childhood development on the recollections of his adult patients!

A **case study** is an in-depth biography of a specific individual. The researcher will use a variety of methods of measurement often including observation, self report and standardized tests. This design allows for a much more extensive set of data about an individual.

Cross-Cultural Research Designs

Cross-cultural designs are used for research comparing the behavior patterns of different cultures. All of the methods of measurement we have discussed may be used. For example, a recent study compared the performance of American teens on a standardized math test with the performance of teen students in six other countries. The American students performed worst and Korean students performed best. Interestingly enough, the American students were the most likely to believe they were good in math while the Koreans were the least likely to hold such beliefs.*

---

* Krauthammer, C. (1990). Education: Doing bad and feeling good. *Time* (Feb. 5, 1990), 78.

Evaluation Research Designs

Evaluation of educational, therapeutic, and social programs is an important part of the research process. **Evaluation research designs** are much more prevalent today than in the past. It was not uncommon, a few years ago, for governmental, educational and other kinds of programs to be introduced with little or no attempt made to evaluate the efficacy or cost-effectiveness of the program. For example, about 15 years ago I was employed to evaluate a social services program that had been operating for several years. It was designed to help severely handicapped individuals learn basic skills of daily living. I discovered quite quickly that when the program had initially been designed, there were no provisions made for evaluation. In other words, the program developers failed to build into the program any methods of measuring whether goals were being met or not. No systematic data collection occurred. I was forced to inform the administrators that their program's success or failure in meeting its goals could not be evaluated.

Quite recently, on the other hand, I was asked to be an evaluation consultant for a program that was not yet developed. This permitted me to be involved in the initial planning of the program, thereby ensuring that appropriate measures would be taken to allow for future evaluation of the program's effectiveness. Psychologists and sociologists are finding themselves more and more frequently acting as evaluation consultants.

Using Computers in Statistics

Computer technology has been a real boon to statisticians. It is a rare researcher who analyzes data by hand these days. Even hand-held calculators are sophisticated enough to do a wide variety of analyses. Many of you probably own calculators and now is a good time to go back to your instruction booklet and learn how to use the various functions of your calculator. Most medium priced calculators will sum a list of numbers, sum the squares of those numbers, calculate means and standard deviations, and run a simple t-test and correlation test.

For many of you the first step in using a computer to help with statistical analyses is to learn how to use a **spread sheet**. A spread sheet is an elaborate electronic calculator that can do an enormous number of arithmetic and statistical manipulations, almost instantaneously. You enter the data and you create formulas to do certain things and you use the built-in functions to do other things. Once a formula is created the spread sheet will automatically perform the arithmetic indicated in the formula.

Let's look at a simple example of what a spread sheet might be used for. Imagine I have the scores of ten students who took a statistics test with a maximum obtainable score of 65. Here are the data.

Raw Scores/65
52
15
50
29
25
59
23
22
25
19

Let's put these data into a spread sheet.* We will have it perform a variety of arithmetic manipulations on these numbers including computing the class average, converting each score into percentage, determining the highest and lowest score, and counting the number of scores. All of the above manipulations, with the exception of converting to percentage, are built-in functions that most spread sheets already know how to do. I used a formula to tell the spreadsheet how to convert the raw scores into percentage scores. Here is the spread sheet showing the actual formulas and functions that will be performed.

Table 1-1 Example of a spread sheet: formulas and functions

July 10 90

Column A	B	C
1		
2	Raw Scores/65	%
3	52	=B3/65*100
4	15	=B4/65*100
5	50	=B5/65*100
6	29	=B6/65*100
7	25	=B7/65*100
8	59	=B8/65*100
9	23	=B9/65*100
10	22	=B10/65*100
11	25	=B11/65*100
12	19	=B12/65*100
Average	=Average(B3:B12)	=Average(C3:C12)
Total number	=Count(B3:B12)	=Count(C3:C12)
Top score	=Max(B3:B12)	=Max(C3:C12)
Bottom score	=Min(B3:B12)	=Min(C3:C12)

---

* Microsoft Works

The information in boldprint was first entered into the spread sheet. Under the % sign I instructed the program to find the number in Row 3-Column B. You can see that number is 52. The formula continues to instruct the program to divide that number by 65, the maximum on the test, and multiply the ratio by 100 to give percentage. On the lower left of the table are the built-in functions I used. For example, to compute the class average all I had to do was indicate which values are to be included in the computation. You can see that the program will compute the average of all the scores found in column B from Row 3 to Row 12. Once these formulas and functions are in place, it's a matter of a key stroke to get the results. Here is the spread sheet showing the solutions to everything I asked for.

Table 1-2   Example of a spread sheet: calculations

Column A Row	7/10/90 B Raw Scores/65	C %
3	52	80.00
4	15	23.08
5	50	76.92
6	29	44.62
7	25	38.46
8	59	90.77
9	23	35.38
10	22	33.85
11	25	38.46
12	19	29.23
Average	31.9	49.08
Total number	10	10
Top score	59	90.77
Bottom score	15	23.08

Even with such a small set of data a spreadsheet is very useful. With large data sets, it is invaluable. It isn't possible here to teach you how to use a spread sheet but it is well worth your time learning to do so. Knowing how to use a spread-sheet gives you a lot of flexibility in custom-tailoring the analyses you want to do on a set of data.

Many statistical analyses are standard techniques that don't vary from one set of data to another and there are commercially available programs you can use. Not long ago the best statistics packages would only run on a main-frame computer. The most popular ones include SPSS (Statistical Package for the Social Sciences), SAS (Statistical Analysis System) and MINITAB.

There are versions of these programs available today for most micro-computers. In addition to these packages there are numerous smaller statistics programs. It may well be worth your time to learn about the programs available. Which one you choose of course depends on your needs as well as the type of micro-computer you own or use. I own a MacIntosh SE/30 and I use two statistics programs regularly. One is called StatWorks. I seldom work with large sets of data and this program suits my needs quite well. The second program I use is called SYSTAT and is more sophisticated than StatWorks. The statistical package available with this text book, MYSTAT, is a version of SYSTAT. In Appendix C are several problems set up to be solved with your MYSTAT program.

FOCUS ON RESEARCH

A cross-cultural study of marital communication and marital distress was reported by Halford, Hahlweg, and Dunne (1990).* They examined the problem-solving behaviors of happily married and unhappily married couples from Germany and from Australia.

The Data
The couples were rated on a variety of categories during a ten-minute problem-solving discussion. The content of the utterance (verbal interaction) and non-verbal cues such as facial expression and tone of voice were used to rate the interactions between couples.

The Variables
The rating categories included the following:
DE: Direct expression such as expression of feelings, constructive proposals etc.
AA: Acceptance of spouses utterance and agreement with spouse.
NI: Neutral information such as neutral question or request for clarification.
CR: Critique such as personal criticism.
RF: Refusal such as denial of responsibility or disagreement.

The Analyses
An initial descriptive analysis of the type of interactions by culture and marital satisfaction was performed. Some of the results are presented below.

It was found that unhappy couples engaged in higher rates of negative behaviors than happy couples. Some cultural differences were apparent with the German sample showing higher rates of negative verbal behaviors such as criticism and refusal than the Australian sample. The researchers concluded that important cultural differences exist in the types of interactions between married couples.

---

* Halford, W.K., Hahlweg, K., and Dunne, M. (1990). The Cross-Cultural Consistency of Marital Communication associated with Marital Distress. *Journal of Marriage and the Family*, 52, 487–500.

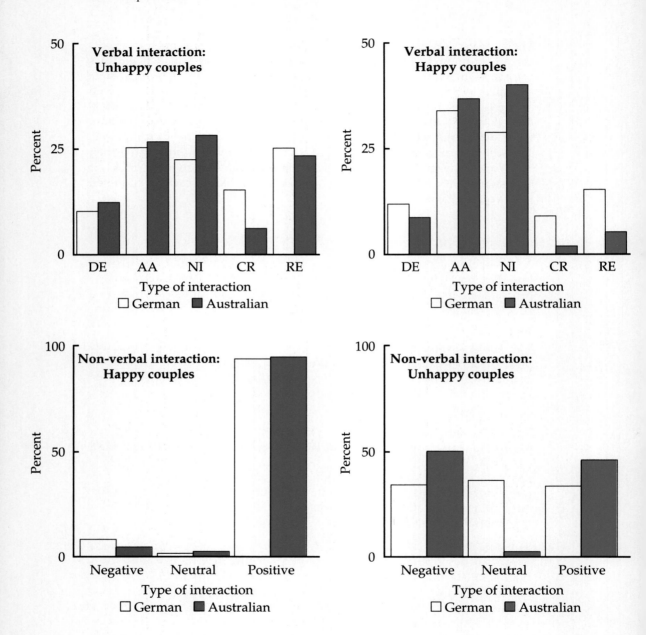

Figure 1-1 Type of interaction by culture and marital satisfaction

Source: Adapted with permission from Halford, Hahlweg, and Dunne (1990). Copyright 1990 by the National Council on Family Relations, 3989 Central Ave. N.E., Suite 550, Minneapolis, MN 55421.

SUMMARY OF TERMS AND CONCEPTS

Descriptive statistics describe the characteristics of an entire set of data, called a **population**.

Inferential statistics use **sample** data to make inferences about populations.

Relationship and **predictive statistics** describe the relationship between X and Y or predict Y from X.

Variables take on more than one value but **constants** take on only one value.

Independent variables are **experimental variables** used by the experimenter to cause changes in **dependent variables**.

Continuous variables may have an infinite number of values but **discrete variables** have a finite set of values.

Nominal variables have values which differ in name only, whereas **ordinal variables** have values that are ordered with respect to quantity.

Interval variables have equal intervals between values and an arbitrary zero point.

Ratio variables are like interval variables with real zero points.

X refers to a set of scores as in the X distribution.

N is the total number of scores in a distribution.

f refers to the frequency of a score in a distribution.

Σ is a summation sign. It is an instruction to sum a set of scores as in ΣX.

Research in the behavioral sciences is conducted both in the **field** and in the **laboratory**.

Researchers gather much of their data through **observation**, **self report**, and **standarized tests**.

A research study is **internally valid** if the outcome was dependent upon the specific variables involved in the study. A research study is **externally valid** if the findings generalize to other situations and other subjects.

Factors that affect internal validity include **proactive** and **retroactive history**, **maturation**, **testing**, **attrition**, and **investigator bias**. Factors that affect external validity include **sampling bias** and subject awareness (called the **Hawthorne effect**).

Common research designs include **experimental designs, correlational designs, case studies, cross-cultural designs,** and **evaluation research designs**.

The use of computers and **spread sheets** has greatly facilitated the analysis of statistical data.

EXERCISES

1. DATA: $X_1, X_2, X_3, \ldots, X_N$

   Describe what you can say about these data if they were measured on a(n):
   a. nominal scale of measurement
   b. ordinal scale (in order from low to high)
   c. interval scale (in order from low to high)
   d. ratio scale (in order from low to high)

2. In a horse race, *Two and a Juice* came first, *Dynamite* came second, and *Beetlebomb* came third.
   a. What scale is involved?
   b. If we report that *Two and a Juice* won by a length and *Dynamite* beat *Beetlebomb* by three lengths, what kind of scale do we have?
   c. If we report the time to run the race for the three horses, what kind of scale do we have?
   d. If we report the post position of each horse, what kind of scale do we have?

3. For each of the following, indicate which category of statistics is most likely involved. Choose from descriptive, inferential, correlational, and predictive.
   a. A researcher wonders if higher income Canadians are more likely to be in favor of free trade with the United States than lower income Canadians. In other words, she wonders if income and attitude about free trade are related.
   b. A researcher wonders how Albertans feel about the free trade issue. He interviews a selected group of Alberta residents.
   c. A researcher is interested in whether being abused as a child has an effect on whether that person later abuses his own children. He gathers data about the childhood experiences of abusing parents and non-abusing parents.
   d. A researcher stationed in a local mall asked every tenth person who passed her whether he or she bought anything that day and from which shop. She wants to compare the popularity of the various shops in the mall.
   e. A professor has given the first midterm exam in his first-year anthropology course and wants to present the results to his students.
   f. A researcher is hired as a consultant to help with the screening of applicants to police training school. She uses a standard psychological test to determine emotional and psychological health.

4. Label each of the following as a variable or a constant.
   a. the highest temperature of the day in Toronto (as measured at the airport) on July 18, 1991
   b. the number of children delivered in 1990 at the Royal Victoria Hospital in Montreal
   c. the religious affiliation of students at the University of New Brunswick
   d. student gender at a preparatory school for boys
   e. species of bird spotted by the Winnipeg Bird Society's annual Bird Watching Extravaganza

5. For each of the following decide which is the independent and which is the dependent variable.
   a. reaction time slows down with increasing blood-alcohol level
   b. policemen trained in conflict mediation are more effective in domestic crisis control
   c. effective study strategy training improves student grades
   d. political labels influence how people perceive the motives of the politician
   e. babies fed on demand gain weight faster than babies fed on a schedule
   f. aerobic exercise improves physical fitness over no exercise

6. Label each of the following as discrete or continuous.
   a. academic aptitude
   b. number of students in psychology courses
   c. reaction time
   d. temperature
   e. socioeconomic class
   f. academic degree
   g. age
   h. gender
   i. dress size

7. A researcher wants to study the effects of three different brands of pain reliever on perceived pain relief. He gives one of the three brands to different groups of subjects suffering from chronic headache. He asks all subjects to rate the effectiveness of the drug on their headaches. What is the independent variable and what is the dependent variable?

8. Label the following as nominal, ordinal, interval or ratio.
   a. grading system using A, B, C, F
   b. number correct on a quiz
   c. fur colour of dogs
   d. numbers on football jerseys
   e. type of housing in an urban centre

f. gender
g. age
h. psychopathological diagnosis (i.e. neurotic or psychotic or personality disorder)
i. the ten healthiest Canadian cities to live in based on weather, pollution, crime rate etc.

9. Answer the following questions about the distribution of scores below.
DATA: 23, 10, 9, 8, 8, 8, 8, 6, 4, 4, 2
   a. $N = ?$
   b. f for the score value 8 is?
   c. $X_8 = ?$
   d. $X_N = ?$

10. Label each of following according to the measurement method used.
   a. A biologist spends her summers in the outback studying the habits of the ground squirrel.
   b. A sociologist joins a cult to gather information on their practices and rituals without the members being aware of her purpose.
   c. A public health nurse interviews new mothers in their homes to determine the need for more in-hospital education.
   d. A grad student in education sends a questionnaire to city teachers to determine their satisfaction in their jobs.
   e. A researcher in the department of Native Studies gives a standard IQ test to children on a reserve in the far north.
   f. A speech pathologist sits in on a regular class of special needs children to determine the need for formal speech assessment.

11. List any factors that might threaten the internal validity of the research described below and explain how validity might be threatened.
A professor has come to believe that his lectures are boring and need more pizzaz. In particular he thinks he needs to use more humor in the classroom. He decides to conduct an investigation. In his 8:00 am class he continues with his normal lecturing style. In his 11:00 am class he injects several jokes throughout his lecture. Otherwise he treats the two classes the same way. After a few weeks of this, he has his students assess his lectures with an evaluation form.

12. List any factors that might threaten the internal validity of the research described below and explain how validity might be threatened.
An elementary school teacher, having just returned from a seminar in innovative teaching strategies, decides to try out her new skills on her students. She assesses their performance after two weeks of innovative instruction.

13. List any factors that might threaten the internal validity of the research described below and explain how validity might be threatened.

An elementary school teacher, having just returned from a seminar in innovative teaching strategies, decides to try out her new skills on her students. She assesses their performance before and after two weeks of innovative instruction.

14. List any factors that might threaten the internal validity of the research described below and explain how validity might be threatened.

A gerontologist investigated a new drug that purports to improve memory performance. He decides to study three different age groups (40–50 yrs, 60–70 yrs, and 80–90 yrs). He randomly selects fifty people in each age group and randomly assigns half of them to an experimental group and the other half to a control group. The experimental subjects from each of the three age groups are administered daily doses of the drug for a period of two years. The control subjects receive a placebo. None of the subjects know whether they receive the placebo or the drug. Every three months a standard memory test is given to all subjects by an assistant of the gerontologist who is unaware of which group the subject is in.

CHAPTER 2

Organizing and Presenting Data

LEARNING OBJECTIVES

After reading this chapter you should be able to:

1. Describe the difference between a univariate and a bivariate frequency distribution.
2. Describe how a simple frequency distribution is constructed.
3. Construct a simple frequency distribution from a given set of data.
4. Define absolute, relative, and cumulative frequency.
5. Describe the conditions where relative frequency is preferred over absolute.
6. Describe the conditions where cumulative frequency is used.
7. Describe how a grouped frequency distribution is constructed. Construct a grouped frequency distribution from a given set of data.
8. Explain when a grouped frequency distribution is used.
9. Define mutually exclusive interval, mid-point, and width.
10. Describe how a bar graph is constructed. Give an example of the kind of data suitable for depiction in a bar graph.
11. Obtain exact limits for a given score or interval.
12. Describe how a histogram is constructed. Give an example of the kind of data suitable for depiction in a histogram.
13. Describe the difference between a histogram and a frequency polygon.
14. Describe how an ogive is constructed and why it is used.
15. Describe how a scattergraph is constructed and why it is used.
16. Construct a bar graph, histogram, stem and leaf diagram, frequency polygon, ogive, and scattergraph for a given set of data.

17. Describe symmetry in a frequency distribution and provide an example sketch.
18. Describe a positively skewed distribution and provide an example sketch.
19. Describe a negatively skewed distribution and provide an example sketch.
20. Describe the difference between a platykurtic and a leptokurtic distribution and provide an example sketch.

In research, we frequently find ourselves with a great many numbers about some event. Only rarely can we simply "scan" these raw data and make any sense out of them. We must organize our numbers into some form that is consistent and understandable not only to us, as data collectors, but also to anyone else who might be examining the data that we have collected.

Organizing Raw Data

Imagine a researcher who wishes to compare two different high schools in terms of grade 12 student performance on a standardized achievement test. Here are the data.

					97	96	
						94	78
90				76			
	82	75					
		79	70			68	
	69						
65	66						
		64	58				
	63	55					
						62	46

As you can see these data are not easily interpretable!

Options are available to the data collector for organizing these scores. He should, of course, organize first by school. Within each school he can organize by value of the variable. In other words, he can list all the scores, from highest to lowest. Alternatively, he can organize by subject name, or **subject number** if he has assigned numbers to his test participants. As long as his technique is consistent, either method is fine for the initial organization of his data.

Table 2-1 Organizing by value

Holly H.S.	Rally H.S.
97	96
94	78
90	76
82	75
79	70
69	68
65	66
64	58
63	55
62	46

Table 2-2 Organizing by subject number

Subject	Rally H.S.	Subject	Holly H.S.
1	46	1	82
2	75	2	64
3	66	3	90
4	78	4	69
5	76	5	94
6	55	6	62
7	68	7	79
8	70	8	63
9	58	9	97
10	96	10	65

Although the above example has only 20 data points, this initial organization is hard to interpret. We cannot, at a glance, tell which school seems superior. Imagine the chaos if there were hundreds of scores. Clearly, we need ways to organize data to present our findings.

Presenting Raw Data

Often researchers are called upon to report or present their data in journals or at conferences. Psychologists, as well as researchers in other disciplines, have several conventions that they follow for uniformity. This makes it easier for readers of reports and for convention audiences. Raw data that are organized for the purpose of presentation are ordered by values of a variable and by group. We do not present data by subject number in most cases.[1] There are two ways of presenting raw data, by table and by graph.

Presenting Data in a Table: The Frequency Distribution

A frequency distribution is a table indicating the values that a variable can take on and the frequency with which each value occurs.

Types of Frequency Distributions

There are two basic types of frequency distributions. A **univariate frequency** distribution has one variable; each subject contributes one observation. A **bivariate frequency** distribution has two variables; each subject contributes two observations.

Table 2-3 Univariate frequency distributions

Score on Exam	Frequency (f)
90	2
89	0
88	4
87	3
86	1

Notice that two students received scores of 90 and no one received an 89 on the exam.

Table 2-4 Bivariate frequency distributions

		\multicolumn{4}{c}{Score Value Variable One}

		Score Value Variable One			
		71	72	73	74
Score Value Variable Two	9	1	2	0	0
	8	1	0	3	0
	7	3	0	2	2
	6	0	1	4	3
	5	4	4	1	3

Notice that one subject scored 9 on Variable Two and 71 on Variable One, whereas no one got a 71 and a 6.

---

[1] Data are often presented by subject number when the researcher has used a single-subject design rather than a groups design. This is usually the case in the field of psychology called Experimental Analysis of Behavior.

Forms of Frequency Distributions

There are several different forms typically used to present data in a frequency distribution. The particular form a researcher selects will depend on the type of measurement, the number of values, and the purpose for presenting the data. We will look at two basic forms.

Simple Frequency Distributions To construct a **simple frequency distribution,** we list all possible values of the variable in a column and indicate the frequency of each value in a second column to the right. All possible values of the variable must be listed, including those that may not have actually occurred. If the variable is nominal the values may be listed in any order. With ordinal, interval and ratio data the values are listed from highest to lowest. All tables should be labeled with a number and a title and this label placed above the table. These are simply conventions that we follow for uniformity. Table 2-5 is an example of a simple frequency distribution of a hypothetical statistics class for the 1986 semester.

Table 2-5   Simple frequency distribution of statistics grades

Grade	f
9	2
8	0
7	4
6	7
5	8
4	6
3	2

Frequently, we want to compare groups. Perhaps I would like to compare the performance of my class with a class taught by a different instructor. If the two classes are of different sizes, **relative frequency** rather than **absolute frequency** is preferable. If, for example, I have a class of 50 students that I wish to compare with another class of 150 students, it is difficult to do so using absolute frequency. To say that 10 of my students received 9's compared to 20 students in my colleague's class would not tell us very much because of the huge difference in class size. In such a case it is much easier to interpret relative or proportionate frequency. For example, it means much more when I say that 20% of my class earned 9's but only 13% of my colleague's students did so.

> **Absolute frequency:** The number of times a score occurs in a distribution.
>
> **Relative frequency:** The number of times a score occurs in a distribution, divided by the total number of scores.

Relative frequency is extremely useful when we are comparing groups of different sizes. Relative frequency is also preferable when we are describing the performance of a single group of an unusual size. Reporting that 43% of 147 people think that day care should be heavily subsidized by the government is more meaningful than reporting the absolute frequency of 63. Always keep in mind that the purpose of presenting data is to make it easy for your reader or audience to see the trends in your results. The following table shows how we would present my statistics grades using relative frequency reported in decimal form.

Table 2-6 Simple frequency distribution of statistics grades

Grade	Rel f*
9	0.07
8	0.00
7	0.14
6	0.24
5	0.27
4	0.21
3	0.07
Total	1.00

There is a third way to report frequency. **Cumulative frequency** is used when we are interested in determining relative standing at a glance.

> **Cumulative frequency:** Summing frequencies from the bottom of a frequency distribution up for each value or interval.

---

* This column must add up to 1.00

Cumulative frequency distributions add the frequency of each value to the total frequency below. Absolute or relative frequency may be used. Table 2-7 shows my statistics grades reported using absolute cumulative frequency.

Table 2-7 Simple frequency distribution of statistics grades

Grade	cf*
9	29
8	27
7	27
6	23
5	16
4	8
3	2

A quick glance at this distribution tells us that 23 of my 29 statistics students received grades of 6 or less. As you can see, this type of frequency is useful for determining relative standing. A student who received a 6 in the course can see that she performed better than at least 16 of the students.

Reporting the cumulative frequency in relative frequency form produces a relative cumulative frequency distribution. Again we would translate to relative frequency if we were comparing groups or if our group size was unusual. With a cumulative relative frequency distribution we are able, at a glance, to determine what proportion of the group obtained a particular score or below that score. Table 2-8 presents the grades of my statistics class using cumulative relative frequency.

Table 2-8 Simple frequency distribution of statistics grades

Grade	Rel cf**
9	1.00
8	0.93
7	0.93
6	0.79
5	0.55
4	0.28
3	0.07

---

* The top value in the cumulative frequency column must equal the group size.

** The top value in any cumulative relative frequency distribution must always be 1.00 since the entire group must have received the top score or below.

A student who received an 8 in this course sees, at a glance, that he performed as well or better than 93% of the class. This type of distribution, then, is helpful for quickly determining the location of a particular score in a distribution.

Grouped Frequency Distributions Any simple frequency distribution lists all possible values of the variable, even those that did not occur. Often there are too many possible values for a simple frequency distribution to be practical. For example, a typical variable used in schools is percentage. If one student got 0 and another got 100 on a test, a simple frequency distribution of these data would require listing all 101 values in a column. In situations like these we often prefer to group data for the sake of clarity. As a rule of thumb, whenever there are more than 20 values of the variable, or when there are a large number of zero values in our data, a grouped frequency distribution is preferable.

To construct a **grouped frequency distribution,** the values are grouped into equal-sized intervals. These intervals are then listed from highest to lowest. Intervals must be **mutually exclusive**; each score belongs in one interval only.

When selecting an interval **width**, it is helpful to use an odd-sized rather than an even-sized one. This makes finding **mid-points**, which we will do shortly, much easier.

> **Mutually exclusive interval:** Non-overlapping interval in a grouped frequency distribution such that each score belongs in one interval only.
>
> **Width:** The range of each interval in a grouped frequency distribution.
>
> **Mid-point:** The middle value of an interval in a grouped frequency distribution.

The following data (hypothetical) are the number of goals scored by 20 hockey players in a Canadian league in a single season. Let's use these data to construct a grouped frequency distribution. We will do this in a step-by-step manner.

DATA: 64, 63, 57, 56, 55, 54, 47, 46, 45, 45, 45, 44, 43, 37, 36, 34, 34, 23, 23, 15

Step 1. Determine how many *possible* values exist. The span of our data is 50 values (i.e., from 15 to 64). There are too many values for a simple frequency distribution to be practical. We would have a column of 50 numbers if we chose to do this.

Step 2. Decide how many intervals to use. It is conventional to use between 10 and 20 intervals. We will use 10.

Step 3. Determine the interval width. The symbol for width is **i**. We have already decided that we want to have 10 intervals, so we must determine what width will give us 10 intervals. Since we have a range of 50 values, we can see that an interval width of 5 will produce what we want.

Step 4. List the intervals from highest to lowest in a column and the frequencies in a second column.

Table 2-9 Grouped frequency distribution of hockey goals

No. of Goals	f	Rel f	Cum f	Rel cf
60-64	2	0.10	20	1.00
55-59	3	0.15	18	0.90
50-54	1	0.05	15	0.75
45-49	5	0.25	14	0.70
40-44	2	0.10	9	0.45
35-39	2	0.10	7	0.35
30-34	2	0.10	5	0.25
25-29	0	0.00	3	0.15
20-24	2	0.10	3	0.15
15-19	1	0.05	1	0.05

If we look at the cumulative frequency and relative cumulative frequency columns, we can see at a glance that 14 hockey players or 70% of the hockey players scored 49 goals or less. These frequency distributions, then, are useful when we want to determine relative standing or location of a particular score in a distribution.

Presenting Data in a Graph

Frequency distributions can also be presented in graphic form. Many people find it easier to interpret data presented in a graph rather than a table.

Graphing Univariate Frequency Distributions

There are several conventions in graphing. These provide consistency in presentation.

1. Graphs are called figures.
2. The figure number and label are found below the graph.
3. Frequency is indicated on the ordinate (Y axis) and the values of the variable are on the abscissa (X axis).
4. A 3/4 rule is generally used (the ordinate should be 3/4 as long as the abscissa).
5. Break any axes which do not begin at zero.

There are several types of graphs. The one you select will depend upon your purpose and the type of data you have. Absolute, relative or cumulative frequency may be used.

Bar Graph The **bar graph** is used to present discrete data. Separate bars represent each value of the variable and the height corresponds to the frequency with which each value occurred. The bars are separated to indicate that the variable is discrete rather than continuous. Nominal and ordinal data are often presented in a bar graph.

Suppose that I am thinking of going into the dog breeding business. I decide to collect data about the popularity of some breeds of dogs. These data will help me decide what breeds to specialize in. I survey a large neighbourhood and determine the kinds of dogs people own in it. These data are nominal and should be depicted in a bar graph. See Figure 2-1.

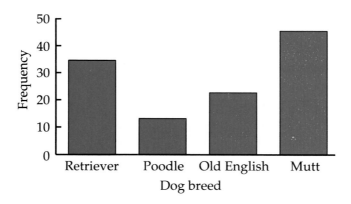

Figure 2-1 Popularity of dog breed

The bar graph can be used to depict ordinal data as well as nominal data. The values of the variable should reflect their natural order. A hypothetical survey of student attitude toward the legalization of marijuana provided the data for the graph in Figure 2-2. As you can see, relative frequency is on the ordinate or Y axis.

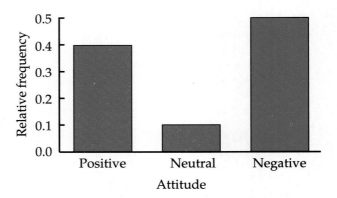

Figure 2-2 Attitude toward legalizing marijuana

Histogram The **histogram** is similar to the bar graph except the bars are attached to indicate that the data are continuous. To construct a histogram we need to learn a new term: **exact limits**. When data are continuous, exact limits are the precise beginning and end points of a score or an interval. To obtain the upper exact limit we add half of the smallest unit of measurement to the score or upper limit of the interval. To obtain the lower exact limit we subtract half of the smallest unit of measurement from the score or lower limit of the interval.

> **Exact limits:** The mathematically precise beginning and end points of a score or interval. Also called real limits.

For example, consider a bathroom scale which weighs to the nearest kg. The smallest unit of measurement, then, is 1 kg. I weigh 55 kg. The exact limits for my weight are 54.5 kg and 55.5 kg. If this procedure seems obscure, remember that my bathroom scale measures to the nearest kg. If, in reality, my weight was 54.62 kg, my scale would report my weight at 55 kg. If I weighed 55.43 kg, my scale would report me at 55 kg. When my scale says I weigh 55 kg, I may, in reality, weigh anything between 54.5 kg and 55.5 kg.

Here are some other examples.

Variable	Smallest Unit	Amount to + and −	Score or Interval	Exact Limits
Weight	1 kg	0.50 kg	56 kg	55.5–56.5 kg
Weight	0.5 kg	0.25 kg	50–53 kg	49.75–53.25 kg
Time	0.1 sec.	0.05 sec.	15.5 sec.	15.45–15.55 sec.

The way a number is written may tell you the precision of measurement. For example consider the numbers below.

$$2$$
$$2.0$$
$$2.00$$

These three versions of the number two indicate different levels of precision. The first version (2) indicates that we can only measure to the nearest whole number so that the exact limits for 2 are 1.5 and 2.5. The second version (2.0) indicates we can measure to the nearest one-tenth and so the exact limits are 1.95 and 2.05. The third version (2.00) indicates measurement to the nearest one one-hundredth and so the exact limits are 1.995 and 2.005. The smallest unit of measurement, then, may sometimes be determined by examining the way the number is written.

When constructing a histogram, the outsides of the bars are the exact limits and the middle of the bar is over the middle (**mid-point**) of the interval. A histogram may report the exact limits or the mid-point on the abscissa. I prefer to use mid-points because I think the graph looks better. Figure 2-3 presents student performance on a statistics exam.

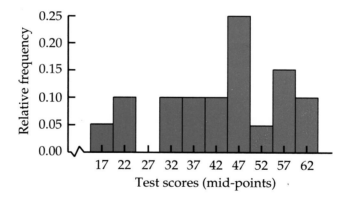

Figure 2-3 Student performance (histogram)

Notice that the abscissa is broken to indicate that the test score variable does not begin at zero. The histogram is a very useful graphing technique for continuous data. Most people have no difficulty interpreting data presented in a histogram.

When constructing a histogram or frequency polygon, mid-points are typically used to mark the abscissa. The bar or point is positioned over the mid-point to indicate the frequency for that interval. The actual raw scores then are not discernable, just the interval within which the scores fall.

Stem and Leaf Diagrams A very simple technique for presenting all the data from a distribution is called a **stem and leaf diagram** developed by Tukey (1977).* As you will see this produces something similar to a histogram.

To construct a stem and leaf diagram we break each score into a stem and a leaf. For example for the number 18, the stem would be 1 and the leaf would be 8. The number 92 would have a stem of 9 and a leaf of 2. Let's construct a stem and leaf diagram for the following data.

80	54	45	25
73	54	41	25
68	52	39	25
66	51	38	24
64	51	38	23
59	50	37	22
58	50	34	20
58	48	30	19
57	46	29	15
55	45	26	15

Since our numbers range from 15 to 80, we will list our stems (the numbers 1 through 8) on the left in a column. The leafs will be placed from left to right next to the appropriate stem. For example, the numbers 64, 66, and 68 all have the same stem so we place the stem (6) on the left and the three leafs (4, 6, and 8) to its immediate right. Here is an example of a stem and leaf diagram for our data.

```
1 | 5 5 9
2 | 0 2 3 4 5 5 5 9
3 | 0 4 7 8 8 9
4 | 1 5 6 8
5 | 0 0 1 1 2 4 4 7 8 8 9
6 | 4 6 8
7 | 3
8 | 0
```

As you read the diagram from left to right starting from the top you simply append each leaf with the stem to the left to find the values. You can see, for example, that we have two scores of 15 and one of 19. We may prefer to repeat the stems. This will spread our diagram out somewhat. We would place leafs from 0 to 4 next to the first stem and the leafs 5 to 9 next to the second stem. If we did that our diagram would look like the following.

---

* Tukey, J.W. (1977). *Exploratory Data Analysis*. Reading, MA: Addison-Wesley.

```
1 | 5 5 9
2 | 0 2 3 4
2 | 5 5 5 9
3 | 0 4
3 | 7 8 8 9
4 | 1
4 | 5 6 8
5 | 0 0 1 1 2 4 4
5 | 7 8 8 9
6 | 4
6 | 6 8
7 | 3
8 | 0
```

Repeating stems serves to stretch the diagram out. If you turn your head 90 degrees to the right, you will see that a stem and leaf diagram looks something like a histogram. It has the advantage that all the data points are readily visible. This technique has a second advantage of being easy for people to understand.

Frequency Polygon Data presented in a histogram may also be presented in a **frequency polygon**. Points are used instead of bars. When data are grouped, each data point is plotted over the mid-point of the interval; when data are in a simple frequency distribution, each point is plotted over the score value. The points are then connected by straight lines. Let's present the student performance data of Figure 2-3 in a frequency polygon.

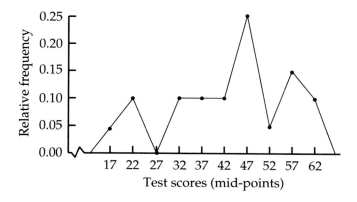

Figure 2-4   Student performance (frequency polygon)

It is customary to drop the line to the abscissa at the mid-point of the adjacent interval at both extreme ends. In this way, the polygon is formed.

Ogive I have seen the **ogive** called a *cumulative frequency polygon* which I find very strange, since it is not a polygon at all. This graph is constructed from a cumulative frequency distribution. It is appropriate for continuous data and is often used when we wish to locate score position. Questions like "How have I done compared to the rest of the group?" and "What score would I have needed to be in the top 10% of the group?" can be answered by inspecting the ogive. Cumulative frequencies are plotted as points directly over the *upper exact limit* of each score or interval and the points are connected by straight lines. The ogive below presents our data in cumulative frequency.

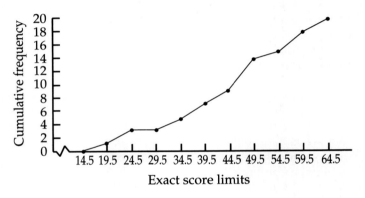

Figure 2-5   Student performance (ogive)

The ogive is useful for determining relative standing. A student who scored 49 on this exam can see, at a glance, that he performed as well or better than 14 of the 20 students in the class.

Graphing Bivariate Frequency Distributions: The Scattergraph

The graph used for bivariate frequency distributions is called a **scattergraph**. Recall that a bivariate frequency distribution has frequencies for two variables. Graphing these data can show us, at a glance, whether or not the variables are related or correlated.

The values of the first variable are located on the abscissa and the values of the second on the ordinate. Each subject contributes one point to the graph. The points are not connected.

As an example, imagine that I have collected sense of humor ratings and popularity ratings (provided by impartial judges) on 10 of my closest friends.

I want to find out whether these two variables are related. In other words, are my friends who are rated the most popular also rated as having a good sense of humor? The data might look something like this:

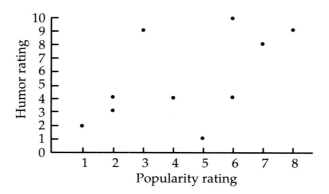

Figure 2-6 Ratings of sense of humor versus popularity

Each point represents the rating a friend got on the two variables. It looks as if there might be some relationship. Except for two individuals, those who are most popular seem also to have a good sense of humor.

A quick inspection of a scattergraph will give some indication of the degree of relationship between variables. There is a statistical technique which quantifies this relationship and we will be studying this in the chapters on correlation.

The Shape of Univariate Frequency Distributions

Univariate frequency distributions have two important shape characteristics: **symmetry** and **kurtosis**.

Symmetry

A **symmetrical distribution** is a mirror image about its center. Some examples of symmetrical distributions used in statistics are the *normal distribution* and the *t-distribution*. Rectangular and U-shaped distributions may also be symmetrical. Figure 2-7 shows what they look like graphically.

In a **skewed** distribution, the bulk of the observations (frequency) lies to one side. One side of the distribution is not a mirror-image of the other. Skewed distributions are described as having a positive or negative skew.

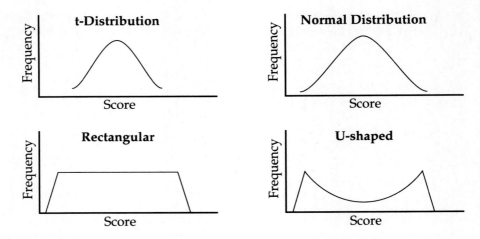

Figure 2-7   Examples of symmetrical distributions

When the extreme end or tail of the distribution points toward the positive side (the right) of the graph, we call this a **positive skew**. When the tail points to the negative or left side of the graph, we call this a **negative skew**. Examples used in statistics are the *Chi-square* and the *F-distribution*, both of which are positively skewed.

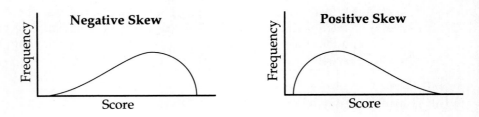

Figure 2-8   Examples of skewed distributions

> **Symmetrical distribution:** One which is a mirror image about its center.
> **Positively skewed distribution:** Graphically presented, a distribution with a tail pointing to the right of the graph.
> **Negatively skewed distribution:** Graphically presented, a distribution with a tail pointing to the left of the graph.

Kurtosis

Kurtosis is a shape characteristic describing the spread or scatter of the observations or scores. If each score has a similar frequency (i.e., occurred the same number of times), the distribution will look flat when it is graphed. Flat distributions are called **platykurtic** (think of the bill of a platypus). Distributions with lots of scores bunched in the middle are called **leptokurtic**.

> **Platykurtic:** Flat compared to the normal distribution.
>
> **Leptokurtic:** More peaked with more area in the tails than the normal distribution.

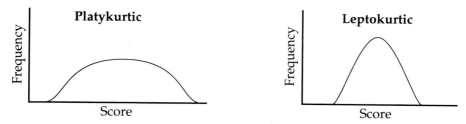

Figure 2-9 Distributions differing in kurtosis

Kurtosis is defined in relation to the normal distribution, which will be discussed later. Basically, a distribution which is flatter or more variable than the normal is platykurtic, and distributions which are less variable, with more area in the tails than the normal, are called leptokurtic.

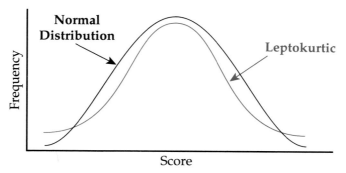

Figure 2-10 The normal distribution versus a leptokurtic distribution

FOCUS ON RESEARCH

Prentice-Hall Canada was about to begin production of the second edition of the statistics text book *Using Basic Statistics in the Behavioral Sciences*. The company sent out a questionnaire to 46 professors using the current edition to find out what kinds of changes should be made in the new edition. Here is a portion of the questionnaire.

Please respond to the following questions regarding your experience with the texbook entitled *Using Basic Statistics in the Behavioral Sciences*. Your input will help us in the preparation of the new edition.

1. What is the major area of study of your students?
   - psychology
   - sociology
   - education
   - political science
   - human resources
   - psychology/sociology combination
   - recreation/parks/tourism
   - physical education
   - nursing
   - general social sciences
   - social work
   - interdisciplinary
   - other

2. Please evaluate each of the chapters in the current textbook by checking the appropriate column below.

Chapter	retain	delete	expand	condense	no response
1					
2					
3					
4					
5					
6					
7					
8					
9					
10					
11					
12					
13					
14					
15					
16					
17					
18					

3. Please give your opinion about the following topics as possible additions to the second edition of the book.

Topic	Add	Don't Add	Don't Know
combinatorics			
design/methodology			
analysis of covariance			
split-plot analyses			
multiple regression			
other			

4. Are you satisfied with the way the current text book is organized?
   Yes   No   No opinion

Data obtained from a questionnaire must first be organized in some systematic way. Prentice-Hall initially counted the number of responses in each of the categories for each question asked.

These are some of the results from the survey.

1. psychology   16
   sociology   10
   education   5
   political science   3
   human resources   1
   psychology/sociology combination   3
   recreation/parks/tourism   1
   physical education   1
   nursing   2
   general social sciences   1
   social work   1
   interdisciplinary   1
   other   1

2. Please evaluate each of the chapters in the current textbook by checking the appropriate column below.

Chapter	retain	delete	expand	condense	no response
1	33	1	10	0	2
2	32	1	9	3	1
3	36	1	6	3	
4	33	1	7	5	
5	32	2	4	7	1
6	28	1	13	4	
7	24	3	11	8	
8	32	1	8	5	
9	37	1	6	2	
10	35	2	5	4	
11	28	2	8	7	1
12	20	7	6	10	3
13	19	5	9	9	4
14	34	1	9	2	
15	20	5	12	72	
16	29	1	14	2	
17	27	1	17	1	
18	31	3	5	3	4

3. Please give your opinion about the following topics as possible additions to the second edition of the book.

Add topic	yes	no	no opinion
combinatorics	6	39	1
design/methodology	21	24	1
covariant analysis	9	37	
split-plot analysis	5	41	
multiple regression	23	23	
other	17	28	1

4. Are you satisfied with the way the current text book is organized?

Yes	No	No opinion
38	7	1

Forty-six people were surveyed in this research. The best way to present the final data might be to use relative or percent frequency rather than absolute frequency as presented above. Some of the data might best be presented graphically. Here is a summary of the Prentice-Hall findings that might be prepared by a statistician.

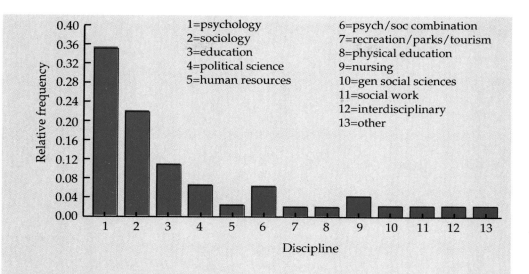

Figure 2-11 Proportion of respondents choosing each discipline (question 1)

2. Percentage of respondents choosing each evaluatory description.

Chapter	Evaluation				
	retain	delete	expand	condense	no response
1	71.74	2.17	21.74	0.00	4.35
2	69.57	2.17	19.57	6.52	2.17
3	78.26	2.17	13.04	6.52	0.00
4	71.74	2.17	15.22	10.87	0.00
5	69.57	4.35	8.70	15.22	2.17
6	60.87	2.17	28.26	8.70	0.00
7	52.17	6.52	23.91	17.39	0.00
8	69.57	2.17	17.39	10.87	0.00
9	80.43	2.17	13.04	4.35	0.00
10	76.09	4.35	10.87	8.70	0.00
11	60.87	4.35	17.39	15.22	2.17
12	43.48	15.22	13.04	21.74	6.52
13	41.30	10.87	19.57	19.57	8.70
14	73.91	2.17	19.57	4.35	0.00
15	43.48	10.87	26.09	15.22	4.35
16	63.04	2.17	30.43	4.35	0.00
17	58.70	2.17	36.96	2.17	0.00
18	67.39	6.52	10.87	6.52	8.70

3. Percentage of respondents in each opinion category. Which topics should be added?

	Yes	No	No opinion
Combinatorics	13.04	84.78	2.17
Design/methodology	45.65	52.17	2.17
Covariant analysis	19.57	80.43	0.00
Split-plot analysis	10.87	89.13	0.00
Multiple Regression	50.00	50.00	0.00
Other	36.96	60.87	2.17

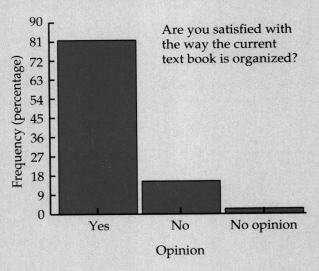

Figure 2-12 Percentage responses on text organization (question 4)

SUMMARY OF TERMS AND CONCEPTS

Raw data are initially organized by **subject number** or from the highest to the lowest value of the variable.

Data are often presented in tables, called **univariate** and **bivariate frequency distributions**.

A **simple frequency distribution** lists all possible values of the variable in a column accompanied by the frequencies with which each value occurred. **Absolute**, **relative**, and **cumulative frequency** may be used.

A **grouped frequency distribution** is used for data which have been grouped into equal sized intervals. The intervals, which must be **mutually exclusive**, are listed in a column accompanied by the total frequency of values within each.

Discrete variables are presented graphically in a **bar graph**. The separation of the bars indicates the discreteness of the data.

Continuous variables may be presented in a **histogram** or a **frequency polygon**.

A **stem and leaf diagram** is easily constructed and similar to a histogram.

The **ogive** is used to present cumulative frequency data and is useful for locating scores, graphically.

Bivariate data are presented in a **scattergraph**. The scattergraph provides a visual display of the relationship between the variables.

Symmetrical distributions have a left side which is a mirror image of the right.

Positively skewed distributions have the bulk of the frequency on the left side; **negatively skewed distributions** have the bulk of the frequency on the right side.

Distributions that are flatter than the normal distribution are **platykurtic**; distributions that are more peaked with more area in the tails than the normal are **leptokurtic**.

EXERCISES

1. DATA: Listed below are the weights of 100 women enrolled in a fitness program.

85	131	122	88	129	86	123	94	136	90
100	119	115	103	117	101	116	109	124	105
105	103	103	108	101	106	104	114	108	110
116	93	90	119	91	117	91	125	98	121
118	108	114	121	106	119	115	127	113	123
128	100	129	131	98	129	130	137	105	133
133	111	96	136	109	134	97	142	116	138
150	130	132	153	128	151	133	159	135	155
154	104	110	157	102	155	111	164	109	159
97	136	116	100	134	98	117	106	141	102

   a. Construct a simple frequency distribution of the data.
   b. Construct a grouped frequency distribution in which the interval width (i) is 5 and the lower limits of the intervals are multiples of 5.

c. From the grouped frequency distribution construct a frequency polygon. Use mid-points on the abscissa and absolute frequency on the ordinate. Label both axes and break the abscissa or ordinate if appropriate.
d. From the grouped frequency distribution construct a histogram. Use mid-points and relative frequency. Label both axes and break them when necessary.
e. From the grouped frequency distribution construct an ogive. Use exact limits and label axes.

2. Twenty-five Canadian cities participated in a crime prevention program designed to educate citizens about ways of protecting themselves against theft. The following data are the average number of thefts reported each week before and after the program was completed.

Before
66, 57, 56, 48, 48, 48, 42, 41, 41, 40, 39, 35, 34, 33, 32, 31, 31, 30, 30, 29, 26, 24, 24, 21, 20

After
50, 46, 41, 40, 40, 40, 39, 39, 33, 31, 30, 29, 28, 26, 25, 25, 24, 24, 23, 22, 22, 20, 19, 18, 17

a. Construct a grouped frequency distribution for the before and after data. Use a width of 3 and the same intervals for both sets of data.
b. Plot the grouped data in a frequency polygon.

3. Construct a simple frequency distribution for the following data. Use absolute frequency.
DATA: 15, 12, 10, 9, 8, 18, 25, 11, 13, 14, 7, 6, 15, 15, 8

4. Construct a simple frequency distribution for the following data. Use relative frequency.
DATA: 90, 89, 84, 83, 79, 75, 72, 84, 80, 77, 77, 72, 71, 71, 71, 70, 70, 88, 78, 71

5. Construct a simple frequency distribution for the following data. Use cumulative frequency.
DATA: 10, 10, 10, 11, 13, 13, 16, 17, 17, 16, 18, 19, 19, 21, 20, 15, 15, 15, 14, 14, 14, 16, 16, 13, 13

6. The following data are the proportion of the student body majoring in each of five disciplines. Use the appropriate graph to present the data.

Major	Proportion of student body
psychology	0.36
sociology	0.32
biology	0.12
mathematics	0.12
anthropology	0.08

7. The following data represent the responses of 100 people asked to indicate their opinion to the following statement on a scale from 1 to 7, where 1 means strongly agree with the statement and 7 means strongly disagree with the statement.

"Mandatory AIDS testing should be carried out on all public school teachers."

1 strongly agree	13
2 moderately agree	16
3 agree somewhat	24
4 indifferent	10
5 disagree somewhat	12
6 moderately disagree	5
7 strongly disagree	20

Present the data in the appropriate graph.

8. Thirty professors were rated by students on two variables: their knowledge of their subject area and their empathy towards their students. Students rated the professors for knowledge of their subject area on a scale from 1 to five according the following scheme.

Knowledge of subject area
1 = excellent
2 = good
3 = fair
4 = poor

Students rated those same professors for empathy towards their students on a scale from 1 to 5 according to the following scheme.

Empathy
1 = very empathetic
2 = moderately empathetic
3 = somewhat empathetic
4 = not empathetic

The final ratings for each professor are provided below. Present these data in a bivariate frequency distribution.

Professor	Knowledge rating	Empathy rating
1	1	1
2	1	1
3	1	1
4	1	1
5	1	2
6	1	3
7	1	3
8	1	3
9	1	1
10	2	1
11	2	1
12	2	2
13	2	2
14	2	2
15	2	3
16	3	2
17	3	2
18	3	2
19	3	3
20	3	3
21	3	3
22	3	3
23	3	4
24	4	1
25	4	1
26	4	1
27	4	2
28	4	4
29	4	4
30	4	4

9. Construct a grouped frequency distribution for the following data in which the interval width (i) = 5 and the upper limits of the intervals are multiples of 5. Use absolute frequency.

   DATA: 50, 44, 36, 12, 23, 14, 8, 10, 5, 45, 36, 9, 9, 9

10. From the grouped frequency distribution in Exercise 9, construct a frequency polygon. Use the mid-points on the abscissa and absolute frequency on the ordinate.

11. From the grouped frequency distribution in Exercise 9, construct a histogram. Use the mid-points and relative frequency.

12. From the grouped frequency distribution in Exercise 9, construct an ogive using the real limits and cumulative frequency.
13. Construct a grouped frequency distribution for the following data. Use an interval width of 7 and relative frequency.

DATA

90	58	47	28
87	57	47	28
84	56	47	27
78	56	46	27
78	53	46	27
68	53	46	25
67	53	45	25
67	53	45	24
67	52	42	24
65	52	41	21
64	51	39	20
64	51	38	18
61	50	38	14
61	50	37	13
60	50	36	13
60	49	36	8
59	49	36	6
59	49	34	4
59	49	30	3
59	48	29	1

14. Construct a histogram of the data in Exercise 13.
15. State the exact limits for each of the following scores or intervals.
    a. 2.0 sec
    b. 2.6 sec
    c. 2–4 sec
    d. 25–29 lbs
    e. 24.5–29.5 lbs
    f. 24.50–29.50 lbs
16. A restaurant owner keeps track of the number of times that each of five dinner entrées is ordered over two 5-day periods, one in mid-winter and one in mid-summer. A total of 59 customers ordered one of the five dishes during this period in the winter and 47 in the summer. Which type of graph should be used to present these data? What measure of frequency should go on the ordinate?
17. Find the mid-point for the following intervals. Construct a frequency polygon using relative frequency.

X	f
23–25	1
20–22	2
17–19	2
14–16	4
11–13	5
8–10	3
5–7	1
2–4	2

18. Construct a scattergraph of the following data.

Subject number	X	Y
1	78	65
2	66	43
3	54	38
4	89	79
5	46	67
6	70	67
7	55	69
8	95	80
9	64	72
10	86	62

19. A researcher asked his twenty students how may hours they studied per week on average. At the end of their first year, the researcher recorded the grade point average (GPA) received by each of the twenty students. Construct a scattergraph of the data.

Subject number	GPA	Study hrs per week
1	9	16
2	9	9
3	8	13
4	8	10
5	8	8
6	8	8
7	8	10
8	7	9
9	7	9
10	6	4
11	6	15
12	6	10
13	6	6
14	5	6
15	5	7
16	4	4
17	3	8
18	3	3
19	2	6
20	1	5

20. A psychiatrist has diagnosed her 65 patients as suffering from a neurosis, a psychosis or a personality disorder. How should she graphically present these data?

21. Construct a stem and leaf diagram for the following data.

10	25	37	46	59	66	75	90
10	26	38	48	59	67	77	90
11	27	39	49	59	67	84	93
15	28	39	49	59	68	85	94
16	31	42	50	61	72	85	95
21	32	42	51	64	73	86	96
23	33	43	52	64	73	87	
23	37	46	58	65	74	88	

CHAPTER 3
Describing the Central Tendency of Distributions

LEARNING OBJECTIVES

After reading this chapter you should be able to:
1. Define the mode, median, and mean.
2. List the assumption that permits calculation of the median by linear interpolation.
3. Determine the mode from a given set of data.
4. Calculate the median and the mean for a given set of data.
5. Define deviation score. Define positive deviation and negative deviation.
6. Describe what is meant by the mean as a balance point in a distribution in terms of the sum of the deviations.
7. Describe the position of the mean, median and mode in a skewed distribution.
8. Describe what is meant by an open-ended distribution.
9. Describe the term combined mean.
10. Calculate the combined mean for a given set of data.
11. Determine the most appropriate measure of central tendency for a given set of data.

Measures of central tendency describe the "average" of a distribution of scores. There are several ways of measuring "average." We will consider the three most commonly used measures: mode, median and mean.

Three Measures of Central Tendency

Mode

The **mode** (**Mo**) is the most frequently occurring value in a distribution. The mode is the score with a higher frequency than any other score in the distribution. It is the "typical" value in a distribution.

Median

The **median** (**Mdn**) is the score point at or below which, exactly 50% of the scores lie. The median divides the distribution of scores in half.

Mean

The **mean** is the arithmetic average obtained by summing all the scores and dividing the sum by the total number of scores in the distribution. The mean is the measure most of us think of when we talk about "average." Statisticians use the symbol μ ("mew") to refer to the mean.

> **Mode (Mo):** The most frequently occurring score in a distribution.
>
> **Median (Mdn):** The score at or below which exactly 50% of the scores lie.
>
> **Mean (μ):** The arithmetic average of all the scores.

Calculating Measures of Central Tendency

Mode

The mode is easy to determine.

For Ungrouped Data

When data are ungrouped or in a simple frequency distribution, the mode is simply the value with the greatest frequency. A distribution may have more than one mode, and some distributions have no mode; differential frequencies must occur before a mode can be determined. The mode must have a higher frequency than other values. The following examples show numerical and graphic representations of various distributions.

	Data	Mo
Unimodal (one mode)	1, 2, 3, 4, 5, 5, 6	5
Bimodal (two modes)	1, 2, 2, 4, 5, 5, 6	2, 5
No mode	1, 2, 3, 4, 5, 6	all values occur an equal number of times.
No mode	3, 3, 4, 4, 5, 5	all values occur an equal number of times.

Here are some examples of smoothed out frequency polygons.

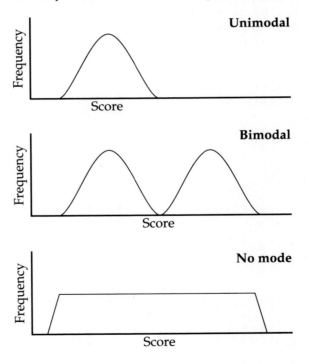

Figure 3-1 Distributions with different types of modes

For Grouped Data
When the data have been placed in a grouped frequency distribution, the mode is the mid-point of the interval containing the highest frequency. The

mode of grouped data is often called the "crude" mode, since the mid-point of the interval may or may not actually be the score value with the highest frequency. The mid-point, however, is used to represent the interval. Here is an example.

X	f	
50–54	3	
45–49	2	
40–44	7	Mo = 42
35–39	4	
30–34	3	
25–29	2	

The interval between 40 and 44 contains the highest frequency and so the mid-point of that interval (42) is the mode. As with ungrouped data, there must be differential frequency before a mode can be determined.

Median

Calculation of the median is complicated by certain conditions.

For Ungrouped Data

Median calculation for ungrouped data is a simple matter if there are no repeated values in the middle. If values are repeated, however, certain assumptions must be made.

Data with No Repeated Middle Values When the scores are arranged from highest to lowest, the median is the middle value, provided there are no other scores with this value. If there is an even number of scores, the median is the value halfway between the two middle values, providing again that these are not repeated. For example:

Data	Mdn
1, 2, 3, 4, 5, 6, 7	4
1, 2, 3, 4, 5, 5, 5	4
1, 2, 3, 4, 5, 6, 7, 8	4.5

Linear Interpolation when Middle Values Are Repeated When repeated middle values occur in a distribution, we must use **linear interpolation** to determine the median. Linear interpolation assumes that repeated values are *evenly distributed* between the exact or real limits of the score. For example, consider a score value of 3 that occurs twice. The exact limits of that score are 2.5 and 3.5. Our assumption requires that we distribute the two scores evenly between these limits. We do this by dividing the interval of one unit into two halves and placing one score in each half. We could draw this the following way:

```
._____X_____._____X_____.
2.5              3.5
```
The X's represent the two scores.

Let's use this method to find the median when we have repeated middle values. Remember, the median is the score value at or below which *exactly* half the scores fall.

DATA: 1, 2, 2	Score	Exact Limits
	1	0.5–1.5
	2	1.5–2.5

Step 1. Draw a line representing the exact limits of the scores.

```
._____._____.
0.5            1.5            2.5
```

Step 2. Divide each interval into as many equal distances as you have scores.

```
._____._____._____.
0.5            1.5           2.5
```

Between 0.5 and 1.5 we have only one score so we do not divide the interval. Between 1.5 and 2.5 we have two scores and so we divide the interval into two equal parts.

Step 3. Place the scores in the middle of each divided portion.

```
._____X_____.___X___.___X___.
0.5         1.5             2.5
```

Step 4. Count exactly half the scores and locate the median.
One half of 3 is 1½.

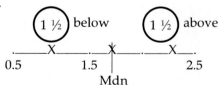

```
._____X_____.___X___.___X___.
0.5         1.5 ↑           2.5
                Mdn
```

Step 5. Add the lower exact limit of the interval containing the median to the exact portion of that interval needed to reach the median.

```
                    1/2  1/2
._____X_____.___X___.___X___.
0.5         1.5 ↑           2.5
```

Mdn = 1.5 + 1/2(1/2)
    = 1.75

We need exactly one quarter of the interval to reach the median. Here are some more examples.

DATA: 1, 2, 2, 2, 3, 4

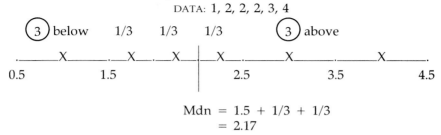

$$Mdn = 1.5 + 1/3 + 1/3$$
$$= 2.17$$

It is not necessary to draw the line representing all the numbers but only that portion where the median lies. Consider the following:

DATA: 5, 7, 8, 8, 8, 8, 8

We need ½ of 7 scores above and ½ below the median. This value must lie in the interval from 7.5 to 8.5.

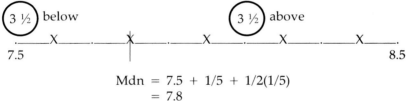

$$Mdn = 7.5 + 1/5 + 1/2(1/5)$$
$$= 7.8$$

Two values are below 7.5. We need 1½ more to reach the median.

For Grouped Data

Linear interpolation is also required to determine the median of grouped data. The procedure is basically the same. We must keep in mind, however, that the interval between exact limits is no longer one unit long. Here is an example.

Interval	f	cf
60–64	1	28
55–59	0	27
50–54	3	27
45–49	5	24
40–44	3	19
35–39	6	16
30–34	5	10
25–29	1	5
20–24	4	4

We have a total of 28 scores in this grouped frequency distribution. The median is the value at or below which exactly 14 scores fall. It lies somewhere in the interval between 35 and 39. We will draw our line to represent the exact limits of that interval.

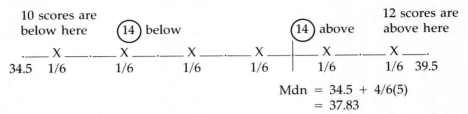

$$\text{Mdn} = 34.5 + 4/6(5)$$
$$= 37.83$$

We need to add 4/6 of the interval to reach the median. The interval is 5 units long in this case and so we need to add 4/6 of 5 units to the exact lower limit of the interval.

Linear interpolation is always required when data are grouped or when ungrouped data have repeated values in the middle. A formula is available that performs the linear interpolation for you.

$$\text{Mdn} = L + \frac{\left[N\left(\frac{50}{100}\right) - f_b\right]i}{f_w} \quad \text{Median}$$

L = lower exact limit of the interval containing the median.
f_b = total frequency below the lower limit of the interval containing the median
f_w = frequency within the interval containing the median. For ungrouped data this is the number of repeated middle values.
i = interval width. For ungrouped data the width is always 1.

Let's use the formula to verify the previous example.

$$\text{Mdn} = 34.5 + \frac{\left[28\left(\frac{50}{100}\right) - 10\right]5}{6}$$
$$= 34.5 + 4/6(5) = 37.83$$

To use the formula you must first find the interval containing the median. The portion of the formula to the right of the plus sign determines the proportion of the interval needed to reach the median. This formula can be used for calculating the median of grouped frequency distributions or for distributions which are ungrouped but have repeated values in the middle.

Mean

For Raw Data
When data are not in a frequency distribution, the mean is calculated by summing all the scores and dividing by the total number of them. The formula for the mean is

$$\mu = \frac{\Sigma X}{N} \quad \text{Mean for Raw Data}$$

X is a general symbol standing for all the scores in the distribution. The ΣX tells us to sum up all the scores in the X distribution. N is the total number of scores. Ready for an example?

DATA: 5, 4, 3, 4, 3, 0, 2

$\Sigma X = 21$
$N = 7$
$\mu = 21/7 = 3$

I don't think we need to belabor this point, do you?

For Data in a Simple Frequency Distribution
When data are in a frequency distribution we must multiply each score by its frequency before we sum and then divide by the number of scores. The formula is

$$\mu = \frac{\Sigma fX}{N} \quad \text{Mean for Data in a Frequency Distribution}$$

Here is an example.

X	f	fX
5	1	5
4	2	8
3	2	6
2	1	2
1	0	0
0	1	0

$$\Sigma fX = 21$$
$$N = \Sigma f = 7$$
$$\mu = 21/7 = 3$$

For Data in a Grouped Frequency Distribution

When we determined the mode of a grouped frequency distribution, we used the mid-point of the interval with the highest frequency as our mode. Similarly, the mean is determined by using the midpoint of each interval to represent that interval.

Interval	Midpt(X)	f	fX
25–29	27	2	54
20–24	22	2	44
15–19	17	4	68
10–14	12	1	12
5–9	7	0	0
0–4	2	1	2

$$\Sigma fX = 180$$
$$N = \Sigma f = 10$$
$$\mu = 180/10 = 18$$

The mean of a grouped frequency distribution will not exactly equal the mean of the raw data because mid-points are used to represent the intervals, not the actual scores. The larger the interval width, the greater the amount of error due to grouping.

Interpreting Measures of Central Tendency

Mode

The mode is interpreted as the "typical" value in a set of scores. If we are interested in the value which occurs more often than any other, then the mode is appropriate. A dress manufacturer, for example, who wants to make dresses of only one size, would sell the most by using the modal dress size. This way he could fit the greatest number of people. The mode is a quick way of describing central tendency. The mode is the only measure of central tendency suitable for nominal data. Median or mean hair color makes no sense, but modal hair color does.

Median

The median is the middle point in a distribution. It divides the number of scores in a distribution exactly in half. If you want to divide a large number of scores into two equal-sized groups, the median would be a good place to do this.

Mean

The mean can be considered the *balance point* of a distribution of scores. The scores below the mean "balance" the scores above the mean. A way to conceptualize the mean is to consider what happens when two children play on a teeter-totter. If one playmate is heavier than the other, he will have to sit closer to the middle of the teeter-totter to balance. If one playmate is lighter, then he must sit further toward the end to balance the board.

The mean acts like the fulcrum of a teeter-totter. The scores represent the weight of the children sitting on the teeter-totter. The distance of the scores above or below the mean represents the distance from the fulcrum that each playmate sits to make the board balance.

The distance between a particular score and the mean of the distribution is its **deviation score**. For example, if a score of 80 comes from a distribution with a mean of 65, then the deviation score for that raw score is 15. The raw score is 15 units away from the mean.

> **Deviation score:** The difference between a score and the mean of its distribution.

The formal way of expressing the mean as a balance point is $\Sigma(X - \mu) = 0$.

This equation says that if all the scores in a distribution are expressed in terms of deviations from the mean, then the sum of all the deviations is zero. For deviations taken about any mean, the sum of the negative deviations is numerically equal to the sum of the positive deviations.

Arithmetic and algebraic proofs of this appear below.

Arithmetic Proof:
DATA: 2, 3, 4, 5, 6
$\mu = 20/5 = 4$
$$\begin{aligned}\Sigma(X - \mu) &= (2 - 4) + (3 - 4) + (4 - 4) + (5 - 4) + (6 - 4) \\ &= -3 + 3 \\ &= 0\end{aligned}$$

Algebraic Proof:
$$\begin{aligned}\Sigma(X - \mu) &= \Sigma X - \Sigma \mu \\ &= \Sigma X - N\mu^* \\ &= \Sigma X - N(\Sigma X/N) \\ &= \Sigma X - \Sigma X \\ &= 0\end{aligned}$$

Let's go back to our teeter-totter analogy. The line below represents the teeter-totter. The fulcrum is the mean. The raw scores and their deviations are indicated.

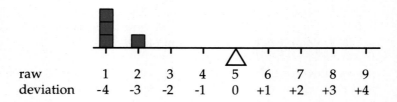

raw	1	2	3	4	5	6	7	8	9
deviation	-4	-3	-2	-1	0	+1	+2	+3	+4

Figure 3-2 The mean as the balance point in distributions

In this example, there are three raw scores with a value of 1. They are 4 deviations below the mean; their total deviation value is -12 units, -4 units for each score. Another raw score is a 2 which is 3 units below the mean; its deviation score is -3. The total of the negative deviations is $(-12) + (-3) = -15$.

To balance we must have equal "weight" above the mean, so we need a total of $+15$ deviations. There are several ways this could occur. For example, we could place 15 scores at the raw score value of 6. This would

---

* The sum of a constant is the constant multiplied by the number of times it appears in the distribution, i.e., N.

produce a total of 15 (+1) = + 15 deviations and the board would balance. Could we balance the board by adding only one score?

Yes: It would have to provide +15 deviations so it would have to be 15 units above the mean. Since the mean is 5, our single score would have a value of 20 to balance the distribution.

The sum of the deviations is determined by their size and frequency. A single score far away from the mean may be balanced by many scores close to the mean, on the other side.

Shape and Measures of Central Tendency

Symmetrical Distributions

Recall that in a symmetrical distribution the right half, the side above the mean, is a mirror image of the left half, the side below the mean. For any symmetrical distribution, the mean and median are equal. If the distribution is also unimodal, the mean, median and mode are equal. Here are some examples.

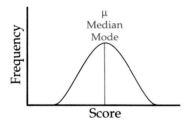 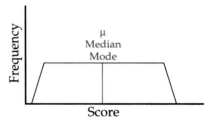

Figure 3-3 The relationship between measures of central tendency in symmetrical distributions

Skewed Distributions

Recall that skewed distributions are labeled on the basis of the direction of the tail. When the tail points to the negative or left side of the distribution, it is called a negative skew. A positively skewed distribution has the tail pointing to the right or positive side. When a distribution is skewed, the mean, mode and median are not equal. The mean always lies closest to the tail. The mode is always at the highest point and the median is always between the mean and mode. Here are some examples.

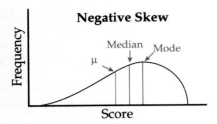 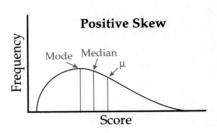

Figure 3-4   The relationship between measures of central tendency in skewed distributions

Comparing Measures of Central Tendency

Choosing which of the three measures of central tendency to use as your "average" depends on your reasons for reporting the measure, the kind of data you have, and what additional measures you will be taking.

Sensitivity to Score Position in a Distribution

The mean is most sensitive to the exact value of each score in a distribution because all the scores are used to compute the mean. If your objective is to reflect all the scores, then the mean is the most appropriate "average" to use. If, however, you do not want your measure of "average" to be "pushed" toward a few very extreme scores, then the median may be a better choice. The median is not sensitive to the exact value of each score but only to the number of scores above and below it. It doesn't matter how far above or how far below those scores are. In the example below, the median is the same although the distributions are clearly different.

Distribution A: 1, 10, <u>100</u>, 1000, 10 000
Distribution B: 98, 99, <u>100</u>, 101, 102

The median of both distributions is 100, but the mean of distribution A is 2222.2 and the mean of distribution B is 100. The median is not sensitive to score value but only to score frequency. The mean, on the other hand, is sensitive to score values because its computation uses each score value. This requires, of course, that we know the value of each score!

Sometimes we find ourselves in a situation where we do not know each score. In these cases the median may be the only "average" we can determine. For example, consider an experiment where 100 rats are timed running through a maze. After the experiment is complete, we find that 12 rats got lost in the maze and didn't finish. If we wish to include those rats in our measure of "average running time," we cannot use the mean. We could, however, compute the median. We would count those 12 rats as taking more time than even the slowest rat. This would produce an **open ended distribution**; there are no values for the extreme end. The median can be calculated for most open-ended distributions since it relies on the number of cases above and below it, not on the distance.

> **Open-ended distribution:** One where the exact upper or lower limit is unknown.

The mode is not sensitive to exact score values either. It is sensitive only to the score with the highest frequency. It is often used as a very quick and somewhat crude measure of central tendency. The mode is the only measure of central tendency appropriate for nominal variables.

Resistance to Sampling Fluctuation

Inferential statistics use samples drawn from a population to make inferences about the properties of that population. We assume that the characteristics of the sample adequately reflect the characteristics of the population from which the sample was drawn. If samples were repeatedly drawn from a population, and the three measures of central tendency computed for each sample, the values of the mean would be more similar than the medians or modes. The mean fluctuates the least from sample to sample. The greatest variation would occur in the modes. The importance of this will become evident in later chapters.

The Mean of Combined Subgroups

Frequently it is necessary to find the overall mean of two or more distributions of scores. For example, by the end of the year my statistics students have written six exams. I always determine the mean on each exam as I record the grades. What if I would like to know the overall mean of the class on the first two exams or all six? If the same number of students wrote each exam, I would simply compute the mean of the means. Unfortunately, even in *my* statistics class, some students drop out during the year and so the number taking each exam often differs. Let's use the data from two exams to illustrate how to compute the **combined mean** of two subgroups.

> **Combined mean:** The grand mean of all the scores in all groups when two or more groups are combined.

If we have the sum of the raw scores for each exam, we would use the following formula to compute the combined mean (μ_c).

$$\mu_c = \frac{\Sigma X + \Sigma Y}{N_x + N_y} \qquad \text{Mean of combined subgroups when the sums are known.}$$

The X distribution will be the scores of the 20 students who wrote the first statistics exam. The Y distribution will be the scores of the 18 who remained to write the second exam.

$$\Sigma X = 1302$$
$$\Sigma Y = 1070$$
$$\mu_c = \frac{1302 + 1070}{20 + 18} = 62.42$$

Let's say that we don't happen to have the sums of the raw scores on the exams but we do have the means for each. In this case we would use the following formula.

$$\mu_c = \frac{N_x \mu_x + N_y \mu_y}{N_x + N_y} \qquad \text{Mean of combined subgroups when the means are known.}$$

The mean on the first exam was 65.10 and the mean on the second exam was 59.44.

$$\mu_x = 65.10$$
$$\mu_y = 59.44$$
$$\mu_c = \frac{20(65.10) + 18(59.44)}{20 + 18}$$
$$= 62.42$$

The mean for each exam was computed using a different number of students. There were 20 students who wrote the first exam, but only 18 wrote the second. We cannot simply average the two means because they were computed on different group sizes. We must first weight each mean by the number of cases that contributed to its calculation, sum these weighted scores, and then divide by the total number of scores. As you can see, this weighting procedure produces the subgroup sums:

$$\mu = \Sigma X/N$$
and by rearranging things
$$\Sigma X = N\mu$$

When the subgroups are equal in size, we don't have to weight the means but simply average the means by adding them and dividing by the number of subgroups. If all 20 students had written the second exam and its mean was 59.44, then we could find the combined mean in the following way.

$$\mu_c = \frac{\mu_x + \mu_y}{2} = \frac{65.10 + 59.44}{2} = 62.27$$

Although this value is close to the value we got when we used the weighted mean formula, it is not exactly the same. The amount of error produced by averaging the means of different-sized groups depends on how different the group sizes are. Larger differences produce larger error.

Measures of central tendency are important techniques for describing the average of distributions. In the next chapter, we will study another important characteristic of distributions: spread or variability.

SUMMARY OF TERMS AND FORMULAS

The **mode (Mo)** is the most frequently occurring value in a distribution.

The **median (Mdn)** is the score value at or below which 50% of the values fall.

The **mean (μ)** is the arithmetic average of all the scores.

Linear interpolation assumes that repeated values are evenly distributed between the exact or real limits of the score.

Deviation score is the difference between a score and the mean of its distribution.

An **open-ended** distribution has no values at the extreme end.

The **combined mean** is the grand mean of all the scores in all groups when two or more groups are combined.

Measure	Formula
Median	$\text{Mdn} = L + \dfrac{\left[N\left(\dfrac{50}{100}\right) - f_b\right]i}{f_w}$
Mean for Raw Data	$\mu = \dfrac{\Sigma X}{N}$
Mean for Data in a Frequency Distribution	$\mu = \dfrac{\Sigma fX}{N}$
Mean for Combined Subgroups	$\mu_c = \dfrac{\Sigma X + \Sigma Y}{N_x + N_y}$ when sums are known
	$\mu_c = \dfrac{N_x\mu_x + N_y\mu_y}{N_x + N_y}$ when means are known
	$\mu_c = \dfrac{\mu_x + \mu_y}{2}$ when $N_x = N_y$

EXERCISES

1. For each set of raw data, calculate the following.

    DATA SET A: 11, 5, 9, 6, 3, 9, 8, 3, 11, 7, 5, 8, 7, 12, 10.
    a. $\Sigma X =$
    b. $N =$
    c. $\mu =$
    d. Mo =
    e. Mdn =
    f. What direction is the skew?

    DATA SET B: 4, 3, 7, 2, 1, 0, 2, 0, 1, 2
    a. $\Sigma X =$
    b. $N =$
    c. $\mu =$
    d. Mo =
    e. Mdn =
    f. What direction is the skew?

2. For each set of raw data, calculate the following.

   DATA SET A:

X	f
10	1
9	3
8	4
7	6
6	3
5	2

   a. N =
   b. ΣfX =
   c. μ =
   d. Mo =
   e. Mdn =
   f. Skew =

   DATA SET B:

Midpoints	f
52	2
47	5
42	2
37	3
32	6
27	3
22	12
17	15
12	11
7	4
2	2

   a. N =
   b. ΣfX =
   c. μ =
   d. Mo =
   e. Mdn =
   f. Skew =

3. Construct a frequency polygon for Data Set B in Exercise 2.
4. Calculate the mean, mode and median for the following set of raw data. What direction is the skew?

   DATA: 10, 5, 8, 7, 3, 5, 9, 8, 3, 8, 11

5. Calculate the mean, mode and median for the following set of raw data. What direction is the skew?

   DATA: 5, 3, 8, 2, 1, 0, 2

6. Calculate the combined mean of the distributions in Exercises 1 and 2.

7. Calculate the mean, mode and median for the following set of raw data. What direction is the skew?

   DATA: 35, 32, 32, 31, 28, 27, 27, 26, 26, 24, 23, 23, 22, 20, 19, 18, 18, 17, 15, 15, 14, 14, 13, 12, 12, 12, 11, 11, 8, 7

8. Calculate the mean, mode and median for the following set of data. What direction is the skew?

X	f
10	3
9	1
8	2
7	2
6	5
5	6

9. Calculate the mean, mode and median for the following set of data. What direction is the skew?

Interval	f
150–154	2
145–149	1
140–144	2
135–139	5
130–134	7
125–129	9
120–124	8
115–119	13
110–114	11
105–109	14
100–104	12
95–99	4
90–94	5
85–89	5
80–84	2

10. For the following data, calculate the mean, mode and median. (N = 30). What direction is the skew?

X	rel f
16–18	0.2
13–15	0.1
10–12	0.2
7–9	0.3
4–6	0.1
1–3	0.1

11. A distribution has a mean of 10. The sum of the positive deviations is +60. If the sum of the negative deviations of all but one score is -45, what is the *value* of the last score?

12. Income is a positively skewed distribution.
    a. Why do you think this is so?
    b. If Statistics Canada wants to impress the world with our standard of living, which measure of central tendency should they use to report average income of Canadians?
13. Sixty gerbils were timed as they ran through a complicated maze, at the end of which was a reward of gerbil treats. The data are presented below. Compute the mean, median, and mode. What direction is the skew?

Interval	f
15.0–15.2	3
14.7–14.9	2
14.4–14.6	1
14.1–14.3	0
13.8–14.0	0
13.5–13.7	4
13.2–13.4	8
12.9–13.1	8
12.6–12.8	7
12.3–12.5	7
12.0–12.2	5
11.7–11.9	10
11.4–11.6	0
11.1–11.3	2
10.8–11.0	2
10.5–10.7	1

14. Which measure of central tendency should be reported for each of the following examples?
    a. A dress manufacturer wants to know the average dress size of women.
    b. A researcher wants to separate people on the basis of a personality test into two groups of equal sizes: a high-anxious group and a low-anxious group.
    c. Students rated a professor using the following scale.
       This professor was an effective instructor.
          1. strongly agree
          2. moderately agree
          3. neither agree nor disagree
          4. moderately disagree
          5. strongly disagree
    d. In a timed problem solving experiment, some of the subjects failed to solve the problem within a reasonable period of time. The experimenter would like to include these subjects in his measure of average time to solve the problem.

CHAPTER 4

Describing the Variability of Distributions

LEARNING OBJECTIVES

After reading this chapter you should be able to:

1. Describe in words the term variability.
2. Define the range.
3. Determine the range from a given set of data.
4. Define the variance.
5. Compute the variance from a given set of data.
6. Define the standard deviation.
7. Compute the standard deviation from a given set of data.
8. Compare distributions with different variances.
9. Compute the variance and standard deviation of combined subgroups.

Chapter 3 dealt with measures of central tendency—methods for indicating the "average" of a distribution. Measures of **variability** provide methods for describing the variation in scores or the amount of scatter around the centre of a distribution. These measures indicate whether scores are clustered closely around the middle of the distribution or whether they are scattered far from the middle. To adequately describe a distribution of scores, a measure of variability as well as a measure of central tendency is required. There are several ways of measuring variations in scores. We will consider three of these: range, variance, and standard deviation.

Three Measures of Variability

Range
The **range** of a distribution is the number of values over which the distribution spans. The range gives us a quick measure of variability.

Variance
The **variance** is the average of the squared deviations of scores from the mean of the distribution. The symbol for the variance is σ^2 "sigma squared."

Standard Deviation
The **standard deviation** is used most often to describe variability. It is the square root of the variance and its symbol is σ "sigma."

Calculating Measures of Variability

Range
The range is by far the easiest measure to determine. It is the difference between the highest and lowest score, plus one. In a distribution of test scores, if someone got 1% and someone else got 100%, then the range would be $100 - 1 + 1 = 100$. In other words, the scores would range over a total of 100 possible values. We determined the range in Chapter 2, when we constructed a grouped frequency distribution. This measure can be thought of as the *width* of the entire distribution.

Variance and Standard Deviation
Calculating these two measures is not difficult; however, it is somewhat tedious. Before we begin, let's examine some symbols and abbreviations.

The previous chapter discussed the mean as a balance point because the sum of the negative deviations equals the sum of the positive deviations. We will need the concept of the deviation score again, this time to calculate variance and standard deviation. We will use a new symbol to stand for deviation score, namely, x.

Defining Formulas
The deviation of a score from its mean is determined by subtracting the mean from the score. This operation can be expressed as $X - \mu = x$.

The variance is the average of the squared deviations of the scores from the mean of the distribution. The formula which defines the variance is:

$$\sigma^2 = \frac{\Sigma x^2}{N} = \frac{\Sigma(X - \mu)^2}{N} \qquad \text{Population Variance: Defining Formula}$$

To use the variance formula we follow:

Step 1. Subtract the mean from each raw score.

Step 2. Square each difference.

Step 3. Sum all the squared differences.

Step 4. Divide this sum by N (the total number of cases).

The result of Step 3 gives us the sum of squared deviations of scores from the mean called, for short, the **sum of squares**. The sum of squares is a term frequently used in statistics. Recall in Chapter 3 that one way to define the mean is the value about which the sum of the deviations is equal to zero. Another way to define the mean is *the value about which the sum of squares is a minimum*. This means that the sum of squared deviations from the mean will be less than the sum of squared deviations taken around any other value. This *least squares* concept will turn up again in Chapter 17.

The standard deviation is simply the square root of the variance and so to determine the standard deviation, we add:

Step 5. Take the square root of the number obtained in Step 4.

The formula which defines the standard deviation is

$$\sigma = \sqrt{\frac{\Sigma x^2}{N}} \qquad \text{Population Standard Deviation: Defining Formula}$$

Let's use an example to show the steps for calculating the variance and the standard deviation of a distribution of scores. Let me remind you again at this point that a population is the entire set of observations of interest to the researcher. Although we think of a population as necessarily being a very large set of observations, this is not necessary from a statistical point of view. It is not its size which makes a population a population, or a sample a sample. Of course, in reality, populations are usually much larger than the examples I give in this book. It's important to recognize, however, that describing large populations is no different than describing little populations. Let's compute the variance and standard deviation for the little population below.

X	x	x^2
1	-9	81
4	-6	36
7	-3	9
13	$+3$	9
16	$+6$	36
19	$+9$	81
$\mu = 10$		$\Sigma x^2 = 252$

$$\sigma^2 = \frac{\Sigma x^2}{N} = \frac{252}{6} = 42$$

$$\sigma = \sqrt{42} = 6.48$$

The middle column of numbers contains the deviation scores for each raw score. These deviations are then squared in the right hand column. The sum of the squared deviations is divided by N for the variance. The standard deviation is the square root of the variance.

Computational Formulas

The defining formulas for these two measures of variability are helpful because they show us exactly what we are doing when we compute a variance or standard deviation. However, they are not used often in calculation. The computational formulas for variance and standard deviation have been derived from the defining ones and are easier to use.

For Raw Data When data have not been organized into a frequency distribution, but appear as single raw scores, the formulas for the variance and standard deviation are

$$\sigma^2 = \frac{\Sigma X^2 - (\Sigma X)^2/N}{N} \qquad \text{Variance for Raw Data}$$

> $$\sigma = \sqrt{\frac{\Sigma X^2 - (\Sigma X)^2/N}{N}}$$ Standard Deviation for Raw Data

ΣX^2 is the sum of the squared raw scores. To calculate ΣX^2:
1. Square all the scores.
2. Sum the squared scores.

$(\Sigma X)^2$ is the squared sum of the raw scores. To calculate $(\Sigma X)^2$:
1. Sum all the scores.
2. Square the sum.

The computational formulas for the variance and standard deviation are, of course, equivalent to the defining formulas. Using either one will produce the same value. I like to use the defining formulas in teaching because they show my students exactly what is being computed, whereas the computational formulas often don't seem so clear. You will notice that the only difference between the defining and the computational formula for the variance and standard deviation is in the numerator of the ratio, the sum of squares. To prove the equivalence of the defining and computational formulas requires that we show that the numerators are algebraically equivalent. The proof for the equivalence of the defining and computational formulas for the sum of squares is as follows:

$$\Sigma(X - \mu)^2 = \Sigma(X^2 - 2X\mu + \mu^2)$$
Rule:
$(X - Y)^2 = X^2 - 2XY + Y^2$

$$= \Sigma X^2 - \Sigma 2X\mu + \Sigma \mu^2$$
Rule:
$\Sigma(X - Y) = \Sigma X - \Sigma Y$

$$= \Sigma X^2 - 2\Sigma X\left(\frac{\Sigma X}{N}\right) + N\mu^2$$
Rule when summing a constant: $\Sigma c = Nc$

$$= \Sigma X^2 - 2\frac{(\Sigma X)^2}{N} + N\frac{(\Sigma X)^2}{N^2}$$

$$= \Sigma X^2 - 2\frac{(\Sigma X)^2}{N} + \frac{(\Sigma X)^2}{N}$$

$$= \Sigma X^2 - \frac{(\Sigma X)^2}{N}$$

Let's go ahead and compute the variance and standard deviation for a distribution of scores using the computational formulas. We will use the data we used earlier when we computed variance and standard deviation with the defining formulas.

$$\begin{array}{cc} X & X^2 \\ 1 & 1 \\ 4 & 16 \\ 7 & 49 \\ 13 & 169 \\ 16 & 256 \\ \underline{19} & \underline{361} \\ \Sigma X = 60 & \Sigma X^2 = 852 \end{array}$$

$$\sigma^2 = \frac{\Sigma X^2 - (\Sigma X)^2/N}{N}$$

$$= \frac{852 - 60^2/6}{6} = 42$$

$$\sigma = \sqrt{42} = 6.48$$

For Data in a Simple Frequency Distribution When data have been organized into a frequency distribution, the computational formulas for the variance and standard deviation are

$$\sigma^2 = \frac{\Sigma f X^2 - (\Sigma f X)^2/N}{N}$$ Variance for Data in a Frequency Distribution

$$\sigma = \sqrt{\frac{\Sigma f X^2 - (\Sigma f X)^2/N}{N}}$$ Standard Deviation for Data in a Frequency Distribution

When we calculated the mean for data in a frequency distribution, we multiplied each score by its frequency. We must do the same here.

To calculate $\Sigma f X^2$:

1. Square each X value.
2. Multiply each square by its frequency.
3. Sum all these products.

To calculate $(\Sigma f X)^2$:

1. Multiply each X value by its frequency.
2. Sum these products.
3. Square the sum.

For Data in a Grouped Frequency Distribution When calculating the variance and standard deviation of data in a grouped frequency distribution, we represent each interval by its midpoint just as we did earlier when computing the mean. This procedure is somewhat crude and does not always produce the same result as the raw data. Since the extensive use of calculators this method may be obsolete. I include it because there may be occasions when you do not have access to the original data. Here is an example.

Interval	M.P.	f	fX	X²	fX²
155–159	157	1	157	24 649	24 649
150–154	152	2	304	23 104	46 208
145–149	147	1	147	21 609	21 609
140–144	142	7	994	20 164	141 148
135–139	137	4	548	18 769	75 076
130–134	132	5	660	17 424	87 120
125–129	127	3	381	16 129	48 387
120–124	122	2	244	14 884	29 768
115–119	117	1	117	13 689	13 689
		26	3552		487 654

$$\sigma^2 = \frac{\Sigma fX^2 - (\Sigma fX)^2/N}{N}$$

$$= \frac{487\ 654 - (3552)^2/26}{26}$$

$$= 92.16$$

$$\sigma = \sqrt{92.16} = 9.60$$

Interpreting Measures of Variability

Range

The range indicates the total number of possible values over which the raw scores span. Since the range uses only the highest and lowest scores in its calculation, it is a relatively crude measure of variability. When the median has been used as the measure of central tendency of a distribution, the range may be the most appropriate measure of variability.

Variance

The variance is a number reflecting the "average" squared distance or deviation of scores from the mean of the distribution. Since the deviations are squared, the variance can be hard to interpret because it is not in the same arithmetic units as the raw scores.

Standard Deviation

Like the variance, the standard deviation indicates the "average" distance or deviation of the scores from the mean. Because the standard deviation is the square root, it is in the same units as the raw scores and is easier to interpret. A standard deviation of 6, for example, means that, on the average, the scores are located 6 points from the mean.

The standard deviation is a quick way of locating the bulk of the scores in a distribution. In any distribution, regardless of the shape, at least 75% of the scores are within two standard deviations of the mean and at least 89% are within three standard deviations of the mean. A distribution, then, with a standard deviation of 6, has at least 75% of its scores between 12 points below and 12 points above the mean, and 89% between 18 points below and above the mean.

For a fairly symmetrical distribution, more than 90% of the observations fall within two standard deviations of the mean and almost all the observations are within three standard deviations of the mean.

For a normal distribution, which we will study further in later chapters, the following is true:

$$\mu \pm 3\sigma = 99.74\%$$
$$\mu \pm 2\sigma = 95.44\% \quad \text{In the Normal Distribution}$$
$$\mu \pm 1\sigma = 68.26\%$$

This means that in a normal distribution, 99.74% of the scores fall between three standard deviations above and below the mean; 95.44% of the scores are within two standard deviations; 68.26% of the scores are within one standard deviation of the mean. These facts will provide a basis for several statistical techniques that we will study in the chapters on inference.

Whenever we describe a distribution of raw scores, we should include a measure of variability along with a measure of central tendency. It is not sufficient to state the "average" only. For example, two distributions may have the same "average" but may be very different in terms of spread. Figure 4–1 shows two distributions of scores whose means are identical. The A distribution, however, has scores clustered around the centre, whereas the B distribution has scores spread far from the centre. To adequately describe these two distributions, we must include some measure of spread as well as a measure of central tendency.

When the median has been used as the measure of central tendency, it is customary to report the range as the variability measure. When the mean is used, the standard deviation usually accompanies it.

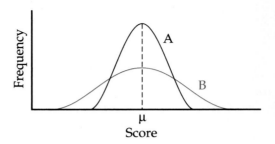

Figure 4-1 Distributions with the same mean but different variability

The Variance and Standard Deviation of Combined Subgroups

When we studied central tendency, we discovered that finding the combined mean of two or more groups is often not as simple as taking the average of the means of each group. Finding the overall variance and standard deviation of several subgroups is no easy task either. In fact, it can be downright complicated.

Variance and standard deviation are measures of spread around the mean of a distribution of scores. To find the variance or standard deviation of combined subgroups, we must determine the average spread of *all the scores around the combined mean*. We cannot simply average the subgroups' variances or standard deviations because each refers to the spread of group scores around the mean of that group. Rather, we must determine the spread of *all* the scores from *all* the distributions around the mean of *all* the scores to find the **pooled variance** or **pooled standard deviation.** The formula for determining the pooled variance of three groups (w, x, and y) is presented below. This formula may be modified for any number of subgroups. The square root of the pooled variance gives the pooled standard deviation.

Combined or pooled variance

$$\sigma^2_c = \frac{N_w\sigma_w^2 + N_x\sigma_x^2 + N_y\sigma_y^2 + N_w(\mu_w - \mu_c)^2 + N_x(\mu_x - \mu_c)^2 + N_y(\mu_y - \mu_c)^2}{N_w + N_x + N_y}$$

Each subgroup variance must be weighted by the number of scores in the group and the squared deviation of each subgroup mean from the combined mean must also be weighted by the group size. To illustrate this, let us determine the pooled variance for the following data:

$$\mu_w = 8 \quad \sigma_w^2 = 2 \quad N_w = 10$$
$$\mu_x = 6 \quad \sigma_x^2 = 1 \quad N_x = 12$$
$$\mu_y = 10 \quad \sigma_y^2 = 3 \quad N_y = 15$$

The first step is to determine the combined mean discussed in Chapter 3. With three groups the formula for the combined mean is

$$\mu_c = \frac{N_w \mu_w + N_x \mu_x + N_y \mu_y}{N_w + N_x + N_y}$$

$$= \frac{10(8) + 12(6) + 15(10)}{10 + 12 + 15}$$

$$= 302/37 = 8.16.$$

Now we can go ahead and compute the combined variance.

$$\sigma_c^2 = \frac{N_w \sigma_w^2 + N_x \sigma_x^2 + N_y \sigma_y^2 + N_w(\mu_w - \mu_c)^2 + N_x(\mu_x - \mu_c)^2 + N_y(\mu_y - \mu_c)^2}{N_w + N_x + N_y}$$

$$= \frac{10(2) + 12(1) + 15(3) + 10(8 - 8.16)^2 + 12(6 - 8.16)^2 + 15(10 - 8.16)^2}{10 + 12 + 15}$$

$$= \frac{77 + 107.03}{37} = 4.97$$

Notice that the combined variance is *not an average* of the subgroup variances. Rather it is a measure of the spread of *all* the subgroup scores around the combined mean.

> **Pooled variance and standard deviation:** The variance and standard deviation of all the scores in all groups around the combined mean when two or more groups are combined.

FOCUS ON RESEARCH

Philippe Rushton, of the University of Western Ontario, has been engaged in some controversial research regarding the relationship between race and crime. He suggests that social organization requires rule-following behavior that can be evaluated in terms of marital functioning, mental durability and law abidingness (Rushton, 1990)*. He reported that on these measures Mongoloid populations are the most socially stable, Negroid populations the least stable and Caucasoid populations somewhere in between, at least within American populations and possibly cross-culturally as well. His research has led him to suggest that genetic influences may be in part responsible for these differences. His position has been attacked by various groups. Some of the data he reported which led him to suggest a genetic hypothesis are presented here. These data are international crime rate statistics from 71 countries in 1984 and 88 countries in 1986. Each country has been classified by primary racial composition as Mongoloid such as Indonesia, Caucasoid such as Latin America, or Negroid such as Sudan.

Table 4-1 Crime rates per 1 000 000 populations for countries categorized by predominant racial type

1984	Homicide		Rape		Serious assault		Total	
	Mean	SD	Mean	SD	Mean	SD	Mean	SD
Mongoloid	8.0	14.1	3.7	2.6	37.1	46.8	48.8	50.3
Caucasoid	4.4	4.3	6.3	6.5	61.6	66.9	72.4	72.5
Negroid	8.7	11.8	12.8	15.3	110.8	124.6	132.3	139.3
1986								
Mongoloid	5.8	10.9	3.2	2.7	29.4	40.2	38.4	42.7
Caucasoid	4.5	4.6	6.2	6.3	65.7	91.2	76.4	95.4
Negroid	9.4	10.6	14.4	15.9	129.6	212.4	153.3	223.8

Source: As reported in Rushton (1990).

Descriptive statistics for data such as these properly include means and standard deviations. Examination of the means shows that for the crimes of rape and serious assault the mongoloid<caucasoid<negroid trend is present. Whether or not this is a significant trend can only be answered by further analyses. Note that the standard deviations are consistently high, in most cases higher than the mean, indicating extreme positive skews. This extreme variability makes interpretation of the means more difficult. Although not reported, it might be more appropriate to use medians rather than means.

---

* Rushton, J.P. (1990). Race and Crime: A Reply to Roberts and Gabor. *Canadian Journal of Criminology*, 32, 315–34.

SUMMARY OF TERMS AND FORMULAS

Measures of **variability** describe the spread or scatter of the scores in a distribution.

The **range** measures the span of the distribution. The **variance** and **standard deviation** measure how far, on the average, the scores are from the mean of the distribution.

The sum of squared deviations of scores from the mean is often called the **sum of squares**.

When the **mean** is used as the measure of central tendency, the **standard deviation** usually accompanies it as the measure of variability. When the **median** is used, it is usually accompanied by the **range**.

Pooled variance and **pooled standard deviation** are measures of spread around the combined mean of all scores from two or more groups.

Measure	Computational Formula	Defining Formula
Range	$H - L + 1$	
Variance for Raw Data	$\dfrac{\Sigma X^2 - (\Sigma X)^2/N}{N}$	$\dfrac{\Sigma(X - \mu)^2}{N}$
Variance for Data in a Frequency Distribution	$\dfrac{\Sigma fX^2 - (\Sigma fX)^2/N}{N}$	
Standard Deviation for Raw Data	$\sqrt{\dfrac{\Sigma X^2 - (\Sigma X)^2/N}{N}}$	$\sqrt{\dfrac{\Sigma(X - \mu)^2}{N}}$
Standard Deviation for Data in a Frequency Distribution	$\sqrt{\dfrac{\Sigma fX^2 - (\Sigma fX)^2/N}{N}}$	

Pooled Variance for Three Combined Subgroups

$$\sigma^2_c = \frac{N_w \sigma_w^2 + N_x \sigma_x^2 + N_y \sigma_y^2 + N_w(\mu_w - \mu_c)^2 + N_x(\mu_x - \mu_c)^2 + N_y(\mu_y - \mu_c)^2}{N_w + N_x + N_y}$$

EXERCISES

1. For each set of raw data, calculate the following.

   DATA SET A
   13, 15, 21, 12, 45, 30, 10, 19, 28, 7
   a. $\Sigma X =$
   b. $\Sigma(X - \mu) =$
   c. $\Sigma(X - \mu)^2 =$
   d. $N =$
   e. $\mu =$
   f. $\sigma^2 =$
   g. $\sigma =$

   DATA SET B
   12, 12, 8, 7, 6, 3, 1
   a. $\Sigma X =$
   b. $\Sigma(X - \mu) =$
   c. $\Sigma(X - \mu)^2 =$
   d. $N =$
   e. $\mu =$
   f. $\sigma^2 =$
   g. $\sigma =$

2. For each set of data, calculate the following.

   DATA SET A
   10, 9, 7, 7, 5, 3, 1
   a. $\Sigma X =$
   b. $\Sigma X^2 =$
   c. $\mu =$
   d. $(\Sigma X)^2 =$
   e. $(\Sigma X)^2/N =$
   f. $\sigma^2 =$
   g. $\sigma =$

   DATA SET B

X	f
10	3
9	1
8	2
7	2
6	5
5	6
4	4
3	2
2	0
1	1

   a. $\Sigma fX^2 =$

b. $\Sigma fX =$
c. $\mu =$
d. $(\Sigma fX)^2 =$
e. $(\Sigma fX)^2/N =$
f. $\sigma^2 =$
g. $\sigma =$

3. For the following distributions, determine the deviation scores for each raw score.

   X: 2, 4, 6, 7, 4, 3, 2
   Y: 12, 23, 50, 35, 20

4. Use the defining formulas to calculate the variance and standard deviation of the following data. What is the range?

   DATA: 10, 8, 4, 4, 8, 5, 2

5. Use the defining formulas to calculate the variance and standard deviation of the following data. What is the range?

   DATA: 6, 4, 8, 2, 1, 0, 0, 3

6. Use the computational formulas to calculate the variance and standard deviation for the following data. What is the range?

   DATA: 6, 4, 8, 2, 1, 0, 0, 3

7. Use the computational formulas to calculate the variance and standard deviation for the following data. What is the range?

X	f
10	3
9	1
8	2
7	2
6	5
5	6

8. Calculate the variance and standard deviation for the following grouped frequency distribution.

X	f
23–25	1
20–22	2
17–19	2
14–16	4
11–13	5
8–10	3
5– 7	1
2– 4	2

9. For the data in Exercise 3, compute the pooled variance and standard deviation.

10. In which of the following distributions of test scores would you prefer to be with a score of 112? Explain your reasons.

    Distribution A   Mean = 98   Standard Deviation = 4
    Distribution B   Mean = 98   Standard Deviation = 16

11. The following data are the test results for two different groups of students. Compute the mean, median, and standard deviation for each group. Provide a rough sketch of the two distributions to show how they differ.

    Group 1
    25, 25, 25, 25, 25, 25, 25, 25, 25, 25, 25, 25, 25, 25, 24, 24, 24, 24, 24, 24, 24, 24, 24, 24, 24, 24, 24, 23, 23, 23, 23, 23, 23, 22, 22, 22, 22, 22, 22, 21, 21, 17, 16

    Group 2
    25, 25, 25, 25, 24, 24, 24, 24, 24, 24, 24, 24, 24, 23, 23, 23, 23, 23, 22, 22, 22, 22, 22, 22, 21, 21, 21, 21, 21, 21, 21, 21, 21, 21, 20, 20, 20, 19, 18, 15, 12, 8

12. Compute the mean and standard deviation for the following data.

    60, 82, 58, 51, 49, 22, 40, 35, 55, 59, 95, 50, 41, 45, 46, 41, 32, 43, 85, 66, 40, 32, 43, 71, 42, 47, 27, 78, 38, 48, 62, 77, 38, 22, 39, 58, 41, 19, 90, 41, 19, 85

13. Compute the mean and standard deviation for the following data. Plot the data in a histogram. What is the skew?

    9, 9, 9, 9, 8, 8, 8, 8, 8, 8, 7, 7, 7, 7, 7, 7, 7, 7, 6, 6, 6, 6, 6, 6, 6, 6, 6, 6, 6, 6, 5, 5, 5, 5, 5, 5, 5, 4, 4, 4, 4

CHAPTER 5

Describing the Position of Scores in Distributions

LEARNING OBJECTIVES

After reading this chapter you should be able to:

1. Define the term derived score.
2. Define percentile and provide an example.
3. Define percentile rank and provide an example.
4. Compute percentiles from a given set of data.
5. Compute percentile ranks from a given set of data.
6. Define the term Z-score.
7. Calculate Z-scores for a given set of data.
8. List the properties of a Z-distribution.
9. Use Z to locate the position of scores in a distribution.

Frequently, we wish to describe the **location** of one score in a distribution of many scores. We will examine two techniques that are commonly used to do this.

Percentiles and *percentile ranks* use percentage to describe score position. After taking a test, you may wish to know how well you did compared to the rest of the class. You might find, for example, that your performance on a test was as good or better than 80% of the class. Your test score would have a percentile rank of 80.

Alternatively, you might ask "What score did I need to be in the top 10% of the class?" You might find that to be in the top 10% you would have had to score 78 points on the test. The score of 78, then, would be the 90th percentile.

These techniques rely on how many cases are above and below certain points in the distribution of scores. Recall that the median also does this by indicating the point at or below which half the cases fall; the median is the 50th percentile.

Another way of locating the position of a score is to compare that score with the mean of the distribution. *Z-scores* do this by indicating how far above or below the mean a particular raw score value lies. Z-scores rely on distance from the mean; percentiles and percentile ranks rely on number of cases.

Percentile ranks and Z-scores are **derived scores** since they involve numbers which are derived from the raw scores in the distribution. They help us determine the relative standing of a particular score in a distribution of scores.

> **Derived scores:** Scores obtained by transforming raw scores.

Percentiles and Percentile Ranks

Percentiles

A **percentile** is a *score point* at or below which a particular percentage of cases fall. P_{PR} is the abbreviation for percentile. The subscript indicates the % value at or below which an unknown score falls. A percentile can range over the possible values in the distribution. For example, P_{80} is the score value in a distribution at or below which 80% of the cases fall. P_{50} is the score value at or below which 50% of the cases fall. P_{50} is also the median of a distribution.

Percentile Ranks

The **percentile rank** (PR_x) of a score is a number indicating the percentage of cases falling at or below a particular score value. It is a *percentage value* and can only range from 0 to 100. The subscript x is the score value and the PR indicates what percentage of the distribution is at or below that score value. For example, if the percentile rank of a score of 115 is 65 ($PR_{115} = 65$), then we know that 65% of the cases lie at or below the score of 115. Alternatively, we could say that 115 is the 65th percentile ($P_{65} = 115$).

Earlier, we found that we could divide a distribution exactly in half using the median or the 50th percentile. Similarly, we could divide a distribution into quarters using the 25th, 50th, 75th and 100th percentiles. This would produce four equal-sized groups. This is a common technique and these four percentiles are often called **quartiles**.

Calculating Percentiles and Percentile Ranks

Percentiles

The general formula for computing percentiles from a grouped frequency distribution is

$$P_{PR} = L + \frac{\left[N\left(\frac{PR}{100}\right) - f_b\right]i}{f_w} \quad \text{Percentile}$$

where L is the lower exact limit of the score or interval containing the percentage of cases of interest; N is the total number of cases in the distribution; f_b is the number of cases below the score or interval containing the percentile; f_w is the number of cases within the interval containing the percentile; and i is the width of the interval.

This formula is almost the same as the one we used for calculating the median because the median is the 50th percentile. The procedure we will follow is the same as we used when computing the median. Ready for an example?

Below is a grouped frequency distribution.

Interval	f	cf	
155–159	1	25	
150–154	0	24	
145–149	2	24	P_{90}
140–144	2	22	
135–139	3	20	
130–134	4	17	
125–129	6	13	
120–124	4	7	
115–119	2	3	
110–114	1	1	

Let's determine P_{90}. When we were finding medians the first step was to determine where half the cases fell. To determine P_{90}, we must find where 90% of the cases fall.

Step 1. Determine what 90% of the total is. 90% of 25 is 22.5.

Step 2. Find the interval containing the 22.5th score. Looking at the cf column, we see that this score is in the interval 145–149.

Step 3. Determine the lower limit of this interval and substitute into the formula.

$$P_{90} = 144.5 + \frac{\left[25\left(\frac{90}{100}\right) - 22\right]5}{2}$$

$$= 144.5 + \frac{(22.5 - 22)5}{2}$$

$$= 145.75$$

Therefore, 145.75 is the point in the distribution at or below which 90% of the scores fall.

Earlier we calculated the median by formula and by linear interpolation. Since the median is a percentile, we can use linear interpolation to find any other percentile. Using the above example, let's verify that the 90th percentile is 145.75.

$$\underset{144.5}{\overset{\fbox{22.5} \text{ below}}{\bullet\text{\_\_\_\_\_X\_\_\_\_\_}\bullet\text{\_\_\_\_\_X\_\_\_\_\_}\bullet}} \quad \underset{149.5}{\overset{\fbox{2.5} \text{ above}}{}}$$

$$P_{90} = 144.5 + 1/4(5) = 144.5 + 1.25 = 145.75$$

We can see that there are two scores within the interval containing the 90th percentile. We need exactly one half of one of these scores so that there are 22.5 below and 2.5 above. We need, then, one quarter of the entire interval which is 5 units long. This method can be used to determine any percentile for a grouped frequency distribution.

Percentile Ranks

The formula for determining the percentile rank of any score is

$$PR_x = \frac{\left[f_w \frac{(X - L)}{i} + f_b\right]100}{N} \quad \text{Percentile Rank}$$

where X is the score value whose rank you wish to determine; L is the lower exact limit of the interval in which the score falls; f_w is the number of scores in that interval; f_b is the number of scores below that interval; i is the interval width; and N is the total number of scores in the distribution.

To illustrate this, let's use the same example we used earlier. Recall that the 90th percentile was 145.75. This means that the percentile rank of 145.75 must be 90. Let's use our percentile rank formula to prove that this is true.

$$PR_{145.75} = \frac{\left[\frac{2(145.75 - 144.5)}{5} + 22\right]100}{25}$$

$$= \frac{\left[\frac{2.50}{5} + 22\right]100}{25}$$

$$= 22.5(4) = 90$$

Percentile ranks are derived scores that provide information about relative standing. They indicate the percentage of cases that are found at or below a particular score value. They do not, however, indicate the distance of the scores from the score in question. For example, a score with a percentile rank of 80 indicates that 80% of the cases were at or below that score but not how far below those cases were. A derived score, which indicates the actual distance a raw score is from the mean of a distribution, measured in units of standard deviation, is the Z-score.

The Z-Score

The **Z-score** (pronounced Zee in the U.S. and Zed in Canada) is a derived score that indicates how many standard deviations a raw score is from the mean and in what direction. This derived score is often more meaningful that the percentile rank of a score because it tells us how far above or below the mean the score value is. A raw score value above the mean will have a positive Z-score. A raw score below the mean will have a negative Z-score. A Z-score of -1.00, for example, tells us that the raw score equivalent was exactly one standard deviation unit below the mean of the distribution.

Calculating Z-Scores

The general formula for determining the Z-score equivalent of any raw score is

$$Z = \frac{x}{\sigma} \quad \text{Z for a Raw Score}$$

where $x = X - \mu$.

This formula simply divides the deviation score by the standard deviation of the distribution. In this way the Z value tells us whether the raw score was above or below the mean and exactly how far in standard deviation units.

Consider the distribution below. Its mean is 50 and its standard deviation is 7. Each raw score has been translated into its Z-score equivalent, using our formula.

Raw Scores	x	Z
68	18	2.57
54	4	0.57
51	1	0.14
50	0	0.00
50	0	0.00
48	−2	−0.29
48	−2	−0.29
46	−4	−0.57
45	−5	−0.71
40	−10	−1.43
		0.00

$\mu = 50$
$\sigma = 7$

Notice that a raw score of 40 is nearly 1 1/2 standard deviation units below the mean. A score of 54 is more than 1/2 a standard deviation above the mean. Since Z indicates distance from the mean, a score which is equal to the mean, in this case 50, will always have a Z-score equivalent of zero, regardless of the standard deviation. Notice that the sum of the Z-scores is zero. This is true of any distribution of Z-scores. You will recall that the sum of the deviations about any mean is zero; since Z-scores are deviation scores divided by the standard deviation (a constant), their sum must also be zero.

Properties of a Z-Distribution

A **Z-distribution** is a distribution where all raw scores have been converted to their Z-score equivalents. All Z-distributions have certain unchanging properties.

The Mean

The mean of any Z-distribution is zero. This makes sense because the mean of the distribution does not deviate from itself. Formally, then:

$$\mu_z = 0 \quad \text{Mean of a Z-Distribution}$$

The Variance and Standard Deviation

The variance and standard deviation of any Z-distribution are always equal to 1. Formally:

$$\sigma_z^2 = \sigma_z = 1 \quad \text{Variance and Standard Deviation of a Z-Distribution.}$$

The Shape

When a distribution of raw scores is converted to Z-scores, its shape does *not change*.

This is not true of all derived scores. The "dreaded" stanine system, used in many colleges and universities, changes the shape of the raw score distribution to a bell-shaped curve. The grading scheme used at my college changes the shape of the raw score distribution to a negatively skewed curve. Converting to Z, however, has no effect on the shape.

Using Z to Locate Scores in a Distribution

The Z-score is extremely useful for indicating the location or the relative standing of a score in a distribution of scores. Let's consider an example. Elmer obtained 80% on his psychology midterm exam. He was quite pleased with this grade. He was not so pleased, however, when he received 40% on his anthropology midterm. Although, at first glance, it is tempting to believe that 80% is the better grade, we are statistically sophisticated enough now not to jump to conclusions. First we must ask a couple of questions. We need to know the mean and standard deviation of each exam. Consider the following data:

Psychology Midterm
$\mu = 70\%$
$\sigma = 20$
Elmer's score = 80%

Anthropology Midterm
$\mu = 35\%$
$\sigma = 2$
Elmer's score = 40%

On the anthropology test, most of the students were clustered around the mean and few got high marks. On the psychology test, the students scores were much more variable. Several students got high marks. It is difficult to evaluate Elmer's grades by glancing at the data. Certainly, he was above the mean in both cases, but how far? This question can be answered by converting his raw scores to Z scores.

$$Z \text{ in psychology} = \frac{X - \mu}{\sigma} = \frac{80 - 70}{20} = +0.5$$

$$Z \text{ in anthropology} = \frac{40 - 35}{2} = +2.5$$

In the anthropology test, Elmer was 2 1/2 standard deviations above the class mean. In his psychology test, he was only 1/2 a standard deviation above the mean. Clearly, Elmer's performance, compared to his classmates', was far superior on the anthropology test.

Consider another example. Elmer got 80% in a math test and 80% in a chemistry test. The class average was 60% on both tests. It would be tempting to conclude that Elmer performed equally well on both tests, but we know better. The data on each test were as follows:

Math Test	Chemistry Test
$\mu = 60\%$	$\mu = 60\%$
$\sigma = 15$	$\sigma = 5$
Elmer's score = 80%	Elmer's score = 80%

These two distributions might look like the following:

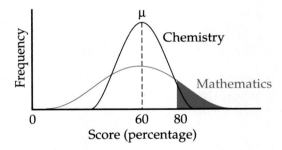

Figure 5-1 Position of a score in two distributions with the same means but different variability

As you can see, the standard deviations differ considerably. In the math exam several students got 80% and higher but in the chemistry test very few students did as well as Elmer. Converting Elmer's grades to Z-scores we find:

$$Z \text{ (in math)} = \frac{80 - 60}{15} = +1.33$$

$$Z \text{ (in chem)} = \frac{80 - 60}{5} = +4.00$$

Elmer's score of 80% on the chemistry test was 4 standard deviations above the mean; his score on the math test was 1 1/3 units above the mean. It is necessary to know both the central tendency and the amount of spread in a distribution to determine relative standing.

SUMMARY OF TERMS AND FORMULAS

The measures discussed in this chapter are useful for determining the **location** of a score in a distribution.

The **percentile** is a score value at or below which a certain percentage of the scores fall. The **percentile rank** is a value indicating the percentage of scores at or below a particular score value.

Because the 25th, 50th, and 100th percentiles divide a distribution into four equal-sized groups, they are known as **quartiles**.

The **Z-score** indicates the distance, above or below the mean of a distribution, that a particular scores falls in units of standard deviation. A **Z-distribution** is a distribution where all raw scores have been converted to Z scores.

Percentile ranks and Z-scores are examples of **derived scores.**

Measure	Formula
Percentile	$P_{PR} = L + \dfrac{\left[N\left(\dfrac{PR}{100}\right) - f_b\right]i}{f_w}$
Percentile Rank	$PR_x = \dfrac{\left[f_w \dfrac{(X - L)}{i} + f_b\right]100}{N}$
Z-Score	$Z = \dfrac{X - \mu}{\sigma}$

EXERCISES

1. Determine the 50th, 75th, and 90th percentiles for the following frequency distribution.

Interval	f
135–139	3
130–134	12
125–129	9
120–124	10
115–119	15
110–114	7
105–109	2
100–104	2

   What is the percentile rank of 117?

2. John got a 45 on his spelling test. If the class mean was 57 and the standard deviation was 6, what was John's Z score?

3. For the following data, determine the Z-scores for each raw score.
   DATA: 4, 6, 8, 9, 11, 3

4. Maria got 87% on her grammar test and 76% on her math test. Using the following data determine if she did better on her grammar test than on her math test.

GRAMMAR TEST	mean = 85	standard deviation = 2
MATH TEST	mean = 70	standard deviation = 4

5. It is possible for a score to have a percentile rank of 65 and a negative Z-score. What kind of distribution must this score come from?

6. The percentile rank of a score of 89% is 62. Describe this in words.

7. Dan got 80% on an English test for which the mean was 70. He got 70% on a French test for which the mean was 80. The standard deviation for both tests was 10 and the median for both was 65. Which of the following is undeniably true?
   a. The English test was easier.
   b. The two distributions differ in skew direction so we can't make comparisons.
   c. Dan's absolute Z-score for both tests is 1.00. Therefore his relative position in the two classes is the same.

8. A distribution of scores on a statistics test has a mean of 54 and a standard deviation of 3. What raw score would you need to be three standard deviations above the class mean?

9. A student received a Z-score of +1.30 on her history exam. If the class mean was 64% and the variance was 9, what was her raw score on the test?

10. a. Compute P_{30}, P_{45}, and P_{85} for the data below.

Interval	f	cf
96–100	1	40
91– 95	3	9
86– 90	1	36
81– 85	5	35
76– 80	7	30
71– 75	7	23
66– 70	1	16
61– 65	2	15
56– 60	4	13
51– 55	5	9
46– 50	4	4

b. Determine the precentile rank of 83, 54, and 78.
c. Compute the mean and standard deviation.
d. Convert the midpoints to Z-scores.

11. Below is the grouped frequency distribution for Chapter 2 Exercise 1 (b).

Apparent Limits	Exact Limits	M.P.	f	rel f	cum f	rel cf
160–164	159.5–164.5	162	1	0.01	100	1.00
155–159	154.5–159.5	157	5	0.05	99	0.99
150–154	149.5–154.5	152	4	0.04	94	0.94
145–149	144.5–149.5	147	0	0.00	90	0.90
140–144	139.5–144.5	142	2	0.02	90	0.90
135–139	134.5–139.5	137	6	0.06	88	0.88
130–134	129.5–134.5	132	10	0.10	82	0.82
125–129	124.5–129.5	127	7	0.07	72	0.72
120–124	119.5–124.5	122	6	0.06	65	0.65
115–119	114.5–119.5	117	13	0.13	59	0.59
110–114	109.5–114.5	112	7	0.07	46	0.46
105–109	104.5–109.5	107	12	0.12	39	0.39
100–104	99.5–104.5	102	12	0.12	27	0.27
95– 99	94.5– 99.5	97	6	0.06	15	0.15
90– 94	89.5– 94.5	92	6	0.06	9	0.09
85– 89	84.5– 89.5	87	3	0.03	3	0.03

Calculate the following.
a. P_{30}
b. P_{95}
c. PR_{27}
d. PR_{139}

12. Construct an ogive for the following data using relative cumulative frequency on the ordinate. Determine the percentile rank of a raw score of 130 using dotted lines from the score up to the curve and across to the ordinate value. Confirm your result with the formula. Using solid lines, indicate the value of the median. Confirm this with the formula.

Interval	f
145–149	2
140–144	4
135–139	6
130–134	13
125–129	16
120–124	7
115–119	2

13. For the data below, calculate the following.

    DATA: 28, 35, 28, 38, 40, 40, 39, 27, 40, 37, 40, 38, 39, 38, 21

    a. $\Sigma X =$
    b. $\Sigma X^2 =$
    c. $N =$
    d. $(\Sigma X)^2 =$
    e. $\mu =$
    f. $(\Sigma X)^2/N =$
    g. $\sigma^2 =$
    h. $\sigma =$
    i. list the Z-scores
    j. $\Sigma(\text{Z-scores}) =$

14. For the following provide a rough sketch of what the two distributions might look like.

    a. Spencer got 60 on his first statistics test and 74 on his second. The mean and standard deviation for the first test were 56 and 12, respectively. The mean and standard deviation for the second test were 68 and 15, respectively. On which test did Spencer do better?
    b. Ben of Baltimore makes $45 000 a year. Tom of Toronto makes $42 500. If the mean income in the United States is $28 000 with a standard deviation of $6000 and the mean income in Canada is $30 000 with a standard deviation of $4000, who is richer? What might the two distributions look like?

CHAPTER 6

Introduction to Inference: The Normal Curve

LEARNING OBJECTIVES

After reading this chapter you should be able to:
1. Describe the difference between empirical and theoretical distributions.
2. List the properties of the normal curve.
3. Find areas under the normal curve given Z-scores.
4. Find Z-scores given areas under the normal curve.
5. Find areas given Z-scores with normal distributions.
6. Find Z-scores given areas with normal distributions.

The **normal curve** is a bell-shaped relative frequency distribution. This curve is a very useful model for many statistical procedures. Many variables, including height, weight, and IQ distribute themselves according to this bell-shaped curve. A normally distributed variable has few observations at either extreme end; the bulk of the observations lie in the middle.

Empirical vs Theoretical Frequency Distributions

Empirical means "data-based." **Empirical frequency distributions** contain actual observations and the distribution has a fixed size. **Theoretical** means based on theory or hypothetical observations. **Theoretical frequency distributions** are composed of theoretical observations and may have an infinite number of terms. The normal curve is a theoretical distribution.

> **Empirical:** Based or founded on real data or observations.
>
> **Theoretical:** Based on theory or hypothetical observations.

The Normal Curve

The normal curve is not a single distribution but rather a family of curves. Just as the mathematical function of a circle describes a family of circles, the mathematical function of the normal curve describes a family of curves.

> **Standard normal curve:** Theoretical bell-shaped distribution. Often simply called normal curve.

Many statistical procedures rely on the normal curve and, therefore, the curve has been standardized and should, more properly, be called the **standard normal curve**. The standard normal curve has Z-scores along the abscissa and relative frequency along the ordinate. In this form, all normal curves are identical.

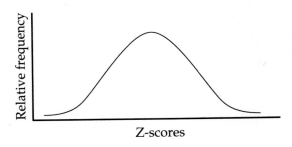

Figure 6-1 The standard normal curve

The Equation for the Standard Normal Curve

The standard normal curve is defined by a mathematical function. It is included here for your interest.

$$Y = \frac{1}{\sqrt{2\pi\sigma^2}} e^{-(X-\mu)^2/2\sigma^2}$$

where Y is the height of curve at point X
X is any point on abscissa
μ is the mean
σ² is the variance
π is a constant = 3.1416...
e is the base of Napierian logarithms = 2.71828

This equation produces a curve with several unchanging properties.

Properties of the Standard Normal Curve

The standard normal curve has the following properties.

1. It is symmetrical.
2. It is unimodal; the mean, median, and the mode are equal.
3. The values along the abscissa are continuous.
4. The curve is asymptotic to the abscissa; because there are an infinite number of terms in the distribution, the curve never touches the abscissa.
5. The mean is zero.
6. The variance and standard deviation equal 1.
7. The area under the curve has a relative frequency of 1.00.

The entire area under the curve contains 100% or 1.00 of the frequency. Since the curve is symmetrical, 0.50 of the area is on each side of the mean. Because these properties don't change, we can solve problems with the standard normal curve. Examine the normal curve below.

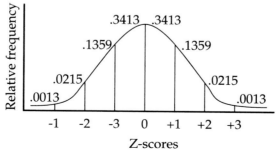

Figure 6-2 Areas under the normal curve

You can see that .3413 of the total area lies between a Z-score of +1 and the mean of the curve. Because the curve is symmetrical, the same proportion of the area, i.e. .3413, lies between a Z of −1 and the mean. Areas under the curve corresponding to any two points have been computed allowing us to use the normal curve to solve problems.

Using the Normal Curve to Solve Problems

Table B-1 in Appendix B near the back of this book contains two columns that provide exact areas under the standard normal curve. The first column provides areas between the mean of the curve and any particular Z-score. The second column provides areas beyond a particular Z-score. Only positive Z-scores are given because the curve is symmetrical. The area beyond a Z of +1.00, for example, is the same as the area beyond a Z of −1.00.

Finding Areas under the Curve

If we are given a particular Z-score, we can use Table B-1 in Appendix B to find out how much of the area lies between it and the mean; and how much of the total area lies beyond that score. When solving problems with the normal curve, first draw a rough picture. This will help you see exactly what you are doing. Ready for some examples?

Example A How much of the total area under the curve lies between the mean and a Z-score of +1.05? We will solve these problems in steps.

Step 1. Draw a curve and shade in the area of concern.

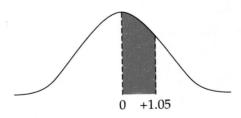

Step 2. Go to Table B-1 and look up the area between the mean and a Z-score of +1.05. Use the first column of the table.

$$\text{Area} = 0.3531$$

Approximately 35% of the total area is found between a Z of 0 (the mean) and a Z of +1.05.

Example B How much of the total area under the curve is found between the mean and a Z-score of −1.74?

Step 1. Draw a curve and shade in the area of concern.

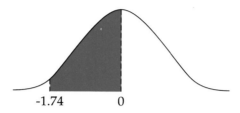

Step 2. Look up the area in Table B-1. Because the curve is symmetrical, we can ignore the minus sign.

$$\text{Area} = 0.4591$$

Approximately 46% of the total area is found between a Z of −1.74 and the mean of the distribution.

Example C How much of the area is found beyond a Z-score of 3.24?

Step 1. Draw a curve and shade in the area of concern.

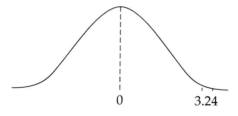

Step 2. Now we need to use the second column of Table B-1. Look up the area beyond a Z of 3.24.

$$\text{Area} = 0.0006$$

As you can see, very little of the area is found beyond a Z of 3.24.

Example D How much of the area is found between the Z-scores of −1.74 and +3.24? This problem illustrates the importance of drawing a curve first.

Step 1. Draw a curve and shade in the area of concern.

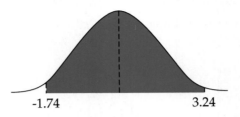

Step 2. We have already determined that 0.4591 of the area lies between a Z of −1.74 and the mean. Look up the area between the mean and a Z of 3.24. There is 0.4994 of the area between these points.

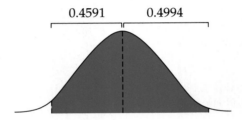

We can add these two areas together to solve our problem. There is 0.9585 or about 96% of the total area between these two scores.

As long as you have specific Z-scores, you can always determine exact proportions of the total area under the curve.

Finding Z-Scores with the Curve

We can also solve problems when the Z-score, not the area, is the unknown.

Example E What Z-score has 0.1915 of the total area between it and the mean? Our step-by-step procedure is as follows:

Step 1. Draw a curve and shade in the area of concern.

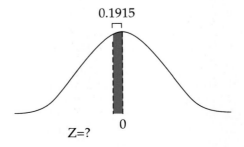

I have shaded the area below the mean. This is arbitrary. There are, of course, two Z-scores, one positive and one negative, which will solve our problem.

Step 2. Look in the first column of Table B-1 for the area of 0.1915. Look across to the left for the Z value. Either the positive or the negative value is appropriate, since both solve the problem.

$$Z's\ are\ +\ or\ -0.50$$

There is 0.1915 of the total area between either Z value and the mean.

Example F Let's find the two Z-scores which cut off the middle 95% of the area from the extreme 5%.

Step 1. Draw a curve and shade in the area of concern.

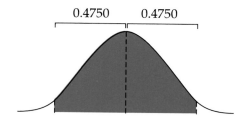

To separate the middle 95% from the extreme 5%, we need half of 95% (0.4750) on either side of the mean.

Step 2. Look up the Z which has 0.4750 between it and the mean. Z = 1.96. Since the curve is symmetrical, we know that 95% of the total area is between the Z-scores of −1.96 and +1.96.

Because the standard normal curve has unchanging properties, we can always determine exact areas when we have Z-scores, and we can find Z-scores when we have exact areas. Whenever we have a real distribution, which is normal in shape, we can use these procedures.

Working with Empirical Data That Are Normally Distributed

If we know that a particular distribution of scores is normal in shape, we can use the standard normal curve. We simply translate our data into Z-score form and then use the normal curve table to solve problems about our specific distribution.

Imagine that we have a distribution of IQ scores, which is normal in shape, with a mean of 100 and a standard deviation of 15.

Example G Let's find the proportion of scores or area below an IQ of 95.

Step 1. Draw a curve and shade in the area of concern.

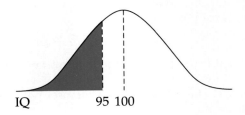

Step 2. Find the Z-score. We must transform our raw score into a Z-score so that we can use Table B-1. Recall that the formula for converting a raw score to a Z-score is

$$Z = \frac{X - \mu}{\sigma}$$

Our Z-score is $$Z = \frac{95 - 100}{15} = -0.33$$

Step 3. Look up the area beyond a Z of -0.33.

$$\text{Area} = 0.3707$$

Approximately 37% of the distribution of IQ scores is below an IQ of 95.

Example H What proportion of the IQ scores lies between 95 and 115?

Step 1. Draw a curve and shade in the area of concern.

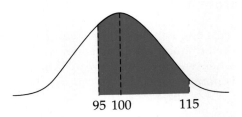

Step 2. We already know that 0.3707 of the area lies below 95, so we can just subtract this from 0.50 to find the area between 95 and the mean of 100. This is 0.1293. Next, we need to translate the score of 115 into a Z-score.

$$Z \text{ of } 115 = \frac{115 - 100}{15} = 1.00$$

Step 3. Looking up the area between the mean and a Z of 1.00, we find it is 0.3413.

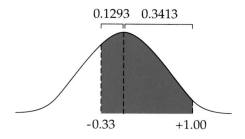

We add these two areas together and we find that 0.4706 of the area is found between the scores of 95 and 115.

Example I   Now, let's find the proportion of IQ scores between 115 and 130.

Step 1. Draw a curve and shade in the area of concern.

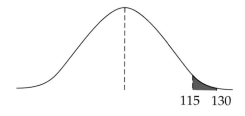

Step 2. Translate the scores into Z-scores.

$$Z \text{ of } 115 \text{ is } +1.00$$
$$Z \text{ of } 130 = \frac{130 - 100}{15} = +2.00$$

Step 3. There are several ways to solve this problem. Let's look up the area between the mean and a Z of +2.00. Then we subtract the area between the mean and a Z of +1.00 from that value.

Area between mean and Z of 2.00 is 0.4772
Area between mean and Z of 1.00 is 0.3413

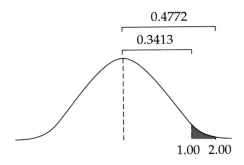

By subtraction, we find 0.1359 (i.e., 0.4772 − 0.3413) of the area is between the Z's of 1.00 and 2.00. Approximately 14% of the scores lies between IQs of 115 and 130.

Example J To continue, let's find the two IQ scores which separate the middle 90% of the distribution from the extreme 10%. We have the area and must find the scores.

Step 1. Draw a curve and shade in the area of concern.

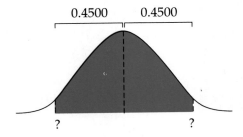

Step 2. Look up the Z score which has 0.4500 of the area between it and the mean.

$$Z = + \text{ or } - 1.645$$

We have the two Z values and we now convert them to the raw scores.

Step 3. Rearrange the Z formula so that X is the unknown.

$$X = \mu \pm Z\sigma$$
$$= 100 \pm 1.645(15)$$
$$= 124.75 \text{ and } 75.25$$

We find that 90% of the scores lies between the values of 124.75 and 75.25 and 10% lies outside these two values.

Example K What two IQ scores cut off the middle 95% from the extreme 5%?

Step 1. Draw a curve and shade in the area of concern.

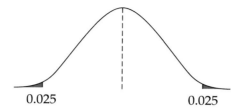

0.025   0.025

Step 2. Look up the appropriate Z-scores.

$$Z = \pm 1.96$$

Step 3. Convert the Z-scores to raw scores.

$$X = 100 \pm 1.96(15) = 129.40 \text{ and } 70.60$$

Between IQs of 129.40 and 70.60, we find 95% of the distribution.

Whenever we have a distribution of scores that we know is normally distributed, we can use the standard normal curve as a model to solve problems about our distribution. We only need the mean and standard deviation of our distribution to use the normal curve table. Many "real" distributions are similar in shape to the normal curve, and so the normal curve table is a very useful device for solving a variety of problems.

SUMMARY OF TERMS AND CONCEPTS

The normal curve is an extremely useful tool for many statistical procedures because it has certain unchanging properties.

Empirical frequency distributions consist of actual observations and the distribution has a fixed size. By contrast, **theoretical frequency distributions** consist of theoretical observations and may have an infinite number of terms.

The **standard normal curve** is a **symmetrical** distribution with a mean, median and mode of zero. The observations along the abscissa of the curve are **infinite** and **continuous** and consist of **Z-scores.**

Because the area under the normal curve represents **relative frequency** and is equal to 1.00, the curve can be used as a model for solving a variety of problems about normally distributed variables.

EXERCISES

1. Determine the area under the normal curve between $Z = \pm 2.50$.
2. Determine the area under the normal curve between $Z = \pm 1.87$.

3. Determine the area under the normal curve beyond $Z = 1.96$.
4. Find the two Z-scores which separate the middle .90 of the area from the extreme .10.
5. Find the Z-score below which .90 of the area lies.
6. Determine the percentile rank of each of the following Z-scores. (Hint: area under the curve can be converted to percentage.)
   a. -2.58
   b. -1.96
   c. 0
   d. 1.64
   e. 2.33
7. Assume you have a normal distribution of 5000 test scores with $\mu = 72$ and $\sigma = 12$.
   a. What percentage of the scores are greater than a score of 80?
   b. What percentage of the scores are below 66?
   c. Between what two test scores do the middle 60% of the scores lie?
   d. Beyond what score does the lower 5% of the scores fall?
   e. How many scores lie below the score in part (d) above?
   f. What score is exceeded by only 4 students (round to the nearest whole number)?
   g. What test score is at the 25th percentile? (Hint: what exactly is a percentile, what does it tell you?)
8. In a normal distribution with a mean of 50 and standard deviation of 10, find PR_{63}.
9. Find the score at the 20th percentile for the distribution in Exercise 8.
10. In a normal distribution with a mean of 112 and a variance of 144, what proportion of the area lies between the scores 70 and 150?
11. A distribution of 10 000 test scores is normally distributed with a mean of 550 and a standard deviation of 60. Determine the two Z-scores that separate the middle 9 000 scores from the extreme 1000 scores.
12. For the distribution described in Exercise 11, determine the two raw scores that separate the middle 90% from the extreme 10% of the distribution.
13. For the distribution described in Exercise 11, find the raw score below which only 50 scores fall.
14. For the distribution described in Exercise 11, determine how many raw scores fall between scores of 500 and 600.

CHAPTER 7

Introduction to Inference: Probability

LEARNING OBJECTIVES

After reading this chapter you should be able to:
1. Define the term simple probability.
2. Solve simple probability problems.
3. Describe conditional probability.
4. Define and catergorize events as dependent and independent.
5. Solve conditional probability problems.
6. Determine the probability of A and B for a given example.
7. Determine the probability of A or B for a given example.
8. Define and categorize events as mutually exclusive .
9. Describe the difference between permutation and combination.
10. Use the formula to determine permutations in a given example.
11. Use the formula to determine combinations in a given example.
12. Describe and provide an example of a dichotomous variable.
13. Use the formula to determine probability with a binomial distribution.
14. Describe how a frequency distribution can be seen as a distribution of probabilities.

Assume for the moment that I am going to toss a coin and bet with you about the outcome. If I bet on heads, how many heads in a row would I have to toss before you started getting suspicious? Let's say I toss the coin three times and all three times it comes up heads. Would you accuse me of trickery? How about five heads in a row? Now would you start to doubt my honesty? What if I tossed the coin ten times and it came up heads each time? What would you have to say about that? Probably most people would be quite doubtful that a fair coin would turn up heads ten times in a row. Most people would think that this is too much for coincidence. What they are really deciding is that it is highly *improbable* that a fair coin would turn up heads as many as ten times in a row *by chance alone*. A betting person would probably conclude that the coin was not fair at all! Now, it is possible that a fair coin could behave this way, but if I had money on it, I think I would be better off rejecting such a hypothesis. It seems much more reasonable to conclude that something fishy is going on.

This simple example demonstrates the underlying logic of all statistical inference. Statistical inference involves determining the probability that a particular outcome (e.g., ten heads in a row) occurred by chance alone given a specific hypothesis about the nature of things (e.g., a fair coin was used). To understand statistical inference thoroughly, it is essential to have an understanding of basic probability.

Simple Probability

The **probability** of a particular **event** or **outcome** occurring is the number of ways that that event can occur, divided by the total number of possible outcomes that could occur in a situation where all outcomes are equally likely.

$$p(A) = \frac{\text{number of ways A can occur } (\#A)}{\text{total number of outcomes } (\#O)} \quad \text{Simple probability}$$

In a single toss of a coin, the probability of getting a head is the number of ways a head can occur (1) over the total number of outcomes possible (2).

$$p(H) = \frac{1}{2}$$

In the roll of a die (one of a pair of dice) the probability of rolling a four is the number of ways a four can occur (one) over the total number of possible outcomes (six).

$$p(4) = \frac{1}{6}$$

Both of these examples have outcomes that are equally likely. In a single toss of a fair coin, a head is as likely to occur as a tail. With a fair die, the likelihood of rolling a four is the same as for a 1, 2, 3, 5 or 6.

What would be the probability of obtaining an even number on a single roll of a fair die? Using the same approach we would determine the number of ways that an even number could occur over the total number of outcomes. There are three ways an even number could show up (i.e., 2, 4, 6) and the total number of outcomes remains the same (six).

$$p(\text{even number}) = \frac{3}{6}$$

If we rolled a die many times then, we would expect to get an even number half the time *on the average* since the probability on a single roll is one half.

Conditional Probability

When the probability of a given event is *dependent upon* or *influenced by* the occurrence or non-occurrence of a previous event, it is called **conditional probability**. The likelihood of a given event occurring is conditional upon what went on before.

Let's determine the probability of drawing a jack from a well-shuffled deck of playing cards. Since all cards are equally likely to be drawn we can determine the probability of drawing a jack by using our simple probability formula.

$$p(J) = \frac{\text{\# of ways a jack can be drawn}}{\text{total number of outcomes or cards}}$$

There are four jacks in a deck of 52 cards and so,

$$p(J) = \frac{4}{52}$$

Now let's draw a second card from our deck without putting the first one back. What is the probability of drawing another jack if the first card drawn was a jack? Since there are only three jacks left, the number of ways we can draw a second jack is 3 and the total number of cards is only 51.

$$p(\text{jack given the first card was a jack}) = \frac{3}{51}$$

This is an example of conditional probability since the outcome (jack on second draw) is conditional upon or dependent upon what happened in the first draw. The general formula for this kind of probability is

$$p(B/A) = \frac{\text{\# ways B can occur given A has occurred}}{\text{total number of outcomes given A has occurred}} \quad \text{Conditional probability}$$

In our example: $$p(J/J) = \frac{3}{51}$$

What if a jack was not drawn the first time? The probability of getting a jack on the second draw, given a jack was not drawn on the first draw, would be the number of ways to draw a jack (four, since all four are still in the deck) over the total number of outcomes (51, since one card was already drawn and not replaced).

$$p(jack/non\text{-}jack) = \frac{4}{51}$$

Dependent events are events where the occurrence of one alters the probability of occurrence of the other. Conditional probability involves dependent events. By contrast, **independent events** are those where the occurrence of one does not affect the probability of occurrence of the other. In our example, had we returned the first card drawn to the deck, the probability of drawing a jack on the second draw would have been unaffected by the outcome of the first draw. In this case, the probability of drawing a second jack would be a matter of simple probability, the number of ways of drawing a jack (four) over the total number of outcomes (52).

$$p(\text{jack on second draw given the first drawn jack was replaced}) = \frac{4}{52}$$

These two events are independent because the outcome of the second draw is not influenced by what happened on the previous draw. Conditonal probability refers only to dependent events. By replacing our first drawn card we have made the second draw independent of the first and, therefore, not a conditional event. We could describe this situation of independent events using our formula. When events are independent then the probability of event B occurring, given A has already occurred, is the same as the probability of B.

If $p(B/A) = p(B)$ then the events are **independent**.

This underlies the "gambler's fallacy." Many gambling games (e.g., roulette) involve independent events. The fact that the ball has just stopped on the 34 has absolutely no effect on its next stopping place. I am, of course, assuming a fair roulette wheel, which may be naive! Unfortunately, many gamblers think these events are dependent, and they have a multitude of schemes for trying to determine probabilities. It's really very simple. If a roulette wheel has 36 numbers the probability of the ball stopping on the number 34 is 1/36 (i.e. the number of ways a 34 can occur, 1, over the number of possible outcomes, 36), no matter what numbers have previously occurred. I should mention that this knowledge has never stopped me from betting on my favorite number 7!

> **Dependent events:** Occurrence of one alters the probability of occurrence of the other.
>
> **Independent events:** Occurrence of one has no effect on the probability of occurrence of the other.

Probability of Compound Events

Probability of A and B

Many situations involve questions about the probability of two or more specified events occurring rather than just a single event. This is called the **probability of A and B**. We may wonder what the probability might be of obtaining a jack on the first draw and another jack on the second draw from our deck of 52 cards. The general formula for the probability of two specified events both occurring is

> $p(A \text{ and } B) = p(A) \cdot p(B/A)$ Probability of A and B: dependent events

The probability of both A and B occurring is the product of the probability of A and the probability of B given A has occurred. We use a dot to indicate multiplication because large brackets are somewhat messy looking. We can now determine the probability of getting two jacks in a row drawn without replacing the first one from a deck of 52 cards:

$$p(J \text{ and } J) = p(J) \cdot p(J/J)$$
$$p(J \text{ and } J) = \frac{4}{52} \cdot \frac{3}{51} = 0.0045$$

On the first draw, the probability of a jack is simply the number of ways a jack can occur (4) over the total number of outcomes (52). On the second draw there are only three ways to get a second jack out of a total of 51 cards because the first jack was not replaced.

If we had replaced the first jack, making the two events independent, then the probability of the second jack would not be affected by the first draw and the probability of getting two jacks in a row would be

$$p(J \text{ and } J) = p(J) \cdot p(J)$$
$$p(J \text{ and } J) = \frac{4}{52} \cdot \frac{4}{52} = 0.0059$$

The general formula for the probability of two independent events occurring is

$$p(A \text{ and } B) = p(A) \cdot p(B) \qquad \text{Probability of A and B: independent events}$$

This procedure can be used for more than two events as well. If all events are independent then the probability of all of them occurring is the product of their individual probabilities. Recall the coin toss experiment from the beginning of this chapter. I wondered how many heads in a row I could toss before you became suspicious about the fairness of my coin, and suggested that 10 heads in a row would cause most people to doubt me. We can now determine what the probability really is of obtaining 10 heads in a row with 10 tosses of a fair coin. This is just the probability of getting a head *and* a head *and* a head etc.

$$p\begin{bmatrix}10 \text{ heads} \\ \text{in a row}\end{bmatrix} = p(H) \cdot p(H) \cdot p(H) \cdot p(H) \cdot p(H) \cdot p(H) \cdot p(H) \cdot p(H) \cdot p(H) \cdot p(H)$$
$$= \frac{1}{2} \cdot \frac{1}{2} \cdot \frac{1}{2} \cdot \frac{1}{2} \cdot \frac{1}{2} \cdot \frac{1}{2} \cdot \frac{1}{2} \cdot \frac{1}{2} \cdot \frac{1}{2} \cdot \frac{1}{2}$$
$$= \frac{1}{1024} = 0.00098$$

As you can see this is a mighty unlikely series of events!

Probability of A or B

We have seen how to determine the probability of two (or more) events occurring together. We can also ask questions about the probability of either of two events occurring. This is called the **probability of A or B** and the general formula is

$$p(A \text{ or } B) = p(A) + p(B) - p(A \text{ and } B) \qquad \text{Probability of A or B}$$

Let's go back to our deck of playing cards. What would be the probability of drawing a jack or a red card in a single draw from our deck of 52? Half of the deck (26) is red and two of the cards are black jacks, so the number of ways to get a jack or a red card must be 28 out of the total number of outcomes (52). Let us use our general formula to verify this.

$$p(J \text{ or } R) = p(J) + p(R) - p(R \text{ and } J)$$
$$= \frac{4}{52} + \frac{26}{52} - \frac{2}{52} = \frac{28}{52} = 0.54$$

This formula is always used when two events can occur together. We needed to subtract the p(R and J) so that we didn't count the red jacks twice. A red card can also be a jack so these events can occur together. When two events cannot occur at the same time, they are said to be **mutually exclusive**. Drawing a jack or a queen, for example, would be mutually exclusive events since you cannot draw a jack and a queen in one draw. If one event has occurred, the other cannot have occurred.

> **Mutually exclusive events:** Two events that cannot occur at the same time.

In the case of mutually exclusive events, the last term in the above formula is zero, since A and B cannot occur at the same time. The probability of drawing a jack or a queen in a single draw is simply the sum of their individual probabilities.

$$p(J \text{ or } Q) = p(J) + p(Q)$$
$$= \frac{4}{52} + \frac{4}{52} = 0.1538$$

The general formula, then, for determining the probability of one event or the other event occurring when events are mutually exclusive is:

> $p(A \text{ or } B) = p(A) + p(B)$ Probability of A or B: mutually exclusive events

The examples we have looked at have been quite simple. We began by learning that the probability of occurrence of a given event (A) is found by dividing the number of ways A can occur by the total number of outcomes possible. The total number of outcomes and the number of ways A can occur are easy to determine when you are dealing with dice, coins, or a couple of draws from a deck of playing cards. What if I ask you to determine the probability of being dealt a royal straight flush (i.e., A, K, Q, J, 10 all in the same suit) from a deck of 52 cards? Could you do it?

It's not too tricky to figure out how many ways you could get a royal straight flush. There are four suits, so there are only four ways, one for each suit. However, determining the total number of 5-card hands possible would daunt most of us! Luckily, we have methods for doing just this sort of thing without the necessity of enumerating every possibility.

Methods of Counting

Permutations

A **permutation** is an **ordered sequence** of things, objects or events. A different order of the same objects is a different permutation of those objects. Consider a relay swim team whose members are Hewey, Dewey, and Susan. There are several ways we could arrange our three swimmers in terms of position.

	\multicolumn{6}{c}{Teams}					
	1	2	3	4	5	6
First swimmer	Hewey	Hewey	Dewey	Dewey	Susan	Susan
Second swimmer	Dewey	Susan	Hewey	Susan	Hewey	Dewey
Third swimmer	Susan	Dewey	Susan	Hewey	Dewey	Hewey

There are six different arrangements that could be made with our three swimmers. We are simply arranging our three objects (swimmers) into different orders or permutations.

What would happen if we added one more swimmer (Lewey)? We would end up with a whole lot more possibilities, 24 to be exact. As you can imagine it would get quite tedious to delineate all possible arrangements. Fortunately, we have a formula to do this work for us. The formula is

$$_nP_r = \frac{n!}{(n-r)!} \qquad \text{Permutations}$$

We will use the letter **n** to stand for the total number of objects we have to work with, and the letter **r** to stand for the number of objects we need in a single arrangement. The number of ordered sequences of r objects that can be selected from a total of n objects is symbolized by $_nP_r$. The symbol $_nP_r$ can be read as the number of permutations of n objects taken r at a time.

The exclamation mark means **factorial**, which I have always thought was a somewhat mysterious operation. Here is how it is done.

$$n! = n(n-1)(n-2)(n-3)\ldots 1$$

$$\text{e.g., } 6! = 6(5)(4)(3)(2)(1) = 720$$

At this point it is important to mention that 0! *is always* 1. Just accept this on faith.

To illustrate this, let's select four objects which we will cleverly call A, B, C and D. We can determine how many different ordered sequences of two objects can be selected from our total of four in the following way:

Objects	Sequences of 2 at a time
A, B, C, D	AB, AC, AD
	BA, BC, BD
	CA, CB, CD
	DA, DB, DC

Note that AB and BA are *different permutations*. The different order of objects makes them different permutations.

By counting up our sequences, we can see that there are 12 permutations of 4 objects taken 2 at a time. We can use our formula to verify this.

$$_4P_2 = \frac{4!}{(4-2)!} = \frac{4 \cdot 3 \cdot 2 \cdot 1}{2 \cdot 1} = 12$$

Let us look at a more useful example. Those of you interested in horse racing may find this profitable. What is the probability of selecting the first, second, and third in a race involving a field of 10 horses? In horse-racing terminology this is called picking the win, place, and show horse. Our general approach tells us that we must divide the number of ways we could pick first, second, and third by the total number of outcomes in such a race. Clearly, there is only one way of selecting the first three horses in the correct position. However, the total number of possible sequences of three horses from a field of 10 is not so obvious. We can use our formula to solve this problem.

$$\text{total number of outcomes} = {_{10}P_3} = \frac{10!}{(10-3)!} = 720$$

There are 720 ordered sequences of 10 horses selected in threes. The probability, then, of picking the winning three horses in the correct order can now be determined.

$$p \text{ (picking win, place and show)} = \frac{\text{\# ways to pick 1st, 2nd and 3rd}}{\text{total \# of outcomes}}$$

$$= \frac{1}{720} = 0.00139$$

You might want to consider this the next time you gamble on a Trifecta! Of course, it is important to point out that the above example assumes we are randomly choosing the three horses from the field. Most of us, I am sure, never behave so frivolously when it comes to betting on horse races. We use important information, such as the attractiveness of the horses' names and their colour, to determine our choices!

Combinations

A **combination** is a **set** of things, objects or events. Order is not important. AB and BA *is the same combination*. The formula to determine the number of combination of n objects taken r at a time is

$$_nC_r = \frac{n!}{(n-r)!r!} \qquad \text{Combinations}$$

Using our four objects (A, B, C, and D) we can determine the number of combinations of two objects that can be selected.

Objects	Combinations of 2
A, B, C, D	AB, AC, AD
	BC, BD, CD

There are only *six combinations* but there were *twelve permutations*. For every one combination, then, there were two permutations. **In any situation, there will be r! permutations for every one combination.** This is why you find r! in the denominator of the combinations formula.

We can verify our example by using the combination formula for 4 objects selected 2 at a time.

$$_4C_2 = \frac{4!}{(4-2)!2!} = \frac{4 \cdot 3 \cdot 2 \cdot 1}{(2 \cdot 1)(2 \cdot 1)} = 6$$

Again, using our four objects, let us determine the number of combinations and permutations of three objects that can be selected.

Objects	Combinations of three	Permutations of three
A, B, C, D	ABC, ABD, ACD, BCD	ABC, ABD, ACD, BCD
		ACB, ADB, ADC, BDC
		BAC, BAD, CAD, CBD
		BCA, BDA, CDA, CDB
		CBA, DBA, DCA, DBC
		CAB, DAB, DAC, DCB

We have 24 permutations but only four combinations. There are 6 permutations for every one combination. Note that r! is 6 so there are r! permutations for every one combination.

Using the formulas for the above example:

$$_4C_3 = \frac{4!}{1!3!} = \frac{4 \cdot 3 \cdot 2 \cdot 1}{1 \cdot 3 \cdot 2 \cdot 1} = 4$$

$$_4P_3 = \frac{4!}{1!} = \frac{4 \cdot 3 \cdot 2 \cdot 1}{1} = 24$$

Binomial Probability

When I was an undergraduate student taking statistics, the topic of **binomial probability** almost defeated me. I could not understand why it was important. It is important, however, because many things in this world have only two outcomes, e.g., on/off, yes/no, pregnant/not pregnant. It's really not very complicated at all.

A special case in probability exists when we are trying to determine the number of combinations when there are only two outcomes of interest for each of several trials. A variable having only two outcomes of interest is also called a **dichotomous variable**. Consider penny tossing again. You may be wondering if all statisticians spend a lot of time tossing pennies. Well... some do and some don't.

In a penny tossing experiment there are only two outcomes of interest, heads and tails. If I were to toss a penny ten times in a row what would be the probability of obtaining exactly two heads? This is a case of binomial probability. We are talking about combinations not permutations, since the question does not specify the order in which the events must occur. We are specifying that only two of the ten tosses must be heads. To determine the probability of such an event, we must first determine the probability of any one arrangement of two heads and eight tails, and then determine how many such arrangements or sequences are possible.

One sequence which fits our requirements could be the following:

$$H,H,T,T,T,T,T,T,T,T$$

What is the probability of tossing this sequence of ten coins? We learned earlier that the probability of several specified events occurring is the product of their individual probabilities, when the events are independent. The events in the above example are definitely independent; earlier events do not alter the probability of later events occurring. The probability of getting a head in a single toss of a coin is 1/2 and the probability of tossing a tail is also 1/2, so the probability of the above sequence of heads and tails is

$$p(H,H,T,T,T,T,T,T,T,T) = \frac{1}{2} \cdot \frac{1}{2} \cdot \frac{1}{2} \cdot \frac{1}{2} \cdot \frac{1}{2} \cdot \frac{1}{2} \cdot \frac{1}{2} \cdot \frac{1}{2} \cdot \frac{1}{2} \cdot \frac{1}{2} = \frac{1}{2^{10}}$$
$$= \frac{1}{1024}$$

Another sequence of events that would satisfy our requirement of exactly two heads in ten tosses is H,T,H,T,T,T,T,T,T,T. The probability of this sequence occurring is also 1/1024. In fact, the probability of *any* particular sequence of two heads and eight tails is 1/1024.

Now that we know the probability of any one sequence occurring, we need to figure out how many sequences fit our requirement of two heads and eight tails.

The number of sequences of two heads in ten tosses of a coin is simply the number of combinations of ten things taken two at a time. Using our combinations formula:

$$_{10}C_2 = \frac{10!}{(10-2)!2!} = 45$$

There are 45 different ways that we can get exactly two heads in ten tosses of a coin. Each way has a probability of occurring of 1/1024. The probability, then, of getting two heads in ten tosses of a coin is

$$p(\text{exactly 2H in 10 tosses}) = 45 \cdot \frac{1}{1024} = 0.0439$$

This may seem like a rather long and drawn out way to solve a seemingly simple problem. It is! Fortunately we have a formula for determining binomial probabilities.

In a sequence of **n** independent trials with only two outcomes of interest (we call them "success" and "failure"), where **p** is the probability of success and **q** is the probability of failure, the probability of exactly **r** successes is

$$_nC_r p^r q^{n-r} = \frac{n!}{(n-r)!r!} p^r q^{n-r} \qquad \text{Binomial Probability}$$

Success and failure are mutually exclusive events. **p** is the probability of success and **q** is the probability of failure. **q** *always equals* **1 − p**. The terms success and failure are really quite arbitrary. In general, success is the event in which you are interested. In our example above, a success is getting a head. p is the probability of getting a head in one trial (i.e., 1/2). q is the probability of not getting a head (i.e., a failure) and in our case that probability is also 1/2. The probability of a success does not have to equal the probability of a failure; their individual probabilities must add up to 1, however (i.e., they must be mutually exclusive events).

Back to our coin tossing experiment. We have already determined the probability of getting exactly two heads in ten tosses of a coin. Now let's verify this with our formula.

$$p(2H \text{ in } 10 \text{ tosses}) = {_{10}C_2} p^r q^{n-r}$$

$$= \frac{10!}{2!(10-2)!} \left(\frac{1}{2}\right)^2 \left(\frac{1}{2}\right)^8$$

$$= 45 \cdot \left(\frac{1}{2}\right)^{10} = \frac{45}{1024} = 0.0439$$

As you can see we ended up with the same number. So now you can go ahead and determine the probability of getting exactly 13 heads with 54 tosses of a fair coin, or 43 heads with 100 tosses of a fair coin, or...

Frequency Distributions as Probability Distributions

Any frequency distribution can be viewed as a distribution of probabilities. Below are the final grades for one of my statistics classes. The grades range from 9 through 1, where grades of 3, 2 and 1 are considered failing.

Grade	f	rel. f
9	2	0.06
8	6	0.19
7	5	0.16
6	6	0.19
5	3	0.09
4	3	0.09
3	5	0.16
2	2	0.06
1	0	0.00
	N = 32	

Viewing this distribution as a probability distribution we can see that the probability of a *randomly selected* student receiving a grade of 7 is .16. Further, the probability of a student receiving a grade of 6 or better would be p(6) + p(7) + p(8) + p(9) = .60.

The normal curve can be viewed as a probability distribution as well. With continuous variables, such as Z-scores, the probability of an event A is found by:

$$p(A) = \frac{\text{area under the curve associated with A}}{\text{total area under the curve}}$$

Suppose we have a normal distribution of scores with a mean of 100 and a standard deviation of 10. Let's determine the probability of randomly selecting a score of 112 or higher. We have already learned how to solve problems like this in Chapter 6. The only difference here is the terminology. In Chapter 6, we would have phrased the question as, "what proportion of the area lies beyond a score of 112?" Using the same procedure, we first convert the raw score to a Z-score and then look up the proportion of the total area beyond that Z-score.

$$Z = \frac{112 - 100}{10} = +1.2$$

$$\text{Area} = .1151$$

The probability, then, of randomly selecting a single score of 112 or greater is 0.1151.

If we were to randomly select a single score from this distribution, what is the probability that it is between 90 and 110? We could write this problem in the following way

$$p(90 \leq X \leq 110) = ?$$

Using our usual procedure,

$$Z = \pm 1$$
$$\text{Area} = .6826$$
$$p(90 \leq X \leq 110) = 0.6826$$

The probability, then, of randomly selecting one score between 90 and 110 is 0.6826. About two-thirds of the time, if we were to repeatedly draw a single score, with replacement, we would expect it to fall between these two values.

Any frequency distribution can be viewed as a probability distribution. This underlies some important procedures we will study later.

SUMMARY OF FORMULAS

Simple Probability	$p(A) = \dfrac{\#A}{\#O}$
Conditional Probability	$p(B/A) = \dfrac{\#B/A \text{ has occurred}}{\#O/A \text{ has occurred}}$
Compound Probability	
Dependent events	$p(A \text{ and } B) = p(A) \cdot p(B/A)$
Independent events	$p(A \text{ and } B) = p(A) \cdot p(B)$
Not mutually exclusive	$p(A \text{ or } B) = p(A) + p(B) - p(A \text{ and } B)$
Mutually exclusive	$p(A \text{ or } B) = p(A) + p(B)$
Permutations	$_nP_r = \dfrac{n!}{(n-r)!}$
Combinations	$_nC_r = \dfrac{n!}{(n-r)!r!}$
Binomial Probability	$_nC_r p^r q^{n-r} = \dfrac{n!}{(n-r)!r!} p^r q^{n-r}$

EXERCISES

1. Which of the following pairs of events are mutually exclusive?
   a. rolling a six: rolling an odd number in one roll of a die
   b. drawing an Ace: drawing a red card in one draw from a deck
   c. flipping a head: flipping a tail in one flip of a coin
   d. being pregnant: not being pregnant

2. Which of the following pairs of events are independent?
   a. flipping a head on the first flip: flipping a head on the second flip of a coin
   b. drawing an ace first: drawing a red card second in two draws from a deck without replacement
   c. drawing an ace first: drawing a red card second in two draws from a deck with replacement
   d. being accepted by the University of Alberta: being accepted by the University of Ottawa

3. Imagine that the probability of your getting married in the next 5 years is 0.80. The probability that you will be a parent withing the next 5 years is 0.70.
   a. What is the probability that you will be a parent and be married?
   b. What are your chances of either being married or being a parent?

4. The probability that a certain (unenlightened) company will hire a woman to be chief executive is 0.15. The probability that this same company will hire an unmarried person is 0.25. What is the probability that this company will hire:
   a. a single woman?
   b. a single man?
   c. either a woman or a married person? (Are these events mutually exclusive?)
   d. a married woman?

5. Sheila wants to move to another city. If Sheila's chance of getting a job in Vancouver is 0.10 and her chance of getting one in Halifax is 0.25, what is the probability that Sheila will be offered both jobs? What is the probability that Sheila will get either the Vancouver position or the Halifax position?

6. My glove compartment contains 3 red fuses, 4 green fuses and 6 blue fuses.
   a. I need a green fuse. What is the probability I will grab a green one if I don't look?
   b. If I grab 3 fuses without looking, what is the probability they are all red?
   c. What is the probability I will grab a green one if I have already grabbed a blue one and not replaced it?

d. What is the probability that in three grabs I will draw one red, one blue and one green fuse in that order?

7. My glove compartment contains 3 red fuses and 5 green fuses. If I draw 6 fuses with replacement, what is the probability of getting exactly 2 red and 4 green fuses?

8. In a horse race with 6 horses and 6 post positions, how many different orders of horses can we have?

9. How many different teams of 5 volleyballers could be made from 8 players?

10. In "Over-the-Line" baseball, there is a pitcher, batter, left fielder and right fielder. If we have 10 players, how many different teams could we have if different positions of the same players is a different team?

11. From a standard deck of shuffled playing cards, you have been dealt the 7, 8, 9, and, 10 of hearts, which you are holding. If you are dealt one more card, what is the probability it will be
    a. the 6 of hearts?
    b. the jack of hearts?
    c. either the 6 or the jack of hearts?
    d. neither the 6 nor the jack of hearts?
    e. any 6?

12. From a standard deck of shuffled playing cards, you have been dealt the 7, 8, 9, and 10 of hearts, which you are holding. If you are dealt two more cards, what is the probability you will get
    a. the 6 of hearts followed by the jack of hearts?
    b. the 6 of hearts and the jack of hearts?
    c. two 6's?

13. Determine the number of possible outcomes for the following.
    a. a pair of dice are rolled
    b. two coins are tossed

14. If a pair of dice are rolled what is the probability of rolling a one and a five?

15. If two coins are tossed what is the probability they will both be heads? What is the probability one is a head and the other is a tail?

16. A six-shooter has been loaded randomly with 2 bullets. You are going to fire the gun twice.
    a. Determine the total number of possible outcomes ($B = bullet$, $E = empty$).
    b. What is the probability of firing both bullets if the barrel is spun after the first shot is made?

17. The following table shows a breakdown of a statistics class in terms of grade received and major.

Grade	Psychology	Pre-Med	Business
9	3	1	0
8	6	4	3
7	15	10	8
6	9	6	10
5	22	12	11
4	2	3	1
3	0	0	0
2	0	1	1
1	1	0	0

a. Determine the total for each row and column.
b. If a student is selected at random from the class, what is the probability that he or she is a psychology major?
c. If a student is selected at random from the class, what is the probability that he or she is a business student with a grade of 7 or better?
d. If 3, 2, and 1 are failing grades, what is the probability of randomly selecting a pre-med student who failed the course?
e. Ignoring major, what is the probability that a randomly selected student passed the course?

18. You are dealt 5 cards from a well-shuffled deck of playing cards. What is the probability of getting:
    a. a flush (5 cards all in the same suit)?
    b. the Ace of spades as your first card?
    c. the Ace of clubs as your second card given you got the Ace of spades as your first card?

CHAPTER 8

Introduction to Inference: The Random Sampling Distribution

LEARNING OBJECTIVES

After reading this chapter you should be able to:
1. Describe the difference between a parameter and a statistic.
2. List the requirements for using descriptive statistics
3. List the requirements for using inferential statistics.
4. Describe how a random sample is selected.
5. List the steps required to construct a random sampling distribution.
6. Define $\mu_{\bar{x}}$ and state its relationship to the population mean.
7. Define the standard error of the mean and state its relationship to the population standard deviation.
8. State the Central Limit Theorem.
9. Use Z for the sample mean to solve problems using the normal curve.
10. Define the mean of the random sampling distribution of the difference and state its relationship to the mean of the population.
11. Define the standard error of the difference and state its relationship to the population standard deviation.
12. Use Z for the difference to solve problems using the normal curve.
13. Define the mean of the random sampling distribution of the proportion and state its relationship to the mean of the population.
14. Define the standard error of the proportion and state its relationship to the population standard deviation.
15. Use Z for the proportion to solve problems using the normal curve.

This chapter introduces the *random sampling distribution*, a distribution which plays a central role in inferential statistics. Although it may seem that we have spent a lot of time introducing statistical inference, it is important to have a thorough understanding of the basic concepts underlying inferential techniques.

Statistical Inference

It is not always practical and often not even possible to collect all the observations in a population. Statistical inference allows us to draw conclusions about values of population **parameters** from the values of **statistics** computed from samples drawn from populations.

> **Parameter:** A characteristic of a population.
> **Statistic:** A characteristic of a sample.

Descriptive vs Inferential Statistics

Descriptive statistics requires:

1. specifying the population of interest;
2. collecting all observations from the population;
3. computing summary values such as the mean and standard deviation;
4. using these summary values to describe the properties of the population.

Technically, since we are examining the entire population, we should not use the word "statistics." Rather, we should talk about "descriptive parameters." However, it has become common to use the term "statistics" even when describing entire populations.

Inferential statistics requires:

1. obtaining one or more samples from the population(s) of interest;
2. computing estimates of parameters from the sample data;
3. making inferences about the corresponding population parameters from which the sample was drawn.

The Random Sample

A **random sample** is drawn so that all observations in the population have an equal likelihood of being included in the sample. The term "random sample" does not define what the sample is like. Rather, it describes *how* the members of the sample were selected. Random sampling is a procedure for collecting observations from a population. It is a common technique in inferential statistics.

> **Random sample:** A sample collected such that all members of the population are equally likely to be included.

Two samples randomly drawn from the same population will rarely be identical. It is a fundamental fact that sample outcomes vary. This is called **sampling fluctuation** or sampling error. Imagine a population of IQ scores of all Canadians. The mean of the population is 100 and the standard deviation is 15. Let's put all these IQ scores in a hat, shake them up, and select 10 scores randomly. We compute the mean of our sample to be 95. If we used this value as our inference about the population mean, we would be wrong. Whenever we make a statistical inference *we may be wrong*!

The key is to discover what values of a statistic would occur, and with what frequency, when sampling repeatedly from the same population. If we know what outcomes are likely to occur, then we can make conclusions about a particular outcome we have found.

The Random Sampling Distribution

The **random sampling distribution** is critical in inferential statistics. It is a *relative frequency distribution* of the values of some statistic calculated for *all possible samples of a fixed size* drawn at random from a given population.

Let's return, for a moment, to the example of the biased coin. How many heads in a row could I toss before you became suspicious about the fairness of my coin? Perhaps you would start feeling doubtful after the sixth head in a row. Let's analyze this situation as a statistician might.

We obtain a coin that we know is fair, toss it six times, and record how many heads occur. If we repeat this experiment enough times, we will get six heads in a row, even though our coin is fair. However, this outcome will be quite rare. If we could determine how often six heads occur in a row with a fair coin, we would know the *probability* of such an outcome in a single experiment of six tosses. If we computed the frequency of all possible outcomes of six coin tosses, we would have a frequency distribution. We could convert this to a relative frequency distribution giving us a random sampling distribution for six tosses of a fair coin, repeated many times.

Let's say that the relative frequency of six heads in a row when the experiment is repeated an infinite number of times is $1/2^6 = 0.016$. This probability is very low. If we find ourselves in a situation where we are betting on the fairness of a coin that came up heads six times in a row, we should put our money on the biased side, not on the fair side. It is extremely unlikely that a fair coin would produce such an outcome.

Random sampling distributions describe the probabilities of outcomes in specified situations. When we know what is likely to occur in a given situation, we are able to make informed decisions about a particular outcome that has occurred.

A random sampling distribution can be constructed for any statistic. The general procedure for constructing a random sampling distribution is the following:

Step 1. Randomly select one (or more) sample(s) of observations of some fixed size from a given population.

Step 2. Calculate some statistic for that sample.

Step 3. Return the sample to the population.

Step 4. Repeat the first three steps until all possible samples have been drawn.

Step 5. Place all statistics in a relative frequency distribution.

A random sampling distribution is named after the statistic of interest. For example, if the statistic calculated on the samples was the median, we would call the relative frequency distribution "the random sampling distribution of the median." If the mode was calculated, it would be the "random sampling distribution of the mode."

In our studies, we will learn about many random sampling distributions. One very useful sampling distribution in inferential statistics is the *random sampling distribution of the mean*.

The Random Sampling Distribution of the Mean

To construct a **random sampling distribution of the mean** we follow these steps:

Step 1. Randomly select a sample of some fixed size from the population of interest.

Step 2. Calculate the sample mean.

Step 3. Return the sample to the population.

Step 4. Repeat steps 1–3 until all possible samples have been drawn.

Step 5. Place the sample means in a relative frequency distribution.

We now have a distribution of sample means. This random sampling distribution of the mean has certain invariable characteristics.

The Mean

Recall that the symbol "μ" stands for the mean of a population of observations. We need new notation to refer to the mean of a sample drawn from a population. We will use $\overline{X}$ (Xbar). The random sampling distribution of the mean is the relative frequency distribution of the means calculated for all possible samples drawn from a population. This distribution of sample means has a mean itself. The symbol for the mean of the sampling distribution of means is $\mu_{\overline{x}}$.

The mean of the random sampling distribution of the mean ($\mu_{\overline{x}}$) equals the mean of the raw score population (μ). To summarize:

μ is the mean of the population.
$\overline{X}$ is the mean of the sample.
$\mu_{\overline{x}}$ is the mean of the sampling distribution of means.
$\mu_{\overline{x}} = \mu$.

The Variance

The symbol for the variance of a population of raw scores is "σ^2." The variance of the sampling distribution of means indicates the variability of the sample means around the mean of the distribution. The symbol for the variance of a random sampling distribution of means is $\sigma_{\overline{x}}^2$. The variance of the sampling distribution of means is *not* equal to the variance of the population. The variability of the means around $\mu_{\overline{x}}$ is less than the variability of the raw scores around μ. In fact, the variance of the sampling distribution ($\sigma_{\overline{x}}^2$) will be less than that of the population by a factor of the size of the sample. We will use lower case **n** to refer to sample size. The variance of the sampling distribution is related to the variance of the population in the following way: $\sigma_{\overline{x}}^2 = \sigma^2/n$. The variance of the sampling distribution is $1/n$ smaller than the variance of the population of raw scores. Note that the variance of the sampling distribution will be less for a distribution constructed from large samples than for a distribution constructed from small samples. As sample size increases, the variance of the distribution of means decreases. To summarize:

σ^2 is the variance of the population.
$\sigma_{\overline{x}}^2$ is the variance of the sampling distribution of means.
$\sigma_{\overline{x}}^2 = \sigma^2/n$ where n is the sample size.

The Standard Deviation

The symbol for the standard deviation of a population is "σ." The symbol for the standard deviation of the random sampling distribution of the mean is $\sigma_{\overline{x}}$. This measure is used so frequently, it has a special name. It is called the **standard error of the mean**. It is easier to say "standard error of the mean" than "standard deviation of the random sampling distribution of means."

> **Standard error:** Standard deviation of a random sampling distribution

Recall that the variance of the sampling distribution is related to the variance of the population by $\sigma_{\bar{x}}^2 = \sigma^2/n$. You can see, then, that the standard error is related to the standard deviation of the population in the following way: $\sigma_{\bar{x}} = \sigma/\sqrt{n}$. The standard error is smaller than the standard deviation of the population by a factor of $1/\sqrt{n}$. To summarize:

σ is the standard deviation of a population.
$\sigma_{\bar{x}}$ is the standard deviation of the sampling distribution of means (called the standard error).
$\sigma_{\bar{x}} = \sigma/\sqrt{n}$ where n is the sample size.

The Shape: The Central Limit Theorem

The **Central Limit Theorem** is likely the most important theorem in inferential statistics. It states the following:

1. The random sampling distribution of means tends toward a normal distribution, irrespective of the shape of the original raw score population.
2. This tendency increases as sample size increases.

In other words no matter what the shape of the original population of raw scores, the relative frequency distribution of means, computed for all possible samples drawn from that population, will approach the normal distribution. Furthermore, the shape will be closer to normal for larger sample sizes.

In Chapter 6, we studied the characteristics of the standard normal distribution. Those same characteristics hold for the random sampling distribution of the mean when the sample size is large enough. The normal curve may be used as a model, then, for a sampling distribution of means when:

1. The original population is normal or close to normal in shape or
2. The original population is not normal but the sample size is large.

The Central Limit Theorem is important because it allows us to solve problems using the normal curve as a model.

> **Central Limit Theorem:** The random sampling distribution of means tends toward a normal distribution, irrespective of the shape of the original raw score population. This tendency increases as sample size increases.

Solving Problems with the Random Sampling Distribution of the Mean

In Chapter 6, we learned how to convert a raw score into a Z-score to solve problems with the normal curve. Recall that the formula to convert a raw score to its corresponding Z is

$$Z = \frac{X - \mu}{\sigma} \quad \text{Z for a raw score.}$$

We were able to find the proportion of the total area under the curve between two Z-scores and to find Z-scores when we knew the area. We learned to use Table B-1 in Appendix B to solve problems with any raw score distribution that was normal in shape.

We know that the random sampling distribution of means is normal in shape under certain conditions; we can use the same table and procedure for solving problems about means of samples that we used for solving problems about raw scores. We need only to convert the sample mean to its corresponding Z-score so that we can use the normal curve table.

Converting a sample mean to a Z-score is done in a similar manner to converting a raw score to a Z-score. The mean of the distribution is subtracted from the corresponding sample statistic and this difference is divided by the standard deviation of the distribution of the statistic. In the case of a sample mean, our formula is

$$Z = \frac{\overline{X} - \mu_{\overline{x}}}{\sigma_{\overline{x}}} \quad \text{Z for a sample mean}$$

We need to know the value of the population mean (μ) and the value of the population standard deviation (σ). We know the mean of the sampling distribution ($\mu_{\bar{x}}$) is equal to the population mean. We can find the standard error ($\sigma_{\bar{x}}$) by dividing σ by $\sqrt{n}$. Ready for an example?

Example A Consider a normal population of raw scores whose mean is 130 and whose standard deviation is 10. Let's randomly select a quantity of samples of 25 observations from this population and compute the mean for each. How often would we expect to get sample means between 128 and 132? We will solve this problem with the same strategy we used in Chapter 6. Remember the following sequence of steps.

$$\text{DATA: } \mu = 130$$
$$\sigma = 10$$
$$n = 25$$

Step 1. Draw a curve and shade in the area of concern.

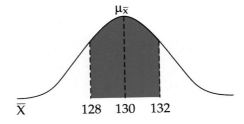

We know that the mean of the sampling distribution is 130 because it is equal to the mean of the population.

Step 2. Convert the sample means to Z-scores.

$$Z_{128} = \frac{\bar{X} - \mu_{\bar{x}}}{\sigma_{\bar{x}}} = \frac{128 - 130}{10/\sqrt{25}} = -1.00$$

$$Z_{132} = \frac{132 - 130}{2} = +1.00$$

Step 3. Look up the area between the two Z values in the normal curve table.

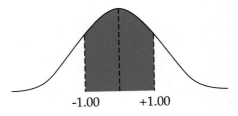

Area between the mean and a Z of +1.00 is 0.3413
Area between the mean and a Z of −1.00 is 0.3413
Area between the two Z values is 0.6826

Therefore, when we draw many samples from this population, we would expect to get means between 128 and 132 about 68% of the time.

Example B Let's try another example. Between what two values would we expect 99% of the means of samples from our population to fall?

Step 1. Draw a curve and shade in the area of concern.

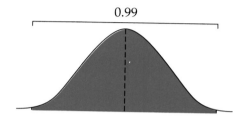

Step 2. Look up the two Z values between which 0.99 of the total area lies, (i.e., 0.4950 on each side of the mean).

$$Z = \pm 2.58$$

Step 3. Rearrange the formula so $\overline{X}$ is the unknown.

$$\overline{X} = \mu_{\overline{x}} \pm Z\sigma_{\overline{x}}$$
$$= 130 \pm 2.58 \, (10/\sqrt{25})$$
$$= 130 \pm 5.16$$
$$= 124.84 \text{ and } 135.16$$

We would expect 99% of the means to fall between 124.84 and 135.16 and the remaining 1% to fall beyond these two points.

Example C How about a third example? How often would we expect to find sample means as large or larger than 145, drawn from our population?

Step 1. Draw a curve and shade in the area of concern.

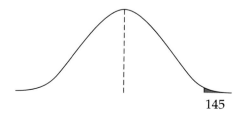

Step 2. Convert the sample mean to a Z-score.

$$Z_{145} = \frac{145 - 130}{2} = 7.5$$

Step 3. The tables don't go this far. Our best answer is that we would never (or hardly ever) expect to get means this large. If a friend told you that she randomly selected 25 observations from a normal population whose mean is 130 and whose standard deviation is 10, and computed a sample mean of 145, your skepticism would be understandable. The probability of such an outcome, given that the information about the population is true, is incredibly low.

However, what if your friend could prove that her calculation of the mean was correct and that she did, in fact, randomly select 25 observations? What can you conclude? Two possibilities come to mind. Either she obtained an amazingly rare outcome; or her information about the population from which she drew her sample is wrong.

Remember the coin toss experiment where 6 heads occurred in a row? Two explanations again come to mind. Either an extremely rare outcome occurred with a fair coin or the coin was not a fair one. In the latter explanation, expectations about how the coin should behave were wrong. This describes the logic of many inferential techniques. Inferences are based on the probability of a particular sample outcome occurring when certain hypotheses are made about the population from which the sample was selected.

The random sampling distribution of the mean is very important in statistical inference. Knowing its properties allows us to make decisions about outcomes of experiments. Another important random sampling distribution involves the differences between means of two populations.

The Random Sampling Distribution of the Difference between Means

The **random sampling distribution of the difference between means** is a relative frequency distribution of the differences between sample means drawn from two populations with equal means. If we draw samples from populations of raw scores having equal means, we would not expect the sample means to be identical. Remember sampling fluctuation? The question we must ask is "How different would we expect sample means to be, when the samples are drawn from populations with equal means?" To answer this question, we need to determine the kinds of differences that would occur. We must construct a random sampling distribution of differences between pairs of means drawn from two populations with equal means. This distribution is constructed in the following manner:

Step 1. Randomly draw two samples, of fixed sizes, from two populations with equal means. (These samples don't have to be equal sizes.)

Step 2. Calculate the mean of each sample and record the mean difference.

Step 3. Return the samples to their respective populations.

Step 4. Repeat steps 1-3 until all possible pairs of samples have been drawn.

Step 5. Place the mean differences in a relative frequency distribution.

The result is a random sampling distribution of the difference between means. This distribution of differences has several invariable properties related to the original populations.

The Mean

If we compute the mean of all the differences we collected, we would find it is zero. This makes sense because we drew our samples from two populations whose mean difference is zero.

Staying with our usual notation:

$\overline{X}_1 - \overline{X}_2$ is the difference between the means of a pair of samples.

$\mu_1 - \mu_2$ is the mean of the population of differences.

$\mu_{\overline{x}_1} - \mu_{\overline{x}_2}$ is the mean of the sampling distribution of the difference.

The means of the raw score populations are equal, so the mean of the distribution of differences is also zero.

$$\mu_1 - \mu_2 = 0$$
$$\mu_{\overline{x}_1} - \mu_{\overline{x}_2} = 0$$

The Variance

Because we have a frequency distribution of values (i.e., differences), we can calculate the variance of that distribution. How much do the differences vary around the mean difference of zero? The variance of the sampling distribution of the difference between means is related to the variances of the populations. It is smaller than in the original populations because we are dealing with sample means, not raw scores. Like the sampling distribution of the mean, as the samples become larger, the variance of the sampling distribution of the difference becomes smaller. The variance of the sampling distribution of the difference is related to the population variances in the following manner:

$$\sigma^2_{\overline{x}_1 - \overline{x}_2} = \sigma^2_{\overline{x}_1} + \sigma^2_{\overline{x}_2} = \frac{\sigma^2_1}{n_1} + \frac{\sigma^2_2}{n_2}$$

Variance of the Random Sampling Distribution of the Difference

When we compute the variance of the sampling distribution of the difference from the sums of squares of the groups, the computational formula is

$$\sigma^2_{\bar{x}_1-\bar{x}_2} = \frac{\Sigma x_1^2 + \Sigma x_2^2}{n_1 + n_2}\left(\frac{1}{n_1} + \frac{1}{n_2}\right)$$

$$\text{or} = \frac{\Sigma x_1^2 + \Sigma x_2^2}{n(n)} \text{ if } n_1 = n_2$$

Computational Formulas for the Variance of the Sampling Distribution of the Difference

where $\Sigma x^2 = \Sigma X^2 - (\Sigma X)^2/n$

If the populations from which the samples were drawn have equal variances as well as equal means, and if the samples were of equal sizes, then the relationship between the population variance and the variance of the sampling distribution is $\sigma^2_{\bar{x}_1-\bar{x}_2} = 2\sigma^2/n$

To summarize:

σ_1^2 is the variance of the first population.
σ_2^2 is the variance of the second population.
$\sigma^2_{\bar{x}_1-\bar{x}_2}$ is the variance of the sampling distribution of differences between means. The relationship between them is

$$\sigma^2_{\bar{x}_1-\bar{x}_2} = \frac{\sigma_1^2}{n_1} + \frac{\sigma_2^2}{n_2}$$

The Standard Deviation

You will recall that the standard deviation of a random sampling distribution is called a standard error. The standard deviation of the sampling distribution of the difference is called the **standard error of the difference between means**. The standard error is simply the square root of the variance. To summarize:

σ_1 is the standard deviation of the first population.
σ_2 is the standard deviation of the second population.
$\sigma_{\bar{x}_1-\bar{x}_2}$ is the standard deviation of the sampling distribution of differences between means.

The standard error is related to the populations in the following way:

$$\sigma_{\bar{x}_1 - \bar{x}_2} = \sqrt{\sigma_{\bar{x}_1}^2 + \sigma_{\bar{x}_2}^2}$$

$$= \sqrt{\frac{\sigma_1^2}{n_1} + \frac{\sigma_2^2}{n_2}}$$

Standard Error of the Random Sampling Distribution of the Difference

or $\quad = \sqrt{\dfrac{2\sigma^2}{n}} \quad$ if $\sigma_1 = \sigma_2$ and $n_1 = n_2$

The computational formulas for the standard error of the difference are

$$\sigma_{\bar{x}_1 - \bar{x}_2} = \sqrt{\frac{\Sigma x_1^2 + \Sigma x_2^2}{n_1 + n_2} \left(\frac{1}{n_1} + \frac{1}{n_2}\right)}$$

or $= \sqrt{\dfrac{\Sigma x_1^2 + \Sigma x_2^2}{n(n)}} \quad$ if $n_1 = n_2$

Computational Formulas for the Standard Error of the Difference

where $\Sigma x^2 = \Sigma X^2 - (\Sigma X)^2/n$

The Shape

Remember the Central Limit Theorem? It governs the shape of the sampling distribution of the difference in the same way it does with the sampling distribution of the mean. This distribution will be normal if the populations are normal or if the samples are reasonably large. We can use the normal curve to solve problems about the sampling distribution of the difference as we did with the sampling distribution of the mean.

Solving Problems with the Random Sampling Distribution of the Difference

Once again, to use the normal curve table, we need to convert our statistic to its Z-score equivalent. The mean of the sampling distribution is subtracted from its corresponding sample statistic, and this difference is divided by the standard deviation of the sampling distribution of the statistic. Since our statistic is the mean difference, the Z-score formula is

146 Chapter Eight

$$Z = \frac{(\overline{X}_1 - \overline{X}_2) - (\mu_{\overline{x}_1} - \mu_{\overline{x}_2})}{\sigma_{\overline{x}_1 - \overline{x}_2}} \qquad \text{Z for the difference}$$

Often the right part of the numerator is omitted since the mean of the sampling distribution of the difference is equal to the mean difference in the population: zero.

We can solve problems about mean differences in the same way we solved problems with single means when the shape of the distribution of mean differences is normal.

Example D Consider two raw score populations with means of 100 and standard deviations of 10. Let us randomly select a sample of 25 observations from each population and compute the difference between the sample means. How often would we expect to get mean differences between 5 and −5? Using the same procedure we applied earlier, we take these steps:

Step 1. Draw the curve and shade in the area of concern.

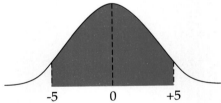

Step 2. Compute the Z scores.

$$Z = \frac{\overline{X}_1 - \overline{X}_2}{\sigma_{\overline{x}_1 - \overline{x}_2}}$$

Since we have drawn equal-sized samples from populations with equal variances, we calculate the standard error by:

$$Z \text{ of } \pm 5 = \frac{\pm 5}{\sqrt{\frac{2(10)^2}{25}}} = \frac{\pm 5}{2.83} = \pm 1.77$$

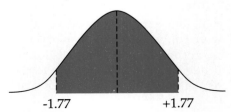

These two Z-scores correspond to mean differences of 5 points or less between the two samples in either direction.

Step 3. Look up the area in the normal curve table (Table B-1 in Appendix B).

Area between the mean of 0 and a Z of ±1.77 is 2(0.4616) = 0.9232

About 92% of the time we would expect to get samples whose means differ by 5 points or less either way, when drawing from such populations. This much sampling fluctuation, then, is quite likely.

Example E Now let's try another question. Beyond what two values would we expect only the extreme 5% of the mean differences to fall, 2½% on either side?

Step 1. Draw the curve and shade in the area of concern.

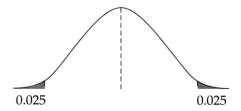

0.025   0.025

Figure 8-7

Step 2. Look up the Z values which separate the middle 95% from the extreme 5% of the area.

$$Z = \pm 1.96$$

Step 3. Convert the Z-scores to mean differences by rearranging the formula.

$$\overline{X}_1 - \overline{X}_2 = (\mu_{\bar{x}_1} - \mu_{\bar{x}_2}) \pm Z(\sigma_{\bar{x}_1 - \bar{x}_2})$$
$$= 0 \pm 1.96(2.83)$$
$$= \pm 5.55$$

We would expect our sample means to differ 5.55 points or more in either direction, 5% of the time.

Solving problems about mean differences follows the same logic as solving problems about single means. The Central Limit Theorem assures us that the shape of the sampling distribution of the difference will be normal if the populations are normal, or close to normal as long as the samples are reasonably large.

The Random Sampling Distribution of a Proportion

Recall our coin toss experiment. In one toss of a coin, only two outcomes are possible. You will recall from Chapter 7 that this is called a *dichotomous variable*. Dichotomous variables are ones where only two mutually exclusive outcomes are of interest. Up to now we have been discussing random sampling distributions where means of samples have been computed. Dichotomous variables can be placed in a random sampling distribution as well. We'll call this **the random sampling distribution of a proportion**. It's easier to say proportion, and any dichotomous variable can be thought of in terms of proportions.

We would construct the random sampling distribution of a proportion in the following manner:

Step 1. Randomly select a sample of some fixed size from the population of a dichotomous variable.

Step 2. Determine the proportion of times the value of interest occurs.

Step 3. Return the sample to the population.

Step 4. Repeat steps 1–3 until all possible samples have been drawn.

Step 5. Place these sample proportions in a relative frequency distribution.

If we were interested in setting up the random sampling distribution of our simple but illustrative experiment of 6 tosses of a coin, we would:

Step 1. Toss the coin 6 times. (Our sample size is 6.)

Step 2. Count the number of times a head occurs and record this as a proportion (e.g., 0.5 or 3/6).

Step 3. Repeat the first two steps an infinite number of times.

Step 4. Place our proportions in a relative frequency distribution.

If you suspect that this distribution has certain invariable properties, you are quite correct.

The Mean

In our coin toss experiment the outcome that will occur most frequently is 3 heads in 6 tosses. With a fair coin, we would expect to get half heads and half tails more often than any other outcome. Occasionally, we will get an unlikely outcome, such as 6 heads in a row, but not often. The mean of the random sampling distribution of a proportion (P_p) is equal to the proportion of times the outcome of interest is expected to occur in the population (**P**). In the case of a coin, we would expect to get heads 50% or 0.50 of the time. This is also the probability of a head; proportions can be thought of as probabilities. (You may recall our discussion of a relative frequency distribution as a probability distribution.) We will use lower case **p** to refer to the proportion of times the outcome of interest occurred in the sample. The mean of all the sample proportions determined from all possible samples is equal to the expected value of the outcome of interest in the population (P). To summarize:

P is the proportion for the outcome of interest in the population or the probability of the outcome of interest.
p is the proportion of times the outcome of interest occurred in the sample.
P_p is the mean of the random sampling distribution of the proportion.
$P_p = P$

The Variance

All the sample proportions vary around the mean of the distribution. The variance of this sampling distribution is

$$\sigma_p^2 = PQ/n \quad \text{Variance of the Sampling Distribution of a Proportion}$$

If we think of P as the probability of the outcome of interest, then Q is the probability of the other outcome. Q is always equal to $1 - P$.

The Standard Deviation

As you might expect, the standard deviation of the random sampling distribution of a proportion is called the **standard error of the proportion**. It is the square root of the variance.

$$\sigma_p = \sqrt{PQ/n} \quad \text{Standard Error of the Proportion}$$

The Shape

Once again the Central Limit Theorem governs the shape of the sampling distribution of a proportion. When the sample size is large, the distribution is normal in shape. Let's repeatedly toss our coin 6 times in a row. Now, let's repeatedly toss the coin 50 times in a row. The relative frequency distribution constructed in the second experiment would be closer to the normal distribution than the one constructed in the first experiment. A rule of thumb is that samples must be about 40 or larger for the sampling distribution to be normal enough to use the normal curve as a model.

Solving Problems with the Random Sampling Distribution of a Proportion

Let's toss our coin 50 times and record the number of heads we get. If we did this over and over again, how often would we expect to get 40 or more heads in 50 tosses? We can solve this problem using the same procedure we used earlier. To use the normal curve table to find areas, we must have a Z-score. Since the general formula for Z is to subtract the mean of the sampling distribution from the sample statistic and divide this difference by the standard error, our Z formula is

$$Z = \frac{p - P_p}{\sigma_p} \quad \text{Z for a Proportion}$$

Now let's apply the procedure.

Example F How often should we expect to get 40 or more heads in 50 tosses of a coin?

Step 1. Draw a curve and shade in the area of concern.

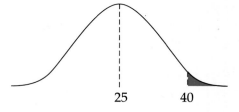

Since we are tossing our coin 50 times, 50 is our sample size. The mean of the sampling distribution of the proportion (P_p) equals the expected proportion in the population. If the coin is fair we would expect to get heads on half of the tosses, or 25 times in 50 tosses, on the average.

Step 2. Compute the Z-score. Our sample proportion is 40/50 or 0.80. The mean of the sampling distribution is 25/50 or 0.50.

$$Z = \frac{p - P_p}{\sigma_p}$$
$$= \frac{0.80 - 0.50}{\sqrt{(0.50)(0.50)/50}}$$
$$= \frac{0.30}{0.07} = 4.29$$

Step 3. Look up the Z value. Once again our Z value is too large for the table. It is extremely unlikely to get 40 heads in 50 tosses of a fair coin. This outcome would occur so rarely that our best bet is that the coin is not fair.

Example G Let's look at a different kind of problem. Remember Mendel's Law? Consider a variety of garden pea where Mendel's Law states that 25% of these peas would be pink in colour and the rest should be green. If we were to randomly select many samples of 400 peas each, how often would we expect to get 79 or fewer pink peas out of the 400 we picked?

Step 1. Draw a curve and shade in the area of concern.

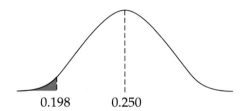

The mean of the sampling distribution is 0.25 because Mendel's Law states that 25% or 100 of the 400 peas should be pink. We are interested in the area under the curve for proportions of 79/400 or 0.198 or less.

Step 2. Compute the Z-score.
$$Z = \frac{0.198 - 0.25}{\sqrt{(0.25)(0.75)/400}} = -\frac{0.052}{0.022} = -2.36$$

Step 3. Look up the area in Table B-1.
$$\text{Area} = 0.0091$$

We would expect to get 79 or fewer pink peas out of 400 less than 1% of the time.

Knowing the shape of the random sampling distribution of a statistic allows us to determine the likelihood of different kinds of sample outcomes. Here we have looked at the normal distribution. Later, we will discuss sampling distributions of other statistics which are not normally shaped.

The procedure will not change, however. When we know the frequency of the expected outcomes, then we can make informed decisions about particular outcomes.

The normal curve is a very useful tool in inferential statistics. It can be used to approximate several different random sampling distributions.

SUMMARY OF TERMS AND FORMULAS

A characteristic of a population is called a **parameter**. A characteristic of a sample is called a **statistic**.

A **random sample** is a sample collected such that each member of the population has an equal likelihood of being included.

Standard error is another name for the standard deviation of a random sampling distribution.

According to the **Central Limit Theorem**, the random sampling distribution of means tends toward a normal distribution, regardless of the shape of the original raw score population. This tendency increases as sample size increases.

Random Sampling Distribution of:	Mean	Variance	Standard Deviation	Z formula
the Mean	$\mu_{\bar{x}}$	$\sigma^2_{\bar{x}}$	$\sigma_{\bar{x}}$	$\dfrac{X - \mu_{\bar{x}}}{\sigma_{\bar{x}}}$
the Difference	$\mu_{\bar{x}_1} - \mu_{\bar{x}_2}$	$\sigma^2_{\bar{x}_1 - \bar{x}_2}$	$\sigma_{\bar{x}_1 - \bar{x}_2}$	$\dfrac{\bar{X}_1 - \bar{X}_2}{\sigma_{\bar{x}_1 - \bar{x}_2}}$
the Proportion	P_p	σ^2_p	σ_p	$\dfrac{p - P_p}{\sigma_p}$

Computational Formulas for the Standard Error of the Difference

$$\sigma_{\bar{x}_1 - \bar{x}_2} = \sqrt{\frac{\Sigma x_1^2 + \Sigma x_2^2}{n_1 + n_2}\left(\frac{1}{n_1} + \frac{1}{n_2}\right)}$$

$$\sigma_{\bar{x}_1 - \bar{x}_2} = \sqrt{\frac{\Sigma x_1^2 + \Sigma x_2^2}{n(n)}} \quad \text{if } n_1 = n_2$$

where $\Sigma x^2 = \Sigma X^2 - (\Sigma X)^2/n$

The Random Sampling Distribution

Relationship between Properties of the Random Sampling Distribution (R.S.D.) and Properties of the Population

R.S.D. of the Mean

$$\mu_{\bar{x}} = \mu$$

$$\sigma_{\bar{x}} = \sigma/\sqrt{n}$$

R.S.D. of the Difference

$$\mu_{\bar{x}_1} - \mu_{\bar{x}_2} = \mu_1 - \mu_2 = 0$$

$$\sigma_{\bar{x}_1 - \bar{x}_2} = \sqrt{\frac{\sigma_1^2}{n_1} + \frac{\sigma_2^2}{n_2}}$$

R.S.D. of the Proportion

$$P_p = P$$

$$\sigma_p = \sqrt{PQ/n}$$

EXERCISES

1. Given the following population of scores calculate the following.
   DATA: 10, 13, 15, 17, 20, 25, 30
   a. $\Sigma X =$
   b. $(\Sigma X)^2/N =$
   c. $N =$
   d. $\Sigma X^2 =$
   e. $\mu =$
   f. $\sigma =$

2. The following data are a population of raw scores.
   DATA: 1, 2, 4, 7, 11
   Compute the mean and standard deviation of this population.

3. Using the population of scores in Exercise 2, list the 25 possible samples of size 2 which can be drawn from this population with replacement. Find the mean of each sample.

4. Place the sample means from Exercise 3 into an absolute frequency distribution. Find the mean of the distribution and the standard deviation of the distribution using the following formulas: (Hint: N=25)

$$\mu_{\bar{x}} = \Sigma f\bar{X}/N$$

$$\sigma_{\bar{x}} = \sqrt{\frac{\Sigma f\bar{X}^2 - (\Sigma f\bar{X})^2/N}{N}}$$

You will find that the mean of the sample means ($\mu_{\bar{x}}$) is equal to the mean of the original population that you computed in Exercise 2 (namely, μ). Check to make sure that the standard deviation or standard error you computed on your distribution of sample means is equal to $\sigma/\sqrt{n}$, where n is the sample size of 2.

5. Using the distribution of sample means from Exercise 4, determine the probability of drawing at random a single sample of 2 scores whose mean is:
   a. equal to 5
   b. > 5
   c. >4 and <6

6. A distribution of scores has a mean of 75 and a standard deviation of 15. If all possible samples were drawn with replacement from this population, calculate the values of $\mu_{\bar{x}}$ and $\sigma_{\bar{x}}$ if:
   a. n = 225
   b. n = 100
   c. n = 25

7. What is the probability of drawing from the population in Exercise 6 a single sample of 25 scores whose mean is between 70 and 80?

8. A normal population has a mean of 100 and a standard deviation of 16. What is the probability of randomly selecting 25 observations from this population and computing a mean
   a. equal to or larger than 112?
   b. between 95 and 105?
   c. equal to or less than 90?

9. Using the distribution described in Exercise 8, determine
   a. between what two means, 95% of the means will lie.
   b. between what two means, 99% of the means will lie.

10. Using the data below solve the following problems. Assume the populations are normally distributed with equal means.

    $$\Sigma x_1^2 = 178 \qquad n_1 = n_2 = 40$$
    $$\Sigma x_2^2 = 156$$

    What is the probability of randomly selecting a sample from each population and getting a mean difference as far or further above zero than indicated in each of the following?
    a. $\bar{X}_1 = 59$ $\quad \bar{X}_2 = 37$
    b. $\bar{X}_1 = 65$ $\quad \bar{X}_2 = 35$
    c. $\bar{X}_1 = 73.9$ $\quad \bar{X}_2 = 26.7$

11. Using the data below solve the following problems. Assume the populations are normally distributed with equal means.

    $$\sigma_1^2 = 16 \qquad n_1 = 36$$
    $$\sigma_2^2 = 25 \qquad n_2 = 50$$

What is the probability of selecting one sample from each population and getting a mean difference as far or further below zero than indicated in each of the following?

a. $\overline{X}_1 = 123.72 \quad \overline{X}_2 = 124.01$
b. $\overline{X}_1 = 124 \quad \overline{X}_2 = 126$
c. $\overline{X}_1 = 122.5 \quad \overline{X}_2 = 123.0$

12. An investigator decides to test a die for fairness. She rolls the die 40 times and counts the number of times a 4 turns up. If the die is fair what is the probability that she will count
    a. ten or more 4s?
    b. six or fewer 4s?
    c. two 4s or less?

13. A sociologist randomly selects 500 Nova Scotian families and categorizes each according to its socio-economic status (SES). Statistics Canada has determined that 75% of the population is middle-upper SES and the rest are lower SES. If Nova Scotians are similar to the rest of the population, what is the probability that the sociologist would find 339 or fewer middle-upper SES families in his sample?

CHAPTER 9

Inference with the Normal Curve

LEARNING OBJECTIVES

After reading this chapter you should be able to:

1. Define the following terms: a priori, post hoc, critical value.
2. List the critical values for one- and two-tailed tests at the .05 and the .01 levels of significance.
3. Indicate the critical values for one- and two-tailed tests at the .05 and the .01 levels of significance on a diagram.
4. Set up the 95% and 99% confidence intervals for a population mean for a given set of data.
5. Set up the 95% and 99% confidence intervals for the difference between population means for a given set of data.
6. Set up the 95% and 99% confidence intervals for the population proportion for a given set of data.
7. Define and provide an example of a conceptual hypothesis.
8. Define and provide an example of a research hypothesis.
9. Define and provide an example of a statistical hypothesis.
10. Describe the difference between an experimental and a correlational research hypothesis.
11. Define and provide an example of a null hypothesis.
12. Define and provide an example of an alternative hypothesis.
13. Describe the difference between a directional and a non-directional alternative hypothesis.
14. List the steps for testing a conceptual hypothesis.
15. List the steps for testing the null hypothesis.
16. Define alpha.
17. Indicate on a diagram the region of rejection and the region of acceptance for one-tailed and two-tailed tests of significance.
18. Run a Z-test for a single mean for a given set of data.
19. Run a Z-test for the difference between means for a given set of data.

20. Run a Z-test for the proportion for a given set of data.
21. Define Type I error, Type II error and power.
22. Determine the appropriate test of significance for a given research problem.

Chapters 6, 7, and 8 discussed topics which are basic to inferential statistics. You now know the properties of the normal curve and several random sampling distributions. You understand probability and how it applies to frequency distributions. It's now time to apply this knowledge to make inferences about populations from samples drawn from them.

Hypothesis Testing and Interval Estimation

Hypothesis testing and **interval estimation** are two inferential techniques which are based on the concept of random sampling distributions. They both use sample statistics to make inferences about population parameters.

In hypothesis testing, we have an **a priori** (before the fact) hypothesis about the value of some parameter or the relationship between parameters. Sample data are used to determine whether or not this hypothesis is reasonable. The sample data are used to "test our guess."

With interval estimation, we do not have any a priori hypotheses about the value of the parameter(s). We use the sample data to infer what the value of the parameter might be. Interval estimation, then, is a **post hoc** (after the fact) technique. Because interval estimation is a simpler technique, it will be discussed first.

> **a priori:** Before the fact.
> **post hoc:** After the fact.

When we use interval estimation with the normal curve, we are asking "What is the value of this population parameter?" or "What is the relationship between parameters?" Interval estimation provides us with a method to set up a *range of values* within which the parameter will likely fall. Although the size of the range of values is arbitrary, most researchers in psychology and related disciplines use two ranges, the 95% and the 99% **confidence intervals**.

Confidence Intervals Using the Normal Distribution

Setting up the Confidence Interval for a Population Mean

In Chapter 8 we saw that a distribution of means, calculated from random samples drawn from a population, distributes itself normally within the limits of the Central Limit Theorem. A single sample mean, if selected randomly, may be viewed as a *single random case* drawn from the distribution of all sample means. Recall that in the random sampling distribution of the mean, 95% of the sample means fall within ±1.96 standard deviations of the mean of the sampling distribution, and 99% of the means fall within ±2.58 standard deviations of the mean of this distribution. These two values, ±1.96 and ±2.58, are called **critical values** in inferential statistics.

> **Critical value:** The value of a statistic corresponding to a given significance level determined by its sampling distribution.

When we know the population standard deviation and the mean of a single random sample, we can estimate where the population mean (μ) is likely to fall. The formulas for setting up the 99% and the 95% confidence intervals (CI) are

---
Confidence Intervals for the Mean

95% CI $\overline{X} \pm 1.96\ \sigma_{\overline{x}}$
99% CI $\overline{X} \pm 2.58\ \sigma_{\overline{x}}$

Let's examine a specific example. Suppose we have drawn a random sample from a population whose standard deviation is 15. We find that the mean of our 25 observations is 100. We wish to determine a range of values within which we are reasonably sure that the population mean will fall. Likely the population mean will not equal 100, since we know that sample means vary somewhat from the population mean. If we claimed that $\mu = 100$, the chances are we would be wrong. To make a better guess, use the two formulas above to provide the 95% and 99% CI's.

Data: $\sigma = 15$
$n = 25$
$\overline{X} = 100$

Before we use the formulas, we need to find the standard deviation of the sampling distribution (the standard error).

$$\sigma_{\bar{x}} = \sigma/\sqrt{n}$$
$$= 15/\sqrt{25}$$
$$= 3$$
$$95\% \text{ CI: } \bar{X} \pm 1.96\sigma_{\bar{x}}$$
$$= 100 \pm 1.96(3)$$
$$= 100 \pm 5.88 = 94.12 \text{ and } 105.88$$

We are 95% confident that the population mean lies between 94.12 and 105.88. In other words, our confidence that the population mean is greater than or equal to 94.12 and less than or equal to 105.88 is .95. This can be expressed in notation:

$$C(94.12 \leq \mu \leq 105.88) = .95$$

If we wanted to be more confident, we could set up a 99% confidence interval by:

$$99\% \text{ CI: } \bar{X} \pm 2.58\sigma_{\bar{x}}$$
$$= 100 \pm 2.58(3)$$
$$= 100 \pm 7.74 = 92.26 \text{ and } 107.74$$

and express this in notation as

$$C(92.26 \leq \mu \leq 107.74) = .99$$

As you can see, the 99% CI sets a wider range of values within which the population mean is likely to fall.

Why do we use the term "confidence" instead of "probability"? This is a good question. When we set up the 95% CI, for example, we know that 95% of the sample means will lie within 1.96 standard error units from the mean of the sampling distribution. Therefore, 5% of the sample means will be further away from $\mu_{\bar{x}}$ than $1.96\sigma_{\bar{x}}$. For these few sample means, the limits set up by our procedure will *not* encompass μ. (Remember that $\mu_{\bar{x}} = \mu$). In other words, 5% of the time, we will obtain a sample mean so far from the mean of the sampling distribution, that our confidence interval will not include μ. *Before* we draw our sample to set up the 95% CI, we can say that the *probability* that our interval will contain μ is .95. However, once the data have been collected and we have set our limits, a given interval *either does or does not* contain μ. Probability is a term that we use to express the likelihood of future outcomes. Once the event has taken place, we cannot use the term probability. A good analogy is one toss of a fair coin. While the coin is still up in the air, we can say the probability of getting a head is 1/2. Once the coin has landed, however, either a head or a tail has occurred. The event has taken place and we can no longer use the term probability. When setting up limits for μ, then, we use the term *confidence* rather than probability.

With any inferential technique, there is some probability of error. When we set up confidence intervals, there is always a possibility that our limits will not encompass the parameter of interest.

Consider a population of raw scores with a mean of 100 and a standard deviation of 20. If we randomly draw all possible samples of 100 observations from this population, and place the sample means in a relative frequency distribution, we will have the random sampling distribution of the mean for a sample size of 100. Suppose we draw a single sample of 100 observations from the population and compute a sample mean of 103. Let's go ahead and set up the 95% CI for this sample mean.

$$95\% \text{ CI} \quad 103 \pm 1.96(20/\sqrt{100})$$
$$= 103 \pm 3.92$$
$$= 99.08 \text{ and } 106.93$$

We are 95% confident that the population mean lies between these two values and justifiably so, since we know that the population mean is 100.

Now, let's draw another sample from the population and compute the mean of the sample. We find it is 95. Now we set up the 95% CI for this sample mean.

$$95\% \text{ CI} \quad 95 \pm 1.96(2) = 91.08 \text{ and } 98.92.$$

We would claim that μ lies between these two values. Are we correct? Not this time. The limits do not include μ. Figure 9-1 illustrates what happened.

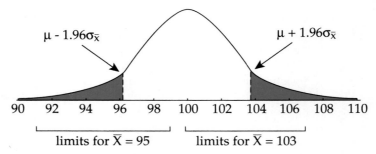

Figure 9-1   Confidence intervals for two sample means

Look at the range of values we set up for the two sample means. You can see that for the mean of 103, our limits included μ, but for the mean of 95, they did not. Whenever a sample mean is further away from the mean of the sampling distribution than $\pm 1.96\ \sigma_{\bar{x}}$, the limits set up by the 95% CI will not contain the population mean. If, on the other hand, the sample mean is within $\pm 1.96\ \sigma_{\bar{x}}$ of $\mu_{\bar{x}}$, the population mean will be included in our interval. We know that 5% of the time a single sample mean will be further away than $\pm 1.96\ \sigma_{\bar{x}}$ of $\mu_{\bar{x}}$, and so 5% of the time we make an incorrect inference about the location of the population mean. Obviously, if we want to be very careful about error, we would use a stricter criterion. The 99% CI is more conservative and we will be in error only 1% of the time.

Setting up the Confidence Interval for the Difference between Population Means

Similarly, confidence intervals can be determined for the difference between population means. The random sampling distribution of the difference tells us what kinds of differences we can expect between sample means when they come from populations with equal means. If we draw two random samples and compute the mean difference, we can set up a range of values between which we are reasonably confident the mean difference in the population lies. The formulas for 95% and 99% confidence intervals for the difference are

---

Confidence Intervals for the Difference between Means

95% CI $\quad (\overline{X}_1 - \overline{X}_2) \pm 1.96(\sigma_{\overline{x}_1 - \overline{x}_2})$

99% CI $\quad (\overline{X}_1 - \overline{X}_2) \pm 2.58(\sigma_{\overline{x}_1 - \overline{x}_2})$

Again, we are simply using the sample statistic, the mean difference, to set up a range of values within which we think the population parameter $(\mu_1 - \mu_2)$ lies. Ready for an example?

In an Introductory Psychology class, 16 students are randomly selected and assigned to two experimental conditions. Both groups of eight students each are given the same 25-item multiple-choice test. Group 1 is given hints on taking multiple-choice tests; Group 2 is not. We want to set up the 99% CI for the difference. Here are the data.

DATA: $\quad \overline{X}_1 = 13.25 \quad \overline{X}_2 = 14.75$
$\quad \Sigma x_1^2 = 43.5 \quad \Sigma x_2^2 = 75.5$
$\quad n_1 = n_2 = 8$

99% CI $\quad (\overline{X}_1 - \overline{X}_2) \pm 2.58(\sigma_{\overline{x}_1 - \overline{x}_2})$

We first need to compute the standard error of the difference. Since the samples are the same size, we can use:

$$\sigma_{\overline{x}_1 - \overline{x}_2} = \sqrt{\frac{\Sigma x_1^2 + \Sigma x_2^2}{n(n)}}$$

$$= \sqrt{\frac{43.5 + 75.5}{8(8)}} = 1.36$$

Now we can go ahead and set up the confidence interval.

99% CI (13.25 − 14.75) ± 2.58(1.36) = −1.50 ± 3.51
= 2.01 and −5.01

We are 99% confident that the true difference in the population lies somewhere between −5.01 and 2.01 or, expressed in notation:

$$C(-5.01 \leq \mu \leq 2.01) = .99$$

Setting up the Confidence Interval for a Population Proportion

We can set up confidence intervals for the proportion using the same logic and procedure. The formulas are

---

Confidence Intervals for the Proportion

95% CI $p \pm 1.96(\sigma_p)$
99% CI $p \pm 2.58(\sigma_p)$

In this case, we are setting up a range of values within which we are reasonably sure that the population proportion lies. Let's do an example.

You have two cards, one red and one black. You randomly select 52 friends and ask each to guess the colour of the card you are holding behind your back. Thirty-eight people guess correctly. You are interested in knowing the proportion of people in the population who would guess correctly. You decide to set up the 95% CI. For each subject, we assume that the probability of guessing correctly is 1/2.

DATA: $p = 38/52 = 0.73$

$$\sigma_p = \sqrt{PQ/n} = \sqrt{(0.5)(0.5)/52} = 0.07$$

95% C.I. = 0.73 ± .1.96(0.07) = 0.59 and 0.83

You are 95% confident that the true percentage in the population is between 59% and 83%, at least under the conditions of your experiment. We might wonder about how you conducted this study, however!

Setting up confidence intervals can be done for many population parameters. All we need is the sample statistic, the standard deviation of the sampling distribution of that statistic, and knowledge of the shape of that sampling distribution. The general formula is

> CI for parameter = statistic ± critical value (standard error)

We use confidence intervals when we have no a priori hypothesis about the value of the population parameter. When we have an hypothesis about some parameter and we wish to test its validity we use a different inferential technique.

Hypothesis Testing with the Normal Curve

In research, we often have hypotheses about events or phenomena. These "educated guesses" may come from theories or from previous research. This section discusses the statistical approach for "testing our guess."

Types of Hypotheses

Three levels of hypotheses can be distinguished in terms of the degree of quantification involved.

Conceptual Hypotheses

A **conceptual hypothesis** is a statement about the relationship between theoretical concepts. Hypotheses like, "Punishment facilitates learning", or "Intelligence is negatively related to sex appeal" are examples of conceptual hypotheses. Punishment, learning, intelligence, and sex appeal are theoretical concepts. They can never be directly tested because they cannot be measured. Conceptual hypotheses must be **operationalized** or made measurable before we can test them.

> **Conceptual hypothesis:** States relationship between theoretical concepts.
> **Operationalize:** To make observable or measurable.

Research Hypotheses

A **research hypothesis** is a statement about the expected relationship between *observable* or *measurable* events. An **experimental research hypothesis** states expected relationships between independent and dependent variables. For example, "Shock, following errors, will decrease the numbers of errors made" is an experimental research hypothesis. A **correlational research hypothesis** states the expected relationship between two or more variables. "The higher the score on a standard IQ test, the lower the rating of sex appeal by 10 male judges" is an example of a correlational research hypothesis. A research hypothesis restates the conceptual hypotheses in observable or measurable terms.

> **Research hypothesis:** States expected relationship between measurable events.
> **Experimental hypothesis:** States expected relationship between an independent variable and a dependent variable.
> **Correlational hypothesis:** States expected relationship between two or more variables.

Statistical Hypotheses

A **statistical hypothesis** states an expected relationship between numbers representing statistical properties of data (e.g., mean, variance, correlation). This type of hypothesis is always a guess about the value of a population parameter or about the relationship between values of two or more parameters, at least in parametric hypothesis testing.

Examples of statistical hypotheses include, "The mean number of errors is the same under shock and no-shock conditions" and "The correlation between IQ and sex appeal rating is zero."

Researchers usually begin with a conceptual hypothesis derived from some theory of published work. They then determine the best way to collect observations or measurements appropriate to their conceptual hypothesis. Data collection follows and statistical procedures commence.

> **Statistical hypothesis:** States expected relationship between statistical properties of data.

The Logic and Procedure for Testing a Conceptual Hypothesis

The steps for testing hypotheses about theoretical concepts are as follows:

Step 1. Restate the conceptual hypothesis as a research hypothesis. (Operationalize the concepts.)

Step 2. Make a statement about expected values of parameters of interest. (State the statistical hypothesis.)

Step 3. Collect and summarize the data.

Step 4. Test the statistical hypothesis.

Step 5. Make conclusions about the conceptual hypothesis.

We will start at Step 2. A statistical hypothesis includes the hypothesis you wish to disprove (*the null hypothesis*) and the hypothesis you wish to confirm (*the alternative hypothesis*).

Null and Alternative Hypotheses

The **null hypothesis** (H_o) is the one you test and hope to prove wrong, reject or nullify. If the null is rejected, the **alternative hypothesis** (H_a) is accepted. The aim of hypothesis testing is to show that the null is false and, thereby, accept an alternative hypothesis. The alternative hypothesis corresponds to the research hypothesis. Confirmation of the research hypothesis lies in *rejecting the null*. For example, if we wish to show that a coin is biased, we must prove *it is not fair*. This may seem to be a pretty strange way of doing things, but it will become clearer to you, I hope!

> **Null hypothesis (H_o):** States expected value of a parameter or expected relationship between parameters.
>
> **Alternative hypothesis (H_a):** States a value or relationship different from the null.

The null hypothesis specifies the expected value of a single population parameter or the expected relationship between two or more parameters. Some examples of null hypotheses are:

$$H_o: \mu = 100$$
$$P = 1/2$$
$$\sigma_1^2 / \sigma_2^2 = 1$$
$$\mu_1 = \mu_2$$

The alternative hypothesis asserts that the value of relationship specified by the null is not true. You test the null hypothesis and if it is rejected, you accept an alternative hypothesis. An alternative hypothesis that simply negates the null is called a **non-directional alternative**. If it specifies the direction of the difference, it is called a **directional alternative**. Some examples are

H_o	Non-Directional H_a	Directional H_a
$\mu = 100$	$\mu \neq 100$	$\mu > 100$ or $\mu < 100$
$\mu_1 = \mu_2$	$\mu_1 \neq \mu_2$	$\mu_1 > \mu_2$ or $\mu_1 < \mu_2$

The type of alternative hypothesis used depends on the research hypothesis. If the researcher's interest is in finding a difference only in a particular direction, then a directional alternative is appropriate. Otherwise, a non-directional alternative hypothesis is used.

> **Non-directional alternative:** Hypothesis that negates the null.
> **Directional alternative:** Hypothesis that specifies the direction of the difference from the null.

Testing the Null

The null hypothesis is tested in a clearly defined series of steps. The steps are

Step 1. Define the H_o and the H_a.

Step 2. Select one or more random samples from the population(s) of interest and calculate the value of the statistic that corresponds to the parameter specified in the null.

Step 3. Determine the probability of getting a sample outcome, by chance alone, that is as far or further from the value hypothesized by the null, as the one you obtained. This is done in reference to the sampling distribution of the statistic specified by the conditions of the null hypothesis.

Step 4. If the probability is low, reject the null and accept the alternative. If the probability is high, do not reject the null.

Let's try to analyze this procedure conceptually. The null hypothesis is the one we want to prove wrong. Suppose we believe that women are more intelligent than men! The null hypothesis might state that women are equal in intelligence to men and the alternative might state that they are more intelligent. (Remember that the alternative corresponds to the researcher's hypothesis.) Let's assume, for the moment, that men and women are equal in intelligence. If this is true, then two random samples, one of men and one of women, should have similar mean intelligence scores. Of course, we wouldn't expect the sample means to be exactly the same because samples do vary. The question is "How much greater does the mean of the female sample have to be in order to conclude that women are more intelligent than men?" To answer this question, we need to find out what kinds of mean differences are likely to occur when we draw two samples from populations with equal means. Then, if our sample difference is much larger than what we would expect by chance alone, we may feel free to conclude that, in fact, the populations do not have equal means.

The null hypothesis, then, provides us with a sampling distribution which *we know a lot about*. We know what kinds of sample outcomes are likely to occur under the conditions assumed by the null. If our sample outcome is very different from what we would expect, we say that the null hypothesis is probably wrong and an alternative hypothesis is true.

Step 4 says that we reject the null if the probability of getting a sample outcome as deviant as the one we got is very low. How do we decide if the probability is low enough?

Decision Criteria

In the behavioral sciences and related disciplines, researchers tend to use two probability values when testing hypotheses. These levels, symbolized by α (alpha) are called **significance levels**. The 1% level of significance (α = .01) allows us to reject the null hypothesis if our sample outcome was likely to have occurred 1% or less of the time if the null were true. The 5% level of significance allows us to reject the null if the probability of our outcome occurring is equal to or less than .05.

> **Significance level:** The level of probability at which we will reject the null.

When we test hypotheses with the normal curve as our sampling distribution, we do not need to determine the exact probability of our sample outcome. We know that the Z-scores of ±1.96 separate the middle 95% of the distribution from the extreme 5%. In other words, Z values lying beyond ±1.96 will occur less than 5% of the time. Once we have calculated our Z value, we only need to compare it to ±1.96. If our Z value is larger numerically than these **critical Z values**, then we know that the probability of occurrence of our outcome is less than .05 and we can reject the null hypothesis.

The same is true for a significance level of .01. The critical values for $\alpha = .01$ are ± 2.58, since these two values separate the middle 99% from the extreme 1% of the distribution. In summary:

Critical Z values: $\alpha = .05$ $Z_{crit} = \pm 1.96$
$\alpha = .01$ $Z_{crit} = \pm 2.58$

Critical values, then, cut off the appropriate areas in the tails of the distribution corresponding to the level of significance selected by the researcher. Any obtained Z value which falls beyond these critical values is said to lie in the **region of rejection** or the **critical region**. Z values falling between the critical values are said to lie in the **region of acceptance**. This is illustrated in Figure 9-2.

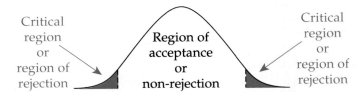

Figure 9-2 Hypothesis testing with the normal curve: regions of rejection and acceptance

---

We reject the null when the obtained Z value lies in the critical region. Otherwise, we *fail to reject the null hypothesis*. We never say accept the null; rather we always state that we have failed to prove it wrong. The term "region of acceptance" implies that we do accept the null. It might be more appropriate to term this area the "region of non-rejection."

Region of rejection: Area beyond the critical value. Outcomes lying in this area lead to rejection of a null.

Region of acceptance: Outcomes in this area lead to non-rejection of the null.

Inference with the Normal Curve

One-Tailed and Two-Tailed Tests

Recall that the alternative hypothesis may be either a non-directional alternative and therefore negate the null or it may be a directional alternative and specify the direction of the difference.

The critical region of a non-directional alternative lies in both tails, and the test of the null is a **two-tailed test of significance**. The critical region of a directional alternative is on one side only and we run a **one-tailed test of significance**. We are interested in one side of the distribution only, because we have specified this in the alternative hypothesis. We may reject the null only if our outcome is in the critical region of that tail.

The critical values given earlier were for a two-tailed test with a non-directional alternative hypothesis. Recall that ±1.96 cuts off 95% of the distribution from the extreme 5% with 2.5% in each tail. These are the critical values for a two-tailed test at $\alpha = .05$. However, if the alternative hypothesis is directional, these critical values won't work.

The significance level of .05 for a one-tailed test requires that the extreme 5% lies in *one tail only*, whichever tail is specified in the alternative. When $\alpha = .01$, we need one Z value which cuts off 99% from the extreme 1% in one tail only. These critical values must be smaller than the corresponding ones for a two-tailed test because all the area is in one tail. Looking in Table B-1, we find that the Z values are + or −1.64 ($\alpha = .05$) and + or −2.33 ($\alpha = .01$).

Figures 9-3 and 9-4 illustrate the critical region for a one-tailed test with alpha levels of .05 and .01, respectively.

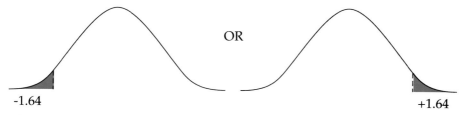

-1.64   +1.64

Figure 9-3   Critical values for a one-tailed test at $\alpha = .05$

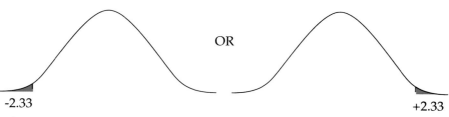

-2.33   +2.33

Figure 9-4   Critical values for a one-tailed test at $\alpha = .01$

In summary:

Critical Z values	α = .05	α = .01
Two-tailed test	±1.96	±2.58
One-tailed test	+ or − 1.64	+ or − 2.33

Notice that the critical values are smaller for a one-tailed test of significance. This means that a smaller Z value is required to reject the null hypothesis. So why don't researchers always do one-tailed tests if it's easier to reject the null?

Part of the answer to this question is that *if our outcome was extremely deviant, but in the wrong direction, we may not reject the null hypothesis!* For example, had we hypothesized that women are smarter than men, and had we found that our female sample mean of IQ scores was very much lower than the mean for the male sample, we would not be able to say that "women are less smart than men." Our outcome was not in the region of rejection specified by the alternative hypothesis. So, although we suspect something is happening here, we may not make the obvious inference, which may be a good thing anyway!

Generally, in research, we use non-directional alternatives unless we have absolutely no interest in finding a difference in the other direction, or unless finding a difference in the opposite direction to that specified by the alternative *has no real meaning*. For example, if we were interested in testing Clare Voyent's claim that she has ESP, we may run a one-tailed test because a finding that Clare performed significantly *lower* than chance level has no meaning. All we could say was that Clare was a pretty poor guesser—poorer than chance level.

Now that we have covered some of the basics, let's put these skills to work.

Testing an Hypothesis about a Population Mean

Mr. Pierre Theroux wants to compare elementary students in Ontario with those in the rest of the country on a test of mathematical achievement. Specifically, he wonders if his special new math program has had an effect on the students' mathematical skills. The national norms for a standardized math test are $\mu = 85$ and $\sigma = 20$. A randomly selected sample of 100 elementary students from Ontario schools is tested and the mean of the sample is 89. Let's use our steps to help Pierre answer his question. We will test the null at $\alpha = .05$.

Step 1. State the null and the alternative. Remember that the null must state that the students are *not* different from the national norm. The alternative states that they are different. The mean of the population on the math test is 85 and so:

$$H_o: \mu = 85$$
$$H_a: \mu \neq 85$$

Step 2. Draw a random sample from the population and calculate the statistic corresponding to the null hypothesis. We have done this and the sample statistic is:

$$\overline{X} = 89$$

Step 3. Determine the probability of getting an outcome as far or farther from the hypothesized value as the one obtained. We don't actually have to do this; rather, we simply compare our value to the critical value. To do this, we need to convert our sample mean to a Z-score so we can compare it to the critical Z value. Recall the Z formula for a sample mean:

$$Z = \frac{\overline{X} - \mu_{\overline{x}}}{\sigma_{\overline{x}}}$$

$$Z = \frac{89 - 85}{20/\sqrt{100}} = 2.00$$

Step 4. If the probability is low enough, reject the null hypothesis. This is the decision step. We can see that our obtained Z value is larger than the critical value, 1.96, so we reject the null hypothesis at $\alpha = .05$. Our sample outcome is **statistically significant**; we have evidence that the Ontario students are *significantly different* from the national norm on the test of mathematical achievement.

> **Statistically significant outcome:** An outcome leading to rejection of the null hypothesis.

What we have really found is that the students in the Ontario sample should not have produced a mean so deviant from the national mean if they were the same as the students in the rest of the country. We conclude that they are not the same. To prove that a sample is from a different population, we must prove that it does not behave in the way a sample from the hypothesized population would, and so it is unlikely to be from the hypothesized population. In this example, we had one sample and we made an inference about the mean of the population from which the sample was drawn. Often, in research, we have two samples and our interest is in the difference between the means of their respective populations.

Summary of Z-Test for a Single Mean

Hypotheses
H_o: μ = specified value
H_a: $\mu \neq$ or $<$ or $>$ specified value

Assumptions
1. Subjects are randomly selected.
2. Population distribution is normal.
3. Population standard deviation is known.

Decision Rules
If $Z_{obt} \geq Z_{crit}$, reject the H_o
If $Z_{obt} < Z_{crit}$, do not reject H_o

Formula
$$Z = \frac{\overline{X} - \mu}{\sigma/\sqrt{n}}$$

Testing an Hypothesis about the Difference between Population Means

To test whether two samples come from populations with different means, we assume a null hypothesis that the samples come from populations with equal means. Even if we drew two random samples from the same population, we would not expect to get identical sample means because samples vary. The question is "How different would we expect sample means to be when they are drawn from populations with equal means?" Once we know what kinds of mean differences to expect under these conditions, we can compare a specific obtained difference with the expected difference. If our sample means differ more than chance alone would predict, we may conclude that our samples come from populations with unequal means. We would reject the null hypothesis and claim a significant difference between the population means from which our samples were drawn.

To find out what kinds of sample mean differences would occur with repeated sampling from populations with equal means, we need the random sampling distribution of the difference between means so that we can compare our obtained difference with that distribution. Recall that this distribution is normal within the limits of the Central Limit Theorem, and so the normal curve is an appropriate model for this test.

If the null hypothesis is true and the population means don't differ, we would expect the mean difference of our two samples to be close to zero. If it is far from zero we would claim the null is false and accept the alternative hypothesis. Hypothesis testing for the difference follows the same general procedure that we have been using. We must compute a Z-score for the difference and compare our obtained Z value with the critical values. The critical values for the test for the difference are the same as those we used for the test for a single mean.

Recall the Z formula for the difference between means:

$$Z = \frac{\overline{X}_1 - \overline{X}_2 - (\mu_1 - \mu_2)}{\sigma_{\overline{x}_1 - \overline{x}_2}}$$

and the formulas for the standard error of the difference:

$$\sigma_{\overline{x}_1 - \overline{x}_2} = \sqrt{\sigma_{\overline{x}_1}^2 + \sigma_{\overline{x}_2}^2} \quad \text{or}$$

$$\sigma_{\overline{x}_1 - \overline{x}_2} = \sqrt{\frac{\sigma_1^2}{n_1} + \frac{\sigma_2^2}{n_2}} \quad \text{or}$$

$$\sigma_{\overline{x}_1 - \overline{x}_2} = \sqrt{\frac{2\sigma^2}{n}} \quad \text{if } \sigma_1^2 = \sigma_2^2 \text{ and } n_1 = n_2$$

Ready for an example? A school board member is interested in the outbreak of "free" high schools where students are given a much more flexible curriculum and allowed to study independently. She decides to select a random sample of 25 students from a "free" school and another sample of 25 students from a traditional high school. All students are given a standardized achievement test which has a standard deviation of 15. The mean score of the "free" school students on this test is 145 and the mean score for the traditional high school students is 148. Let's test the hypothesis that "free" school and traditional school students don't differ in achievement. We will use $\alpha = .01$.

Step 1. State the null and the alternative.
$H_o: \mu_1 = \mu_2$ This is always the null for a test of the difference.
$H_a: \mu_1 \neq \mu_2$ We will use a non-directional alternative.

Step 2. Draw two random samples from the populations and calculate the statistic corresponding to the null hypothesis. We have done this and the sample statistic is:
$$\overline{X}_1 - \overline{X}_2 = 145 - 148 = -3$$

Step 3. Convert the sample statistic to a Z-score and compare it to the critical values. Z_{crit} for a two-tailed test at $\alpha = .01$ is ± 2.58.

$$\sigma_{\overline{x}_1 - \overline{x}_2} = \sqrt{\frac{2\sigma^2}{n}}$$

$$= \sqrt{2(15)^2/25} = 4.24$$

$$Z = \frac{\overline{X}_1 - \overline{X}_2 - (\mu_1 - \mu_2)}{\sigma_{\overline{x}_1 - \overline{x}_2}}$$

$$= \frac{145 - 148 - 0}{4.24} = -0.71$$

Step 4. Make a decision. Our obtained Z value is not larger numerically than the critical value. Because it does not fall in the critical region, we do not reject the null hypothesis. The probability of getting a sample outcome as far or farther from the hypothesized population difference than the one we got is greater than .01. We have no statistical evidence that our samples come from populations with different means. There is no significant difference between "free" school students and students from traditional schools.

Summary of Z-Test for Independent Means

Hypotheses
$H_o: \mu_1 = \mu_2$
$H_a: \mu_1 \neq \mu_2$ or $\mu_1 < \mu_2$ or $\mu_1 > \mu_2$

Assumptions
1. Subjects are randomly selected and independently assigned to groups.
2. Population distributions are normal.
3. Population standard deviations are known.

Decision Rules
If $Z_{obt} \geq Z_{crit}$, reject the H_o
If $Z_{obt} < Z_{crit}$, do not reject H_o

Formula
$$Z = \frac{\overline{X}_1 - \overline{X}_2}{\sqrt{\frac{\Sigma x_1^2 + \Sigma x_2^2}{n_1 + n_2}\left(\frac{1}{n_1} + \frac{1}{n_2}\right)}}$$

where $\Sigma x^2 = \Sigma X^2 - (\Sigma X)^2/n$

Testing an Hypothesis about a Population Proportion

To test an hypothesis about a population proportion we assume, in the null hypothesis, that the population proportion has some specified value and use the same general approach as we used earlier. Let's use our steps to test an hypothesis from Mendelian Law (remember Mendel's peas?). Three hundred garden peas were randomly selected. According to Mendelian Law, 15% of the stock the peas were taken from should exhibit the recessive characteristic of sterility. Of the 300 peas selected, 65 were found to be sterile. Let's test the hypothesis that the peas came from a new hybrid stock. We will use $\alpha = .05$.

Step 1. $H_o: P = 0.15$
$H_a: P \neq 0.15$

Step 2. $p = 65/300 = 0.22$

Step 3. $Z = \dfrac{p - P}{\sqrt{PQ/n}}$

$= \dfrac{0.22 - 0.15}{\sqrt{(0.15)(0.85)/300}} = \dfrac{0.07}{0.02} = 3.5$

Step 4. Our obtained Z value falls in the critical region so we reject the null hypothesis. We have evidence that the stock from which our sample was selected is significantly different from the stock hypothesized in the null.

Testing the null hypothesis involves determining the probability of a particular sample statistic occurring with respect to the sampling distribution of that statistic. The general approach is to calculate the Z value corresponding to the statistic and compare it to the critical values. The general Z formula we use is

$$Z = \dfrac{\text{statistic} - \text{hypothesized parameter value}}{\text{standard error}}$$

In summary:

If $Z_{obtained} \geq Z_{critical}$, then $p < \alpha$ and we reject the null.
If $Z_{obtained} < Z_{critical}$, then $p > \alpha$ and we fail to reject the null.

Summary of Z-Test for a Proportion

Hypotheses
  H_o: P = specified value
  H_a: $P \neq$ or $<$ or $>$ specified value

Assumptions
  1. Subjects are randomly selected.
  2. Sampling distribution of the statistic is normal.
  3. Observations are dichotomous.

Decision Rules
  If $Z_{obt} \geq Z_{crit}$, reject the H_o
  If $Z_{obt} < Z_{crit}$, do not reject H_o

Formula
  $Z = \dfrac{p - P}{\sqrt{PQ/n}}$

Consequences of Statistical Decisions

Whenever we make an inference, there is some probability that we will be wrong! A careful researcher is well aware of the consequences of statistical decisions.

Statistical Significance

The null hypothesis states that a given parameter has some value. When the null is rejected, we claim that the parameter is unlikely to have that value. In other words, there is a *difference between the true population value and the hypothesized population value.*

In practice, any sample outcome that occurs by chance alone 5% (in the case of $\alpha = .05$) or 1% (in the case of $\alpha = .01$) of the time when the null is true, will lead us to conclude that the null is false!

Type I and Type II Errors

A decision as to whether the null is true or false is never made with certainty. A **Type I error** occurs when the null hypothesis is true, but our sample outcome leads us to reject it. In other words, we obtained a rare sample outcome that leads us to make an error. Romeo made a Type I error when he wrongly rejected his hypothesis: "Juliet is alive." His error was tragic. The probability of making a Type I error (i.e., the Type I error rate) is set by α. For example, if the null is true and our α level is .05, we will make a Type I error 5% of the time. If α is .01, we will make a Type I error only 1% of the time. Obviously, to reduce the probability of a Type I error, we need to lower the value of α (from .05 to .01, for example).

Unfortunately, it doesn't stop here! A **Type II error** is made when the null is false but we fail to reject it. In other words, a difference between the true parameter value and the hypothesized value exists, but our test did not discover this. Julius Caesar made a Type II error when he wrongly accepted the null hypothesis: "Brutus is my buddy." Hence his response, "Et tu, Brute?" His error, too, was tragic. The probability of a Type II error (i.e., the Type II error rate) is related to alpha and is called **beta** (β). The exact relationship between α and β is not determined empirically, because the nature of the alternative or true "state of affairs" is unknown, but generally the lower the level of β, the higher the level of α. To reduce the probability of making a Type II error, we need to increase the alpha level (from .01 to .05, for example).

> **Type I error:** Rejecting a null hypothesis that is true.
>
> **Type II error:** Failing to reject a null hypothesis that is false.

The problem is one of balance. By lowering α, we increase β. In preliminary or pilot research, the rule of thumb is to use a higher level of significance like α = .05. In a well developed field, with lots of experimental control, we tend to use stricter, lower, significance levels like α = .01.

In summary:

> As α decreases, p(Type I) decreases and p(Type II) increases.
> As α increases, p(Type I) increases and p(Type II) decreases.

A Type II error is made when the null is false but we do not reject it. This is not a desirable state of affairs since the whole reason for testing hypotheses is to reject the null when it is false. Fortunately, there is another way to reduce β, the probability of making a Type II error.

Increasing the number of observations in the sample(s) reduces β. With larger samples, the standard error (the denominator of the Z formula) tends to be reduced. This is because there is less variability in larger samples. When the denominator is reduced, the Z value tends to increase and so it is more likely that the obtained Z value will be larger than the critical Z value. In other words, by increasing sample size, we increase the probability of rejecting a false null, which is what we are trying to do. When a test of significance has a high probability of rejecting false null hypotheses, it is said to be a **powerful test**.

Power

If β is the probability of *not rejecting a false null*, then clearly, the probability of *rejecting a false null* must be 1 − β. The probability of rejecting a false null hypothesis is called **power**. Power, then, is the capability of our test to reject the null when it should be rejected. In practice, neither β nor power (1 − β) are directly computed. However, increasing the α level (from .01 to .05, for example) or increasing the sample size, increases power.

Figure 9-5 illustrates what can happen when we test hypotheses about population parameters.

The curve on the left represents the random sampling distribution when the null hypothesis is true. The curve on the right represents one of many possible alternative hypotheses. You can see that if the null is true, occasionally we will obtain an outcome in the region of rejection that leads us to reject the null and make a Type I error. This will occur α of the time. Most of the time (1 − α), however, we will not reject a true null and so we make a correct decision. Look at the curve on the right. Here we see what could happen if the null is false and the alternative is true. If our sample outcome

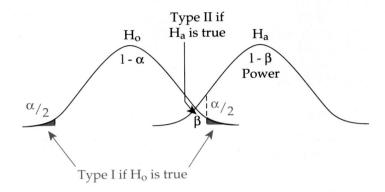

Figure 9-5 Examples of decision outcomes in hypothesis testing

lies in the "region of acceptance," we will not reject the null even though it is false. This will occur β of the time and we will make a Type II error. However, $1 - \beta$ of the time, when the alternative is true, we will get a sample outcome in the critical region, reject the null, and make a correct decision. This is power.

We can summarize this as follows:

Decision	True State of Affairs	
	H_o is True	H_o is False
Reject H_o	Type I $p = \alpha$	Correct Decision $p = 1 - \beta$ (Power)
Do not reject H_o	Correct Decision $p = 1 - \alpha$	Type II $p = \beta$

The concept of power is an important one in hypothesis testing. All researchers want to maximize power when they test hypotheses. We have seen that power is affected by the significance level chosen and by the sample size. Let's look more closely at the relationship between sample size and power. In effect, increasing the number of subjects in the sample serves to decrease the size of the denominator of the Z-ratio. When the denominator of the Z-ratio decreases, the Z value must increase. It is more likely then, that the obtained Z value will be larger than the critical value, resulting in rejection of the null.

The denominator of the Z-ratio, the standard error, is a measure of variability of the random sampling distribution. Recall that the random sampling distribution of the mean, for example, is a distribution of sample means drawn from a population. Sample means vary due to individual differences even when drawn from a single population. This variation is sometimes called error variance. In psychology research the main source of error variance is individual differences between people. People differ in ability, motivation, attention and so on. A small number of people tend to vary more than a larger number of people. The more the people vary, the larger will be the variability of sample means. Anything then that the researcher can do to reduce individual variability will serve to increase the power of his or her statistical procedure. Good research technique is the critical factor here. Many researchers prefer laboratory experiments rather than field experiments because they allow more control over extraneous variables that might increase variability between the subjects. Testing people in a laboratory where distractions can be minimized, for example, will help to reduce variability.

We have learned then that significance level, sample size, and individual differences all affect the power of the test. The most important factor to consider when we talk about power, however, is the effect of the independent variable, the experimental treatment. Clearly an independent variable that has a small effect on the dependent variable, performance, will be harder to detect than an independent variable that has a large effect on performance. A researcher, of course, hopes that the independent variable he has chosen to study will have a large effect on performance but he certainly doesn't know in advance if this is so. If he did he wouldn't be doing the research to begin with! We will look at this dilemma again as we learn more about tests of significance. For now just remember that the significance level chosen, the size of the sample, the inherent differences between subjects, and the effect of the independent variable all influence the power of any statistical test of significance.

Assumptions Underlying Inference with the Normal Curve

Inferential statistical procedures using the normal curve as a model assume certain conditions.

1. The sampling distribution of the statistic is normally distributed.
2. The sample observations have been randomly selected.
3. With two samples, observations have been independently assigned.

We know from the Central Limit Theorem that the sampling distribution will be normally distributed if the population is normal or if the sample(s) is large enough.

The assumptions of random sampling and independent assignment are important ones. In research, we are careful not to violate these assumptions. Random sampling and independent assignment of subjects to groups allow us to use very powerful statistical techniques. When these assumptions have been violated other procedures are available but these are not, usually, as powerful as the techniques we have been studying.

Choosing the Appropriate Test of Significance

Knowing which test to use for a given research problem is the special skill of statisticians. In this chapter three Z-tests were discussed. Deciding which is appropriate is a matter of determining what kind of data are involved and how many groups participated in the experiment. If the data are proportion, frequency, or percentage data, the Z-test for a proportion is called for. If the data are measures where means will be computed then we will choose the Z-test for a single mean for an experiment with one group of subjects and the Z-test for two independent means for an experiment with two groups of subjects. Let's try a few examples.

Example A Suppose the Board of Education has decided to compare students in two different schools using a standardized test of writing competence for which normative statistics are available. A sample is randomly selected from each school and the mean test results are compared. Let's go through the steps involved in choosing the appropriate test of significance.

Step 1. Determine the kind of data collected in the experiment.
In this example, the scores of all the students were collected and the means were computed for each group. A Z-test for a single mean or for two independent means will be used.

Step 2. Determine the number of groups in the experiment.
There were two samples taken, one from each school and so the Board should run a Z-test for two independent means.

Example B The School of Political Science at the University of Manitoba is concerned that its students are not performing at the same level as the rest of the student body. A random sample of the grade point averages of 200 political science students is collected. A comparison is made between the average performance of this group and the performance of the student body at large. Statistics are available for the entire student population.

Step 1. Determine the kind of data collected in the experiment.
The mean grade point average of the political science students is to be compared with the average of the entire student body.

Step 2. Determine the number of groups in the experiment.
Although, at first glance, you might think there are two groups in this study, there is only one randomly selected group. The entire student body is a population and the 200 political science students comprise the sample. A Z-test for a single mean should be used to determine whether the political science students differ from the norm (i.e. the whole university).

Example C A hospital administrator is concerned about the increased length of hospital stay for women having Caesarian sections versus vaginal deliveries. Eighty percent of the women who deliver vaginally stay in hospital two days or less. He selects a random sample of 80 women who had Caesarians and notes the number of women who stayed two days or less. How would he test his hypothesis that Caesarian section increases hospital stay?

Step 1. Determine the kind of data collected in the experiment.

The hospital administrator has simply counted the number of women staying two days or less. He has frequency data that he will use in a Z-test for a proportion.

Developing skills in making decisions about the appropriate test of significance for a given research problem is an important part of learning statistics. With only three tests to choose from, it is not very difficult to decide which one to use. As you learn about other tests of significance, however, you will find it becomes an increasingly more complicated process.

SUMMARY OF FORMULAS

	Hypothesis Testing	Interval Estimation
The Mean	$Z = \dfrac{\overline{X} - \mu_{\overline{x}}}{\sigma_{\overline{x}}}$	$\mu = \overline{X} \pm Z\sigma_{\overline{x}}$
The Difference	$Z = \dfrac{\overline{X}_1 - \overline{X}_2 - (\mu_1 - \mu_2)}{\sigma_{\overline{x}_1 - \overline{x}_2}}$	$\mu_1 - \mu_2 = (\overline{X}_1 - \overline{X}_2) \pm Z\sigma_{\overline{x}_1 - \overline{x}_2}$
The Proportion	$Z = \dfrac{p - P}{\sigma_p}$	$P = p \pm Z\sigma_p$

Formulas for the Standard Error

The Difference	$\sigma_{\overline{x}_1 - \overline{x}_2} = \sqrt{\dfrac{\sigma_1^2}{n_1} + \dfrac{\sigma_2^2}{n_2}}$
The Mean	$\sigma_{\overline{x}} = \sigma/\sqrt{n}$
The Proportion	$\sigma_p = \sqrt{PQ/n}$

EXERCISES

1. The graduating averages of high school students in a large city are normally distributed with a mean of 79 and a standard deviation of 14. A random sample of 25 students from one of the schools has a mean of 85. Use a two-tailed test at $\alpha = .01$ to test the hypothesis that students from this school are at par with the city average.

2. Using the data from Exercise 1, set up the 95% and 99% confidence intervals for the sample of 25 students.

3. Clair Voyent claims to have E.S.P. An investigator tests her with a deck of 52 cards, half red and half black. Clair guesses whether successive cards, turned over out of her sight, are red or black. On 52 independent trials she guesses correctly 29 times. Use a one-tailed test at $\alpha = .05$, to find out if Clair is doing significantly better than chance.

4. A seat belt manufacturer claims that his product has a mean breaking strength of 250 kg with a standard deviation of 3.5 kg. You select a random sample of 49 of his seat belts and compute the mean breaking strength of your sample to be 245 kg. Test the manufacturer's claim at $\alpha = .05$.

5. A realtor claims that more than 75% of retired couples prefer apartment living to single unit housing. A random sample of 100 couples shows that 81 prefer apartment living. Test the claim of the realtor at the 5% level of significance. (Hint: The realtor's claim, that more than 75% prefer apartment living, corresponds to the alternative hypothesis. The null will state that 75% prefer apartment living.)

6. A normal population has a standard deviation of 20. A researcher collects a random sample of 100 scores and computes a mean of 48. Between what two values can the researcher be 99% confident that the population mean lies?

7. A toothpaste company claims that 70% of Canadian dentists use its toothpaste. A random sample of 50 dentists finds that 30 of these use this brand of toothpaste. Test the null hypothesis that the true proportion is 70% at $\alpha = .01$.

8. A total of 173 students were polled for an upcoming election and asked to state their preference for one of two candidates. Candidate A received 98 votes and B got 75. Test at $\alpha = .05$, whether Candidate A is ahead of Candidate B. (Hint: If A is not ahead of B, then what proportion of the total votes would we expect A to get?).

9. The *Friendly Fitness Club* recorded the weights of their members before they began their fitness program. They discovered that the weights were normally distributed with a mean of 145 lbs and a standard deviation of 21. After the fitness program was finished, the director of the

club randomly selected 49 participants and recorded their weights. She found that the mean weight for this group was 138 lbs. Use a one-tailed test at $\alpha = .05$ to determine if the program was effective in reducing weight.
   a. H_o:
      H_a:
   b. Critical Z value =
   c. Obtained Z value =
   d. Decision:
   Put your statistical decision in words.

10. Brad was unprepared for his first exam in statistics. He decides to guess on the multiple-choice exam. Each of the 25 questions had 4 alternatives and Brad got 16 correct. Use a one-tailed test at $\alpha = .01$ to see if Brad was a better than chance guesser.
   a. H_o:
      H_a:
   b. Critical Z value =
   c. Obtained Z value =
   d. Decision:
   Put your statistical decision in words.

11. A Cereal Company advertises that "there is a cup of raisins in each box of Raisin Surprise." You decide to investigate. After contacting the Cereal Company, you find that they claim that the mean is 1.1 cups of raisins with a standard deviation of 0.79. You randomly select 100 boxes of Raisin Surprise and measure the raisin content. You find your sample to have a mean of .90 cups of raisins. At $\alpha = .01$, use a two-tailed test to test the claim of the company.
   a. H_o:
      H_a:
   b. Critical Z value =
   c. Obtained Z value =
   d. Decision:
   Put your statistical decision in words.

12. Set up the 99% confidence interval for the difference with the following data.
   DATA: $\overline{X}_1 = 115$
   $\overline{X}_2 = 118$
   $\sigma_{\overline{x}_1 - \overline{x}_2} = 2$

CHAPTER 10

Inference with the t-Distribution

LEARNING OBJECTIVES

After reading this chapter you should be able to:
1. Define the term "unbiased estimate" of a parameter.
2. Describe the difference between the t-distribution and the normal distribution.
3. Define the term "degrees of freedom."
4. Set up the 95% and 99% confidence intervals for a population mean for a given set of data.
5. Set up the 95% and 99% confidence intervals for the difference between population means for a given set of data.
6. Run a t-test for a single mean for a given set of data.
7. Run a t-test for the difference between independent means for a given set of data.
8. Run a t-test for the difference between dependent means for a given set of data.
9. Describe the difference between an independent groups design and a dependent groups design.
10. Describe the difference between a matched-groups design and a within-subjects design.
11. Determine the appropriate test of significance for a given research problem.

To use the normal curve for estimating the value of population parameters and testing hypotheses about population parameters, a standard score called a Z-score must be determined. To test hypotheses about the value of μ, for example, we used the following to determine Z:

$$Z = \frac{\overline{X} - \mu}{\sigma_{\overline{x}}}$$

This formulation follows the general format for testing the null hypothesis:

$$\text{Standard Score} = \frac{\text{value of statistic} - \text{hypothesized value of the parameter}}{\text{standard deviation of the distribution of the statistic}}$$

To estimate the value of μ from sample data, we used

$$\mu = \overline{X} \pm Z\,\sigma_{\overline{x}}$$

The general formulation, then, for estimating the location of parameter values from samples is

$$\text{Estimate of parameter} = \text{statistic} \pm (\text{standard score})(\text{standard deviation of the distribution of the statistic})$$

Let's look more closely at the two formulas. $\overline{X}$ is determined from the data that we collect. μ is the hypothesized value of the population mean or, in the case of confidence interval estimation, it is unknown. $\sigma_{\overline{x}}$ is the standard deviation of the sampling distribution of means calculated for all possible samples drawn at random from the population of raw scores. We called this the *standard error*. The standard error is determined by its relationship to σ: the standard deviation of the raw score population.

Here is the problem! *Since we don't know enough about the original population to know its mean, how likely are we to know its standard deviation?* Practically speaking, if we don't know μ, we probably don't know σ either!

To determine σ, we would have to look at all the raw scores in the population. If we could we would also know the mean of that population and wouldn't need to make inferences about what it might be. Instead, we would use descriptive statistical techniques, not inferential techniques.

When we do not know the value of σ, we cannot calculate the standard error or use Z to estimate where μ may lie or to test hypotheses about the value of μ.

In most research we do not know the value of σ, and the normal curve cannot be used as a model for making inferences about population parameters. And, as you have probably figured out already, we use a different curve or distribution as our model when we do not know the value of σ.

The t-Distribution and Unbiased Estimates

You will recall that the normal curve is the sampling distribution of the Z statistic. Similarly, the **t-distribution** is the sampling distribution of the t statistic. We use the t-distribution as a model when we do not know the value of the population standard deviation and must estimate its value from our sample data. We use lower case "**s**" to indicate that we are estimating the value of the population standard deviation. In summary:

> **Z-score:** The deviation of a particular value from the mean of its distribution expressed in relationship to the standard deviation of that distribution.

> **t-score:** The deviation of a particular value from the mean of its distribution expressed in relationship to an **estimate** of the standard deviation of that distribution.

The estimate of the population standard deviation used in the t-ratio is the square root of the *unbiased estimate* of the population variance. An **unbiased estimate** of a parameter is one which, on the average, will equal exactly the parameter being estimated. To determine whether an estimate is unbiased:

Step 1. Draw all possible samples of some fixed size from the population.

Step 2. Calculate a statistic for each sample.

Step 3. Compute the mean of the statistics.

If this mean has the same value as the parameter to which it corresponds, then the estiminate is unbiased. Otherwise, it is a biased estimate.

Earlier, we saw that the mean of the sampling distribution of means ($\mu_{\bar{x}}$) is exactly equal to the mean of the population from which the samples were drawn (μ). In other words, the mean of all the sample means ($\bar{X}$'s) exactly equals the population mean. $\bar{X}$, then, is an *unbiased estimate* of μ.

Consider the statistic, **sample variance** (we'll call this S^2). The formula for calculating the variance of a sample is

$$S^2 = \frac{\Sigma(X - \bar{X})^2}{n} \qquad \text{sample variance}$$

If we calculated this S^2 statistic for all possible samples drawn from some population, and computed the mean of all the sample variances, we would find that this mean value is consistently smaller than σ^2. Although the mean of all the sample means will equal the mean of the population, the mean of all the sample variances *will not equal* the population variance. For this reason, we say that sample variance is a *biased estimate* of σ^2. It is biased because it always underestimates σ^2.

Fortunately, we have an arithmetic adjustment to correct this problem. Rather than calculating sample variance by the formula above, we can calculate s^2 as an unbiased estimate of σ^2.

$$s^2 = \frac{\Sigma(X - \overline{X})^2}{n - 1} \qquad \text{unbiased estimate of population variance}$$

As you can see, s^2 uses a denominator of $n - 1$, instead of n. This results in a somewhat larger quotient. Now, if we were to draw all possible samples from a population, calculate s^2 for each sample, and compute the mean of all the s^2's, we would have a value which exactly equals σ^2. This formula, then, produces an unbiased estimate of σ^2 because its expected value is σ^2.

Recall that the t-ratio is the deviation of a value, from the mean of its distribution, expressed in relationship to an estimate of the standard deviation of that distribution. This estimate is always based on the unbiased estimate of the population variance. Some estimates used in inference with the t-distribution are

Estimate	Parameter
$\overline{X}$	μ
s	σ
s^2	σ^2
$s_{\overline{x}}$	$\sigma_{\overline{x}}$
$s_{\overline{x}_1 - \overline{x}_2}$	$\sigma_{\overline{x}_1 - \overline{x}_2}$

Relationship between the Normal and the t-Distribution

Both the normal and the t-distribution:

1. are symmetrical
2. are unimodal
3. have means of zero

Recall that the Z equivalent for a sample mean is

$$Z = \frac{\overline{X} - \mu_{\overline{x}}}{\sigma_{\overline{x}}}$$

Similarly, the t equivalent for a sample mean is

$$t = \frac{\overline{X} - \mu_{\overline{x}}}{s_{\overline{x}}} \qquad \text{t for a sample mean}$$

where $s_{\overline{x}}$ is the estimate of the standard error.

If you drew all possible samples of some fixed size from a population, calculated Z-scores and t-scores for each sample mean, and placed the Z-scores and t-scores in separate frequency distributions, the Z's would follow a normal distribution and the t's would follow a t-distribution.

The difference between the normal and the t-distribution is mainly in the tails. The t-distribution tends to have more area in the tails than does the normal distribution. The Z-distribution is normal in shape because μ and σ are fixed and the sample means are normally distributed or close to it (remember the Central Limit Theorem). Since μ and σ do not change, the distribution of Z values follows the shape of the distribution of the sample means: they are the only values that vary. We know that the distribution of sample means is close to normal, regardless of the shape of the original population, when sample size is reasonably large.

The t-distribution, on the other hand, departs from normality in a regular fashion even though the sample means are normally distributed. μ is fixed but the estimate of $\sigma_{\overline{x}}$ (i.e., $s_{\overline{x}}$) is determined from the sample data and therefore, is a variable differing from sample to sample. The variability of $s_{\overline{x}}$ is directly affected by sample size; smaller samples produce greater variability.

The exact shape of the t-distribution depends on **degrees of freedom (df)**. Recall that the normal curve is a family of curves that has been standardized to the Standard Normal with Z-scores on the abscissa and relative frequency on the ordinate. The t-distribution is also a family of curves the shape of each depending on degrees of freedom. Unless degrees of freedom are infinitely large, the shape of the t-distribution will not be normal. Now, with numerous degrees of freedom, the t-distribution does look close to normal, but with very few degrees of freedom the t-distribution is leptokurtic with respect to the normal curve. Do you remember what that means? You can see from the examples in Figure 10-1 that the t-distribution has more area in the tails than the normal distribution.

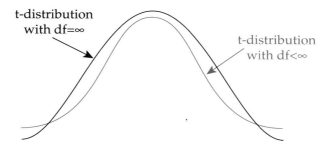

Figure 10-1   Comparing the normal and a t-distribution

Degrees of freedom are related to, but not identical with, sample size. When degrees of freedom are infinitely large, the shape of the t-distribution is normal and the value of the t-ratio equals exactly the value of the Z-ratio. In such cases, there is no *mathematical* distinction between calculating Z and calculating t.

When degrees of freedom are less than infinity, the t-distribution has more area in the tails than does the normal distribution, and the value of the t-ratio will not equal the value of the Z-ratio. When testing the null hypothesis, somewhat larger t values are required to reject the null hypothesis whenever degrees of freedom are less than infinity. The critical values of t are larger than the critical values of Z and depend on degrees of freedom.

Degrees of Freedom when Estimating Parameters

Suppose you overheard a conversation about your performance on a test, between your statistics instructor and her friend Clive. It included the following information: 1. You scored 150 points on your statistics exam. 2. You missed 50 points. 3. A perfect score on the test was 200. You have three pieces of information: your score, the points you missed, and the total number of points possible. Actually, you could have deduced the third piece of information from the first two. Knowing that you scored 150 and missed 50 points is all you need to deduce that the total number of points on the test was 200. In fact, any two of the three values is all you need to obtain the third value. For example, if you heard that you lost 50 points on the test and there were 200 points available you could compute your score by subtraction.

In situations like this, statisticians say that two pieces of information fixed the third. They also say that two of the values are independent and one is dependent. Statisticians tend to state the same thing in as many ways as possible; many statisticians will also say that two values are free to vary and one is fixed.

Degrees of freedom, then, in any particular situation, are determined by the number of values free to vary. This concept is important when we estimate parameter values from sample data. When we estimate σ with our s formula, which we must do to determine the t-ratio for a single mean, we use the sample mean ($\bar{X}$) as an estimate of μ, and by doing so we use up one degree of freedom. In other words, calculating $\bar{X}$ and using it in our computation of s, fixes one value in that it is no longer free to vary.

This point is clear, if we consider the following distribution of scores. The first column provides the original raw scores, and the second column shows the deviation of each score from the mean of the distribution.

X	$(X - \bar{X})$
15	2
14	1
13	0
12	-1
11	-2
$\bar{X} = 13$	$\Sigma(X - \bar{X}) = 0$

You will recall that the sum of the positive deviations must exactly equal the sum of the negative deviations for deviations taken around the mean of any distribution. The mean of this X distribution is 13 and the sum of the negative deviations equals the sum of the positive deviations around 13. How many score values could we change without changing the value of the mean?

Let's change the first value from 15 to 20, the second from 14 to 17, the third from 13 to 10, and the fourth from 12 to 8. Before we go further let's determine the deviation scores. Remember, we cannot change the value of the mean.

X	$(X - \bar{X})$
20	7
17	4
10	-3
8	-5
?	?
$\bar{X} = 13$	$\Sigma(X - \bar{X}) = 0$

Keeping the mean at 13 then, we have a sum of 11 positive deviations [i.e., $(20 - 13) + (17 - 13) = 11$] and a sum of 8 negative deviations [i.e., $(10 - 13) + (8 - 13) = -8$]. Because the sum of the negative deviations must equal the sum of the positive deviations around any mean, our fifth score value must be 3 deviations below the mean. Our fifth value, then, can only be a 10. No other value will do! We have only 4 degrees of freedom. Once four values are changed the fifth value is fixed.

When we estimate the population standard deviation using the sample mean, we constrain the data and use up a degree of freedom. Degrees of freedom are determined by the number of constraints placed on our data by our calculations. When computing a t-score for the mean of a single sample, we estimate the population standard deviation from our sample data; in doing so we use up one degree of freedom. Degrees of freedom, then, are equal to $n - 1$, the number of values free to vary.

When computing a t-score for the difference between means, we estimate population standard deviation using the means of both samples; in doing so, we use up a degree of freedom for each mean calculated. Degrees of freedom, then, are equal to $(n_1 - 1) + (n_2 - 1)$.

When To Use the t-Distribution

Just as the normal curve may be used as a model when making inferences or testing hypotheses about the value of population parameters under certain conditions, so can the t-distribution be used as a model for such procedures under other conditions. The choice depends on whether or not the population standard deviation is known. If it is, the normal curve is the appropriate model. If it must be estimated, then t may be the appropriate distribution. See Figure 10-2.

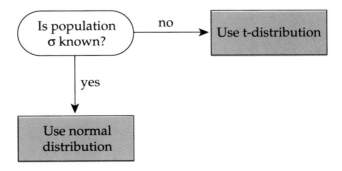

Figure 10-2 Deciding between the normal and the t-distribution

Confidence Intervals Using the t-Distribution

The t-distribution is the sampling distribution of the t statistic. Like Z, t is calculated for all possible samples of some fixed size drawn from a population. Setting up confidence intervals with the t-distribution is essentially the same as it was using the normal curve and Z.

Setting up the Confidence Interval for a Population Mean

You will recall that the normal curve formula for setting up a confidence interval to locate the population mean is

$$\mu = \overline{X} \pm Z_{crit}(\sigma_{\overline{x}})$$

The formula for setting up a confidence interval to locate the population mean using the t-distribution is

---

$$\mu = \overline{X} \pm t_{crit}(s_{\overline{x}})$$ Confidence interval for the mean: t-distribution

---

Rather than using the standard error, we must use an estimate of the standard error. The critical value of t changes with the significance level chosen, as does the critical value of Z, and with the degrees of freedom, unlike Z. So, unless you are going to use the same sample size whenever you do research, I am afraid you are going to have to look up the critical value of t for each confidence interval you set up! Table B-2 in Appendix B, near the back of the book, lists critical values of t depending on degrees of freedom and alpha level.

Ready for an example? The chairperson of the Ski Jump Preparation Committee is in the process of making decisions about the facilities for the next Olympics. She is not sure how long the landing platform should be. She decides to set up the 95% Confidence Interval for the mean length required for landing by world class ski jumpers. (Don't ask me why she didn't confer with the chairperson of the previous Ski Jump Preparation Committee!) She selects a random sample of 25 world class ski jumpers and measures the distance required by each for landing. Here are her data:

Mean Distance: $\overline{X} = 125$ $n = 25$ $df = n - 1 = 24$
$s = 15$ $t_{.05} = 2.064$

The appropriate formula to use is

$$\mu = \overline{X} \pm t_{.05}(s_{\overline{x}})$$

Notice that the estimate of the population standard deviation (i.e., "s") is given. You may recall that in Chapter 9 the standard error was computed by dividing the population standard deviation by the square root of the sample size. We do the same here to obtain the estimate of the standard error. We compute $s_{\bar{x}}$ by dividing s by $\sqrt{n}$.

$$s_{\bar{x}} = s/\sqrt{n}$$
$$s_{\bar{x}} = 15/\sqrt{25}$$
$$= 3.0$$

Now we can proceed to set up the 95% Confidence Interval for μ:

$$\mu = 125 \pm (2.064)(3.0)$$
Limits are: 118.81 to 131.19

Using the "official" format for presenting confidence interval limits:

$$C(118.81 \leq \mu \leq 131.19) = .95$$

The Chairperson of the Ski Jump Preparation Committee can claim, in the next meeting, that her confidence that the average world class ski jumper jumps distances from 118.81 to 131.19 meters is 95%. This may strike you as a ludicrous example, but I hope you get the idea!

Setting up the Confidence Interval for the Difference between Independent Population Means

Setting up confidence interval for the difference between population means follows the same general pattern. The appropriate formula is

$$\mu_1 - \mu_2 = (\bar{X}_1 - \bar{X}_2) \pm t_{crit}(s_{\bar{x}_1 - \bar{x}_2})$$

CI for the difference between independent means

The trickiest part of this procedure is determining the estimate of the standard error of the difference. One formula is

$$s_{\bar{x}_1 - \bar{x}_2} = \sqrt{s_{\bar{x}_1}^2 + s_{\bar{x}_2}^2}$$

This formula is fine if we have already calculated the unbiased estimates of the variance for each sample. If we have not, however, the following computational formula is appropriate:

$$s_{\bar{x}_1-\bar{x}_2} = \sqrt{\frac{\Sigma x_1^2 + \Sigma x_2^2}{n_1 + n_2 - 2}\left(\frac{1}{n_1} + \frac{1}{n_2}\right)} \qquad \text{estimate of the standard error of the difference when } n_1 \neq n_2$$

This formula is appropriate when the two samples are not the same size. When $n_1 = n_2$, the formula simplifies somewhat to:

$$s_{\bar{x}_1-\bar{x}_2} = \sqrt{\frac{\Sigma x_1^2 + \Sigma x_2^2}{n(n-1)}} \qquad \text{estimate of the standard error of the difference when } n_1 = n_2$$

Chas Chauvinist wonders what the difference might be between men and women on a test of creativity he has creatively created. He decided to use a random sample of 15 men and another of 15 women to set up the 99% CI for the difference. Unfortunately, the data from two of the female subjects were lost. Chas decides to continue with the data he has. These are the values he obtained.

Creativity Test Data

For the women: $\bar{X}_1 = 98$ For the men: $\bar{X}_2 = 100$
$n_1 = 13$ $n_2 = 15$
$\Sigma x_1^2 = 30$ $\Sigma x_2^2 = 22$
$df = n_1 + n_2 - 2 = 26$
$t_{.01} = \pm 2.779$

The first thing Chas has to do is to compute the estimate of the standard error of the difference. Since the sample sizes were not the same, he used

$$s_{\bar{x}_1-\bar{x}_2} = \sqrt{\frac{\Sigma x_1^2 + \Sigma x_2^2}{n_1 + n_2 - 2}\left(\frac{1}{n_1} + \frac{1}{n_2}\right)}$$

$$= \sqrt{\frac{30 + 22}{13 + 15 - 2}\left(\frac{1}{13} + \frac{1}{15}\right)}$$

$$= \sqrt{\frac{52}{26}(0.15)} = 0.55$$

Now the 99% CI can be determined.

$$\mu_1 - \mu_2 = (\bar{X}_1 - \bar{X}_2) \pm t_{crit}(s_{\bar{x}_1 - \bar{x}_2})$$
$$= (98 - 100) \pm 2.779(0.55)$$

The limits are -3.53 and -0.47.

Chas may say, with 99% confidence, that the mean difference between men and women on his test of creativity lies between -3.53 and -0.47.

To present these data formally:

$$C(-3.53 \le (\mu_1 - \mu_2) \le -0.47) = .99$$

Hypothesis Testing with the t-Distribution

Testing hypotheses about the value of a population parameter(s), using the t-distribution, follows the same logic and procedure as it does with the normal curve. The general form of the t-ratio is similar to the general form of the Z-ratio.

$$t = \frac{\text{value of statistic} - \text{hypothesized value of parameter}}{\text{estimate of standard deviation of distribution of the statistic}}$$

If $\bar{X}$ is the statistic in question, then

$$t = \frac{\bar{X} - \mu_{\bar{x}}}{s_{\bar{x}}} \qquad \text{t for a single mean}$$

If $\bar{X}_1 - \bar{X}_2$ is the statistic in question, then

$$t = \frac{\bar{X}_1 - \bar{X}_2}{s_{\bar{x}_1 - \bar{x}_2}} \qquad \text{t for the difference between means}$$

Let's go ahead and test some hypotheses using the t-distribution.

Testing an Hypothesis about a Population Mean

A nation wide survey conducted in the 60s reported that young people listened to rock music an average of 3.5 hours per day. Let's hypothesize that the youth of today are not the "rockers of yesterday." We will randomly select a sample of twenty-five 16-year-olds and record the numbers of hours per day each spends listening to rock music over a period of 6 months. Let's use a one-tailed test to test our hypothesis at $\alpha = .05$.

$H_o: \mu = 3.50$ $\overline{X} = 1.89$
$H_a: \mu < 3.50$ $\Sigma X^2 - (\Sigma X)^2/n = 69.36$
$df = 25 - 1 = 24$
$t_{.05} = -1.71$

To use our t formula, we first need to determine the estimate of the standard error. In this example we are given the sum of squares. The computational formula for the estimate of the standard error is

$$s_{\overline{x}} = \sqrt{\frac{\Sigma X^2 - (\Sigma X)^2/n}{n(n - 1)}} \quad \text{Estimate of standard error: computational formula}$$

In our example then,

$$s_{\overline{x}} = \sqrt{\frac{69.36}{25(24)}} = 0.34$$

and our t value is easy to compute.

$$t = \frac{1.89 - 3.50}{0.34} = -4.68$$

Since our obtained t value is larger numerically than the critical value for a one-tailed test with 24 df, we reject the null hypothesis. We conclude that "the youth today don't rock like they used to."

Summary of t-Test for a Single Mean

Hypotheses
H_o: μ = specified value
H_a: $\mu \neq$ or $>$ or $<$ specified value

Assumptions
1. Subjects are randomly selected
2. Population distribution is normal

Decision Rules
df = n − 1
If $t_{obt} \geq t_{crit}$, reject the H_o
If $t_{obt} < t_{crit}$, do not reject H_o

Formula
$$t = \frac{\overline{X} - \mu}{\sqrt{\dfrac{\Sigma X^2 - (\Sigma X)^2/n}{n(n-1)}}}$$

Testing an Hypothesis about the Difference between Independent Population Means

A t-test for the difference between two independent means follows the same general logic and procedure as with the normal curve test. Let's consider the following example.

A psychology professor is interested in knowing whether there is a difference in final exam performance between students who take their introductory psychology course under a personalized system of instruction (PSI) and those who study under more conventional, lecture-discussion, format (L). She selects a random sample of 30 students and randomly assigns 15 of them to each of two groups. One group studies under PSI conditions and the other under L conditions. Unfortunately, two of the PSI students dropped out of school before they wrote the final exam. Nevertheless, she goes ahead and tests her hypothesis.

H_o: $\mu_1 - \mu_2 = 0$
H_a: $\mu_1 - \mu_2 \neq 0$

L condition: $\overline{X}_1 = 75.0$ $\Sigma x_1^2 = 2016$ $n_1 = 15$
PSI condition: $\overline{X}_2 = 86.0$ $\Sigma x_2^2 = 1200$ $n_2 = 13$

df = $n_1 + n_2 - 2 = 26$
$t_{.05} = \pm 2.056$

$$t = \frac{\overline{X}_1 - \overline{X}_2}{\sqrt{\frac{\Sigma x_1^2 + \Sigma x_2^2}{n_1 + n_2 - 2}\left(\frac{1}{n_1} + \frac{1}{n_2}\right)}}$$

$$= \frac{75 - 86}{\sqrt{\frac{2016 + 1200}{15 + 13 - 2}\left(\frac{1}{15} + \frac{1}{13}\right)}} = -2.61$$

Since the obtained value of t is numerically larger than the critical value, she may reject the null hypothesis. She has evidence that there is a significant difference in performance under PSI versus L conditions.

Summary of t-Test for Independent Means

Hypotheses
H_o: $\mu_1 = \mu_2$
H_a: $\mu_1 \neq \mu_2$ or $\mu_1 < \mu_2$ or $\mu_1 > \mu_2$

Assumptions
1. Subjects are randomly selected and independently assigned to groups.
2. Population variances are homogenous.
3. Population distributions are normal.

Decision Rules
df = $n_1 + n_2 - 2$
If $t_{obt} \geq t_{crit}$, reject H_o
If $t_{obt} < t_{crit}$, do not reject H_o

Formula
$$t = \frac{\overline{X}_1 - \overline{X}_2}{\sqrt{\left(\frac{\Sigma x_1^2 + \Sigma x_2^2}{n_1 + n_2 - 2}\right)\left(\frac{1}{n_1} + \frac{1}{n_2}\right)}}$$
where $\Sigma x^2 = \Sigma X^2 - (\Sigma X)^2/n$

Assumptions Underlying Inference with the t-Distribution

The use of the t-distribution in making inferences about population parameters assumes certain conditions. One very important assumption is that the observations were randomly selected from the population(s) of interest. Second, the estimate of the standard error is based on an unbiased estimate of the population variance. Third, the sampling distribution of the statistic (i.e. the sample mean or difference between means) must be normally distributed. You will recall that this will be true (according to the Central Limit Theorem) as long as either the population is normal or the sample size(s) is large enough. A further assumption with t-tests for the difference between means, is that the populations from which the two samples were collected have equal variability. This is called the assumption of **homogeneity of variance.** We want to know if we are sampling from distributions with different means, not different variances. It will probably occur to you that, in real life research, it is unlikely we will know whether the populations are equally variable or not. Not to worry! The t-test is quite insensitive to violations of this assumption as long as our samples sizes are large enough and *approximately equal.*

> **Homogeneity of variance:** Equal variances in populations.

For the t-test for the difference between two independent means we have another very important assumption. It is assumed that the observations have not only been randomly selected but that they have been *assigned randomly* to the two samples. In other words, the samples are independently formed. The observations in the first sample must not be correlated or dependent on observations in the second sample.

There are many occasions in research where we do not have independent samples and for these situations we have another procedure for making inferences with the t-distribution. When samples are dependent or correlated we will use the t-test for dependent samples.

Dependent or Correlated Samples

Probably the major grievance of researchers in the "softer" sciences is the extreme variability of the data. People, for example, do not behave like molecules. Chemists are fortunate. For the most part, when they repeat experiments, they get identical results everytime. Research in psychology and related disciplines is necessarily much less precise.

All statistical inference is really asking the same question. Is our obtained outcome likely to be due to chance? When we obtain a sample outcome that seems highly unlikely to have occurred if the assumptions of the null are true, we say we have a *significant* result. It seems more reasonable to conclude that the null is not true than to conclude we got such an unlikely result by chance alone. In other words, the subjects in our experiment did not behave the way we would expect them to behave if the assumptions of the null were correct. Let's look more closely at the behavior of a subject. Whatever we are dealing with, an animal, an insect or a person, a score for any single subject in a research study reflects at least three factors. We learned in Chapter 9 that those three factors are:

1. Random error.
2. The effects of the experimental variable.
3. The ability of the subject to do the task.

Random error is one of the factors that makes behavioral research so imprecise (I call this the slop factor). We do our best to control this factor by using good experimental techniques.

The effect of the experimental variable on our subjects' behavior is the factor of interest in any experiment. We would like our experimental variable to have a big effect on the subjects' performance.

The third factor, ability, is often the most significant factor contributing to the scores and their variability in research in psychology and related disciplines. Many researchers try to reduce the effects of this factor by using subjects who do not differ much in ability. Many animals, for example, are very close in ability and consequently reveal less variable behavior than do people. Those of us doing research with people, however, must deal with this factor all the time.

Random assignment of subjects to groups is a powerful technique which allows us to assume *initial* "between-group" equality. In other words, if we have randomly assigned subjects to each group in our experiment, we may assume that the groups do not differ in average ability. If, after the introduction of some experimental variable, the groups perform differently, then we may conclude that this difference is due to the variable, not to differences in initial ability. Random assignment of subjects to groups is not the only way to control for between group differences in initial ability. The use of **correlated or dependent samples** is another way of reducing the effect of subject differences on the scores.

Within Subjects Designs

Many studies of the effects of an experimental variable use the same subjects in both the **treatment** (experimental) group and in the **control** group. Measuring performance of subjects before and after they receive some instructional training is an example of a **within-subjects design**. Rather than measuring performance between two groups, one of which receives the training and the other of which does not (a **between-subjects design**), we measure performance of the same subjects under no-training conditions and then under training conditions. This reduces the between-subjects variability because a subject will behave more like himself or herself than anyone else. The effect of this, then, is that the two groups do not differ in initial ability.

> **Treatment group:** The group in an experiment that is exposed to the independent variable.
>
> **Control group:** The group that is not exposed to the independent variable.
>
> **Within subjects design:** The same subjects serve as both the control group and the treatment group.

Matched Groups Designs

Another way of reducing between-subject variability is to **match** subjects on some variable known to be related to the performance measure (usually the dependent variable). Giving subjects a practice-task similar to what they will be doing in the experiment, for example, would allow us to match subjects on initial ability and assign one subject to our control group and another of equal ability to our experimental group. In this way, we would end up with groups of equal initial ability.

> **Matched groups design:** Subjects are matched according to some variable related to the performance measure.

When to Use Dependent Groups Designs

Both the within-subject and the matched-groups techniques serve to reduce the differences in initial ability between groups and, therefore, let us better estimate the effects of the experimental variable on performance. Arithmetically speaking, these procedures reduce the size of the denominator (**error term**) in the t-test. The standard error will be smaller because there is less variability between subjects. With a smaller denominator, the t-ratio will tend to be larger. The dependent samples approach, therefore, may be a more *powerful* test of significance of an experimental variable. You will recall that power is the term we use to describe the ability of the test to reject a false null. I'm sure you are saying to yourself, "why don't we always do dependent sample research?" (Weren't you?) Clearly if the t-ratio tends to be larger with a dependent sample approach, then we are more likely to reject the null . . . right? . . . well, not necessarily!

> **Error term:** the denominator of the significance test ratio.

Nothing is so simple in statistics. It is true that the t-ratio for dependent samples tends to be larger than for independent samples. However, you will recall that the critical value of t, to which we compare our obtained value, depends on degrees of freedom. As degrees of freedom get larger our critical value gets smaller. Remember that for a t-test for two independent samples, the degrees of freedom are $n_1 + n_2 - 2$. With dependent samples degrees of freedom are $n_p - 1$ (number of *pairs* of scores $- 1$).

For example, if we did a study with two groups, ten subjects in each group, we would have 18 df for an independent t-test but *only 9* df for a dependent t-test. Why this is so will become clear to you shortly. But for now realize that, although using a dependent sample approach may increase the value of the obtained t-score, the critical value of t needed for rejection of the null is also increased. On the one hand, we increase the power of our test by reducing the error term. But, on the other hand, we decrease power by losing degrees of freedom. This is why we do not always use a dependent sample approach.

Dependent groups designs are very popular in psychology. In most cases, the effect of between subjects differences is the most significant source of error, and the dependent groups approach is, overall, a more sensitive test of the null in spite of the loss of degrees of freedom. The reduction of the error term, the denominator of the ratio, usually has a greater impact on the outcome of the statistical procedure than does the loss of degrees of freedom.

There are situations, however, where within-subject designs should not be used. Sometimes the performance of the control task carries over to the experimental task. Measuring performance on a problem-solving task before and after instruction on some problem-solving strategy would be an example of such a case. The practice effects of working on the problems first under control conditions may carry over to the experimental condition and thus, mask the effects of the independent variable (i.e. the training). There are other conditions where a within-subjects design may not be desirable, but in many cases this approach is a useful and powerful one.

Matched-groups designs avoid the problem of carryover effects because they use different subjects in each group, matched on some initial measure. It is critical, with this approach, that the matching variable be an important contributing factor to task performance. If it is not, then the t-test will be less powerful than an independent t-test because of the loss of degrees of freedom.

Generally speaking, a matched-groups design will be more powerful than an independent groups design when the variable used to equate subjects is strongly related to performance on the task of interest. If we match subjects on some variable unrelated to performance on the task we are interested in, then we will have a less powerful test of the null hypothesis. For example, say we are interested in the effects of reward on the arithmetic performance of children. We decide to use two groups of children and have them do a whole series of arithmetic problems. One group receives a treat for each correct answer; the other group receives nothing. We count the number of problems solved by each child at the end of the session. Suppose that, for some obscure reason, we believe height may be an important contributing factor to task performance. So, we measure the heights of a group of children and find 20 pairs of children of the same height. We assign one child of each matched pair to the control (no reward) condition and the other child of the same height to the experimental condition (reward). This, somewhat silly, example illustrates a *weak test* of the null hypothesis. Our matching variable is probably unrelated to task performance, so we have not reduced the size of the error term in the t-ratio. Our obtained t-value, then, will be smaller and we have many fewer degrees of freedom (df = 19) than if we had not matched subjects (df = 38). Matched groups designs can be powerful but we must be careful in selecting our matching variable.

If we have matched subjects or used the same subjects under both control and experimental conditions, we will run a dependent or correlated t-test on our data.

t-Test for the Difference between two Dependent Samples

One of the formulas you were given for the standard error used in the denominator of the t-ratio for the difference between means was:

$$s_{\bar{x}_1 - \bar{x}_2} = \sqrt{s_{\bar{x}_1}^2 + s_{\bar{x}_2}^2}$$

Actually, this is not the case!

The real formula for any t-test of the difference whether it be a dependent-groups or an independent-groups test is:

$$s_{\bar{x}_1 - \bar{x}_2} = \sqrt{s_{\bar{x}_1}^2 + s_{\bar{x}_2}^2 - 2\rho s_{\bar{x}_1} s_{\bar{x}_2}}$$

You will appreciate why I didn't show you this earlier! Consider an independent t-test for the difference. This test requires that subjects be independently assigned to groups. If this is done, the performance of the two groups would not be expected to be correlated in any way. A measure of correlation which we will discuss later is symbolized by ρ. With independent samples we expect no correlation between the populations from which the groups were selected ($\rho = 0$). For this reason, we do not include the third term under the square root sign because it is assumed to be zero when samples are independent.

When samples are dependent, however, the correlation will not be zero and the full form of the standard error formula must be used. This formula requires that we determine (actually we estimate) the correlation before we can calculate the standard error. If you do not have a computer handy which will do this for you in no time at all, there is a convenient technique for computing the t-ratio for dependent samples. This technique is called the

direct difference method. The t-ratio follows the same general format we have been using:

$$t = \frac{\overline{D} - \mu_{\overline{D}}}{s_{\overline{D}}} \quad \text{t-ratio for Dependent Means: Direct Difference Method}$$

The differences between the pair of measures for each subject are the data. We take the mean difference between our two groups (i.e., $\overline{D}$) and subtract from that the hypothesized mean difference (i.e., $\mu_{\overline{D}}$) and divide this by the standard error of the difference (i.e., $s_{\overline{D}}$). As with any two-sample t-test, the hypothesized difference stated by the null is zero and so we often leave out the last term $\mu_{\overline{D}}$.

Ready for an example? An administrator at the University of Toronto is interested in the effects of a promotional film on student attitude toward large classes. He assumes that the film will produce more positive attitudes. He decides to measure the attitudes of a random sample of students before and after they view the film. Since the same subjects are tested before and after, he will analyze his data with a dependent t-test. Here are his data:

$H_o: \mu_1 = \mu_2$
$H_a: \mu_1 < \mu_2$
$\alpha = .01$
$t_{.01} = -2.82$
$df = 9$

Attitude			
Before Film	After Film	D	D²
25	28	−3	9
23	19	4	16
30	34	−4	16
7	10	−3	9
3	6	−3	9
22	26	−4	16
12	13	−1	1
30	47	−17	289
5	16	−11	121
14	9	5	25
		$\Sigma D = -37$	$\Sigma D^2 = 511$

$$s_{\overline{D}} = \sqrt{\frac{\Sigma D^2 - (\Sigma D)^2/n}{n(n-1)}} = \sqrt{\frac{511 - (-37)^2/10}{10(9)}} = 2.04$$

$$t = \frac{\overline{D}}{s_{\overline{D}}} = \frac{(-37)/10}{2.04} = \frac{-3.7}{2.04} = -1.81$$

Since the obtained t value does not lie in the critical region, the null is not rejected. The administrator must conclude that he has no evidence that the students' attitudes toward large classes were more positive after viewing the film.

The direct difference method uses difference scores to compute the standard error (denominator) and the mean difference between the groups to compute the numerator of the t-ratio. This technique takes into account the expected correlation.

The example demonstrates why degrees of freedom for a dependent t-test is "number of pairs of scores minus one." We used the ten differences as our data for calculating the t-ratio. The standard error for the dependent samples t-test uses the *mean difference* in the computation of the sum of squares. In our example we had ten differences and we used the mean difference in calculating the sum of squares. Only nine of these differences are free to vary since the mean difference is fixed. Statistically we are operating as if we had only one group of scores: the difference scores. Therefore, the degrees of freedom are equal to the number of difference scores minus one.

Summary of t-Test for Dependent Means

Hypotheses
$H_o: \mu_1 = \mu_2$
$H_a: \mu_1 \neq \mu_2$ or $\mu_1 < \mu_2$ or $\mu_1 > \mu_2$

Assumptions
1. Subjects are randomly selected.
2. Population distributions are normal.
3. Population variances are homogeneous.
4. Repeated measures or matched subjects are used.

Decision Rules
df = $n_{pairs} - 1$
If $t_{obt} \geq t_{crit}$, reject H_o.
If $t_{obt} < t_{crit}$, do not reject H_o.

Formula

$$t = \frac{\overline{D}}{\sqrt{\frac{\Sigma D^2 - (\Sigma D)^2/n}{n(n-1)}}}$$

Power Revisited

Recall the discussion of power concerning hypothesis testing with the normal curve. We learned that the power of a test is affected by the alpha level, the effect of the independent variable, the sample size, and the error variance (the variability between subjects due to inherent individual differences). We learned that power can be increased by using good research techniques that reduce error variance. In this chapter we have seen that a dependent groups design serves to increase power by reducing error variance, either by using the same subjects in both the experimental and the control group or by matching subjects on a variable known to contribute to error variance. The significance level can be selected by the experimenter to increase the power of a test and sample size can be increased as well. So to produce a powerful test we can select the appropriate alpha level, we can increase sample size, and we can use a dependent groups design. All these choices will increase the probability that we will reject the null. But what about the effect of the independent variable? This is the critical factor in any experiment. We want to know if the independent variable has a significant effect on performance. Statistical significance and "real-world" significance are not the same. If we can use these techniques to increase power to the point where the effect of the IV becomes trivial, then we might wonder about the "real-world" significance of our research. For example, it's possible to increase our sample size and therefore power to such an extent that even tiny differences between population means will be detected in our test of significance. Sometimes a "significant" effect is not all that significant!

Statisticians have developed ways of evaluating the magnitude of the treatment effect on the dependent variable, in order to deal with this concern. One measure of treatment effect size is symbolized by $\hat{\omega}^2$. The ω is the Greek letter omega. The formula for $\hat{\omega}^2$ estimated from sample data is

$$\hat{\omega}^2 = \frac{t^2 - 1}{t^2 + df + 1} \qquad \text{Estimate of treatment effect}$$

This formula estimates the proportion of the variance in performance on the dependent measure that can be explained by or is a result of the independent variable manipulation. Clearly this proportion ranges from zero, where none of the variability was due to the treatment, to 1, where all of the variability was due to the treatment. Statisticians differ in their opinions about how large this proportion should be for the effect to be considered "significant" or important.

Imagine that we have conducted a study with an experimental group and a control group and we are going to run a t-test for independent means to test the hypothesis that the population means from which our samples were drawn are equal. We have used 21 subjects in each group. The experimental group mean is 56.9 and the control group mean is 45.8. The critical value of t for a two-tailed test at .05 level of significance is ±2.021. Let's assume that our obtained t was 2.21, which resulted in rejection of the null hypothesis. Lets compute the estimate of the treatment effect.

$$\hat{\omega}^2 = \frac{t^2 - 1}{t^2 + df + 1}$$

$$= \frac{2.21^2 - 1}{2.21^2 + 40 + 1} = \frac{4.88 - 1}{4.88 + 41} = 0.08$$

What does this mean? Well, it means that about 8% of the variability in performance scores can be accounted for by the experimental treatment and the rest, about 92%, is unexplained by the researchers' manipulation. Even though the experimental outcome led us to reject the null and claim a significant effect of the independent variable, we might be wise to pause and consider the importance or meaning of that statistically significant effect.

Choosing the Appropriate Test of Significance

You now have learned about six different tests of significance: three Z-tests (the Z-test for a single mean, for the difference between two independent means, and for a proportion) and three t-tests (t-test for a single mean, for the difference between independent means, and for the difference between dependent means). Let's examine the steps we need to go through to make decisions about the appropriate test of significance. Then we will consider some examples.

Step 1. Determine the kind of data collected in the experiment.

If the data are proportions, frequencies, or percentages, we will use the Z-test for a proportion. If the data are measures which are used to compute means and if there is only one group in the experiment, we go to step 2. If there are two groups, we go to Step 4.

Step 2. Determine whether repeated measures have been taken.

If there is only one group of subjects, then you must determine whether each subject provides one observation or two observations. In other words, you have to determine if repeated measures have been taken. If each subject contributes two data points, you run a t-test for dependent samples. If you have determined that each subject in the group provides only one data point or observation, go to Step 3.

Step 3. Determine if the population standard deviation is known.

You will run a Z-test for a single mean if the population standard deviation is known and a t-test for a single mean if it must be estimated.

Step 4. Determine whether subjects have been matched.

With two groups of subjects, you need to determine whether subjects have been matched (a matched-groups design). If they have, you run a t-test for dependent means. If subjects have not been matched but, rather, have been independently assigned to the two groups, you have one more question to answer.

Step 5. Determine if the population standard deviations are known.

If you know the population standard deviations, you run a Z-test for independent means. If you do not know the population standard deviations, you run a t-test for independent means.

Example A The average performance, on a new test of general nursing practice, of two randomly selected groups of nurses, one group with RN training and the other with BSc training, is compared. Let's go through the steps to determine the appropriate test of significance for this research problem.

Step 1. Determine the kind of data collected in the experiment.

The data are measures from each nurse which will be used to compute the mean performance of each group. Since the data are measures not frequencies, a Z-test for the proportion will not be appropriate. There are two groups, RN's and BSc's, so we go to Step 4.

Step 4. Determine whether subjects have been matched.

The two groups of nurses were randomly selected. A matched-groups design was not used.

Step 5. Determine if the population standard deviations are known.

There was no information in the problem suggesting that the test was standardized with available norms, so we assume the population standard deviations are not known and we run a t-test for independent means.

Example B The Stanford-Binet IQ test has a mean of 100 and a standard deviation of 16. A randomly selected group of teenagers from a Juvenile Offenders program is compared with the norm.

Step 1. Determine the kind of data collected in the experiment.

We can assume that the teen-agers will provide IQ data and the average IQ of the group will be computed. There is one group, so we go to Step 2.

Step 2. Determine whether repeated measures have been taken.

Repeated measures have not been taken. Each teenager provided one data point.

Step 3. Determine if the population standard deviation is known.

Since the Stanford-Binet is a standarized IQ test, the mean and standard deviation are both available. A Z-test for a single mean should be used to compare the juvenile offender group with the general population.

Example C A sociologist has randomly selected a large group of people and collected information regarding SES, annual income, and years of education for each individual. She randomly assigns subjects in pairs to an experimental or a control group, such that each pair is equal in terms of SES, income level, and years of education. The experimental subjects receive special training in mathematical problem-solving. She is interested in the effects of the training on average problem-solving performance.

Step 1. Determine the kind of data collected in the experiment.

The data are mean performance on the problem-solving tasks. There are two groups, so we go to Step 4.

Step 4. Determine whether subjects have been matched.

The subjects have been matched on three variables: SES, income, and education. The experimenter will run a t-test for dependent groups.

Example D With an experimental drug that purports to improve muscle development, a medical researcher injects half of her dogs in the left leg and half of her dogs in the right leg. This procedure continues for six weeks. Muscle mass is measured for both legs of all dogs to see if the drug increased the average amount of muscle tissue.

Step 1. Determine the kind of data collected in the experiment.

Average amount of muscle tissue is measured. There is only one group in the experiment, and so we go to step 2.

Step 2. Determine whether repeated measures have been taken.

The researcher will be comparing left leg versus right leg muscle mass in each of her dogs. This is a repeated measures design since, each subject is contributing two data points. She will run a t-test for dependent samples.

FOCUS ON RESEARCH

A student* in my Principles of Behavior Analysis decided for part of his course requirements to conduct an experiment on his son. He wanted to investigate the effects of self-monitoring and positive reinforcement on nail-biting behavior.

The Data
The son was observed for one hour each night. The hour was divided into 12 five-minute segments and a talley was recorded if nail-biting occurred at any time during the segment. This type of observation is called interval recording. The minimum talley then for one observation session was 0 and the maximum was 12.

The Design
The design was a dependent groups** design with the same subject serving in the control period of ten days and in the treatment period also of ten days.

The Independent Variable
During the control period nail-biting was simply observed. This period is called the baseline in behavior analysis. During the treatment period the subject was provided with a counter to self monitor nail-biting. If a reduction in nail-biting occurred, the experimenter rewarded the subject with the opportunity to engage in a favored activity. This type of treatment is called positive reinforcement in behavior analysis.

The Results
My student who had been studying statistics with me at the same time he was taking the course in behavior analysis decided to put some of his recent knowledge to work. Although researchers using single subject designs rarely conduct statistical significance tests, Ken decided to do so. He chose to run a dependent groups t-test between the control days and the treatment days. With a non-directional alternative and $\alpha = .05$, there was no difference in nail-biting between the control period and the treatment period ($t_{(9)} = 1.9$, $p > .05$).

Although it is perhaps unusual to run a parametric analysis with only one subject in the experiment, there is no statistical reason why this should not be done. Had the outcome been significant the conclusions Ken could make, however, are somewhat limited. Most researchers wish to generalize

---

* Diprose, K. (1990). The Effectiveness of Self-Monitoring and Positive Reinforcement in the Treatment of Fingernail Biting Behavior. Unpublished research paper submitted in partial fulfillment of requirements for a course in his program.

** This is actually a single-subject design typical in behavior analysis research. A dependent groups design usually involves more subjects.

to the population at large. Ken could only generalize to his son's likely behavior under control and treatment conditions. He could not make inferences about nail-biters in general. It is interesting that his outcome came close to significance with only 10 data points in each period. Had he observed and treated for a longer period of time he may well have found a significant difference.

This focus section was included to show you how you can put your knowledge of statistics to work even as an undergraduate student. You don't have to be a seasoned researcher to apply what you have learned and will learn in the course you are taking.

SUMMARY OF FORMULAS

	Hypothesis Testing	Interval Estimation
The Mean	$t = \dfrac{\overline{X} - \mu_{\overline{x}}}{s_{\overline{x}}}$	$\mu = \overline{X} \pm t_{crit}(s_{\overline{x}})$
The Difference Between Independent Means	$t = \dfrac{\overline{X}_1 - \overline{X}_2 - (\mu_1 - \mu_2)}{s_{\overline{x}_1 - \overline{x}_2}}$	$\mu_1 - \mu_2 = (\overline{X}_1 - \overline{X}_2) \pm t_{crit}(s_{\overline{x}_1 - \overline{x}_2})$
The Difference Between Dependent Means	$t = \dfrac{\overline{D} - \mu_{\overline{D}}}{s_{\overline{D}}}$	$\mu_{\overline{D}} = \overline{D} \pm t_{crit}(s_{\overline{D}})$

Computational Formulas for the Estimates of:

Population Standard Deviation

$$s = \sqrt{\dfrac{\Sigma X^2 - (\Sigma X)^2/n}{n - 1}}$$

Standard Error of the Mean

$$s_{\overline{x}} = s/\sqrt{n}$$

$$= \sqrt{\dfrac{\Sigma X^2 - (\Sigma X)^2/n}{n(n - 1)}}$$

**Standard Error
of the Difference**

$$s_{\bar{x}_1 - \bar{x}_2} = \sqrt{s_{\bar{x}_1}^2 + s_{\bar{x}_2}^2}$$

Independent Samples

$$= \sqrt{\left(\frac{\Sigma x_1^2 + \Sigma x_2^2}{n_1 + n_2 - 2}\right)\left(\frac{1}{n_1} + \frac{1}{n_2}\right)} \qquad n_1 \neq n_2$$

$$= \sqrt{\frac{\Sigma x_1^2 + \Sigma x_2^2}{n(n-1)}} \qquad n_1 = n_2$$

where $\Sigma x^2 = \Sigma X^2 - (\Sigma X)^2/n$

Dependent Samples

$$s_{\bar{D}} = \sqrt{\frac{\Sigma D^2 - (\Sigma D)^2/n}{n(n-1)}}$$

Estimate of Treatment Effect

$$\hat{\omega}^2 = \frac{t^2 - 1}{t^2 + df + 1}$$

EXERCISES

1. A group of 23 subjects was given a list of 30 one-word anagrams to solve. Half the solution words were emotionally neutral in meaning and half were unpleasant. Which t-test should you run to determine if affective or emotional meaning of the solution word has any effect on the time to solve the anagrams?

2. A psychologist wanted to find out whether the development of the ability to formulate abstract concepts could be hastened by special training. She selected 10 sets of 5-year old identical twins to be her subjects. The twenty children were given 25 conceptual problems to solve, and it was found that none of them could offer any correct solutions. Following this initial test, one twin in each set was given 30-minute training sessions every day for three weeks. Six months after the training was complete, all 20 children were again given the same set of 25 conceptual problems they had been given earlier. The measure was the number of correct solutions on this second test. Assume that all subjects improved on the second testing. Which t-test should you use to determine if the special training had any additional effect?

3. A school counsellor is interested in the effects of 2 teaching methods in a learning task. She believes, however, that intelligence and gender may be involved. She randomly selects 20 male children all with IQ's over 120. She randomly divides them into two groups, one of which is taught with one method and the other with the second method. She measures amount of time to learn required by each child. Which t-test should be used to determine if teaching method makes a difference in performance?

4. Indicate the degrees of freedom and the critical value of t at $\alpha = .05$ for the following:
   a. two-tailed t-test for independent means
      $n_1 = 18$ $n_2 = 12$
   b. two-tailed t-test for dependent means
      $n_1 = 16$ $n_2 = 16$

5. Sixteen students randomly selected from an introductory anthropology class are assigned randomly to two experimental conditions. Both groups are given the same 25-item multiple choice test on class material. One group (Condition A) is given hints on taking multiple choice tests; the other group (Condition B) is not. At $\alpha = .01$, run a t-test on the data below. Indicate your null and alternative hypothesis and the critical t value. What will be your statistical decision?

Condition A	Condition B
12	16
17	14
15	18
13	19
11	17
10	13
16	11
12	10

6. Fifteen randomly selected students from a political science class at the University of Toronto are given two forms of an attitude questionnaire, one before and the other after listening to a speaker discuss the separation of Quebec from the rest of Canada. Run a t-test on the data below to determine if the speaker had an influence on student attitude regarding separation. Indicate your null and alternative hypothesis and the critical value of t at $\alpha = .01$. What is your statistical decision?

Attitude Score Before Speaker	Attitude Score After Speaker
13	22
17	14
14	23
17	21
23	20
20	26
13	14
25	27
24	20
18	21
17	15
15	29
21	30
19	22
28	28

7. A behavior analyst wants to know if reward has any effect on the learning rate of gerbils. He collected data in the form of number of trials to perfect performance for two randomly selected groups of 10 gerbils each. The reward group received a "gerbil treat" at the end of each trial but the control group received nothing. Unfortunately, four of the gerbils in the control group contracted "gerbil fever" in their home cages and were unable to finish the experiment. Nevertheless, he did a t-test on the remaining data. You do one too on the data below at $\alpha = .05$. Indicate your null, alternative and critical value of t. What is your statistical decision?

Mean Performance	
Control	Reward
12	6
10	5
12	6
20	4
10	3
8	8
	10
	6
	4
	8

8. Set up the 95% C.I. for the difference between means for the following data:

$$\overline{X}_1 = 25 \qquad \overline{X}_2 = 20$$
$$n_1 = 15 \qquad n_2 = 10$$
$$\Sigma x_1^2 = 225 \qquad \Sigma x_2^2 = 200$$

9. Define and give the probability for each of the following:
   a. Type I error
   b. Type II error
   c. Power

10. List three things we can do to increase the power of the t-test.

11. A sociologist uses a standardized test of assertiveness to assess 16 randomly selected students from a class who had completed an assertiveness-training seminar. The normative mean for the test is 28. The sociologist wants to know if the seminar had an effect on the assertiveness of the graduates. Use the data below to answer his question.

$$\overline{X} = 25.75$$
$$\Sigma X^2 = 11290$$
$$\Sigma X = 412$$
$$\alpha = .05$$

   a. H_o:
      H_a:
   b. df =
   c. Critical t value =
   d. s =
   e. Obtained t value =
   f. Decision:
   Put your statistical decision in words.

12. Sixteen students are randomly selected from a class in the philosophy of ethics and are assigned randomly to two experimental conditions. Both groups are given the same aptitude test designed to measure logical decision making. Prior to this test one group is given a lecture on logic and the other group is not. Determine if the lecture affected test performance at $\alpha = .01$.

Group 1	Group 2
13	18
11	14
15	10
10	11
12	17
15	17
12	19
10	16

a. H_o:
   H_a:
b. df =
c. $t_{.01}$ =
d. t =
e. p < or > α?
f. Decision:

Put your decision in words.

13. Ten randomly selected rats are run through a maze before and after being injected with DNA from proven "fast runners". Test the hypothesis that the DNA from the "fast rats" improved running speed. Use $\alpha = .05$.

Rat	Before	After
1	24	22
2	21	23
3	24	21
4	28	26
5	22	22
6	29	28
7	26	21
8	22	23
9	27	23
10	28	24

a. H_o:
   H_a:
b. df =
c. $t_{.05}$ =
d. t =
e. p < or > α?
f. Decision:

Put your decision in words.

14. A behavioral psychologist is interested in the effects of alcohol on the learning rate of gerbils. She collected data in the form of number of trials to perfect performance for two randomly selected groups of 12 gerbils each. The gerbils in the experimental group ingested a small amount of alcohol before testing. Unfortunately, her research assistant lost some of the data. Run a t-test on the remaining data to see if alcohol affected performance. Use $\alpha = .05$.

Alcohol	No-Alcohol
12	10
14	8
16	18
13	12
10	10
17	16
18	14
15	17
	15
	13

  a. H_o:
     H_a:
  b. df =
  c. $t_{.05}$ =
  d. t =
  e. p < or > α?
  f. Decision:
  Put your decision in words.

15. Set up the 95% and 99% CI's for the difference between means for the following data.

$\bar{X}_1 = 21.78$ $\bar{X}_2 = 19.45$
$n_1 = 18$ $n_2 = 11$
$\Sigma x_1^2 = 221.70$ $\Sigma x_2^2 = 197.30$

  a. df =
  b. $t_{.05}$ =
     $t_{.01}$ =
  c. $s_{\bar{x}_1 - \bar{x}_2}$ =
  d. 95% CI =
  e. 99% CI =

CHAPTER 11

Inference with the F-Distribution

LEARNING OBJECTIVES

After reading this chapter you should be able to:
1. List the steps to construct the F-distribution.
2. Describe the shape of the F-distribution.
3. Describe how the total variance is partitioned into three sources of variation in one-way ANOVA.
4. Determine degrees of freedom for each variance estimate in one-way ANOVA for a given set of data.
5. List the means squares for the F-ratio of a one-way ANOVA.
6. Run a one-way ANOVA for a given set of data.
7. Describe the difference between main effects and interaction effects.
8. Describe how the between-groups variance is partitioned in two-way ANOVA.
9. Provide the three F-ratios tested in two-way ANOVA and the degrees of freedom associated with each mean square.
10. Run a two-way ANOVA for a given set of data.
11. Complete an ANOVA summary table for a given analysis.
12. Determine the appropriate test of significance for a given research problem.

The previous two chapters dealt with statistical techniques involving one or two groups of observations or samples. Much scientific research requires statistical analysis of more than two samples. For example, what if we were interested in the recovery rates of patients who had psychoanalysis, behavior modification, or gestalt therapy? Or perhaps we would like to compare the running rates of rats in 10 different kinds of mazes. When we have more than two samples and wish to compare their means, we may find a statistical technique called **analysis of variance (ANOVA)** useful. This is a family of statistical techniques specifically designed for experiments with more than two groups of subjects.

> ANOVA: Analysis of variance.

ANOVA is the appropriate technique for making inferences about population means of two groups or more and uses various measures of variability to do so, hence the name analysis of *variance*. All groups are compared simultaneously and thus, this a very efficient statistical procedure.

You may be wondering why we don't simply compare pairs of samples with several t-tests. This is a good question. Consider an experiment where we gave different doses of an experimental drug to five groups of patients and evaluated the effects on their performance on some motor skills task. We could measure the effect of each dose level by comparing every pair of means using a separate t-test. Remember the formula for the number of combinations of 5 things taken 2 at a time? $_5C_2 = 5!/3!2!$ We would need 10 t-tests. There are several problems with this approach. It would be a lot of work, but there is a statistical problem with it, which is more critical. Running multiple t-tests in a single experiment is inappropriate because the probability of an inferential error is high. We will discuss this in more detail later on.

Recall that inference with the normal curve involved computing Z-scores. Inference with the t-distribution required the computation of t-scores. ANOVA is an inferential technique which uses the F-distribution and requires the computation of F-scores.

The F-Distribution

Just as the normal distribution is the random sampling distribution of the Z statistic and the t-distribution is the random sampling distribution of the t statistic, the **F-distribution** is the random sampling distribution of the F statistic.

In Chapter 10 we saw that when we collect all possible samples from a population, calculate Z and t for each sample mean and place the Z values and the t values in separate relative frequency distributions, the Z values follow a normal curve and the t values follow the t-distribution. We use a similar procedure for setting up the sampling distribution of the F statistic.

Constructing the F-Distribution

The F-distribution is set up a little differently than what you are used to and, as you learn more about ANOVA, the reasons for this will become clearer. The sampling distribution of the F statistic is constructed in the following way:

Step 1. Randomly select two samples of fixed sizes from a population.

Step 2. Calculate an *unbiased estimate of the variance* (s^2) for each sample.

Step 3. Divide the first variance estimate (s_1^2) by the second variance estimate (s_2^2). *This is the F statistic.*

Step 4. Return the samples to the population.

Step 5. Repeat steps 1-4 until all possible pairs of samples have been drawn.

Step 6. Place the F values in a relative frequency distribution.

The F-distribution has certain important properties that allow us to make inferences about population means.

Characteristics of the F-Distribution

The F-distribution is the relative frequency distribution of the F statistic. The F statistic is a ratio between two variance estimates. Since an estimate of the variance cannot be negative (zero variability is as low as it goes), the frequency distribution is limited at zero. The other end of the distribution, however, is not limited and so the distribution is positively skewed.

Notice that the variance estimates are calculated for samples drawn from a single population. On the average, then, we would expect the two estimates to be equal. The expected value of F is approximately 1.00 since

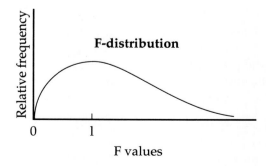

Figure 11-1 An example of an F-distribution

we are computing a ratio between two variance estimates each of which estimates the same population variance. In summary:

The F ratio = s_1^2/s_2^2
The F distribution is positively skewed with a limit at zero.
The expected value of F is approximately 1.00.

The F-distribution, like the t-distribution, is a family of curves whose shape depends on degrees of freedom. Figure 11-1 presents an example of an F-distribution.

Using the F-Distribution

Recall that ANOVA is used to make inferences about the means of the populations from which samples have been drawn. These different samples have been treated differently by the researcher who wishes to know if the treatment or independent variable (IV) had an effect on the dependent variable (DV). If the IV didn't work, we would expect the samples to be similar and their means to be the same, or differ from each other only by chance. In other words, if the IV has no effect, the samples are simply different samples drawn from the same population and their means will differ due to sampling fluctuation only.

If, however, the treatment has an effect, the samples then come from populations with different means and we would expect the sample means to be quite different.

Are you beginning to see why this analysis is called "Analysis of Variance?" ANOVA examines how much sample means vary from each other compared to what would be expected by chance sampling fluctuation.

Null and Alternative Hypotheses

When we made inferences about means with the normal or the t-distribution, the null hypothesis stated that the means did not differ. The same is true when we make inferences about means using the F-distribution. The null hypothesis is

$H_o: \mu_1 = \mu_2 = \mu_3 = ... = \mu_k$

where k is the number of samples in the experiment.

When an analysis compares only two means, we distinguish between directional and non-directional alternative hypotheses. In ANOVA, however, the null hypothesis may be false because two means are different although all the rest are equal, or three means may be different and all the rest the same, for example. ANOVA does not tell us where the difference(s) lies; just that there is a difference between at least two of the means. The alternative hypothesis for ANOVA is

H_a: H_o is false

We do not distinguish between directional and non-directional alternative hypotheses in ANOVA. Once ANOVA has determined that a significant difference exists, we must do further analyses to find out which means are responsible for the outcome of ANOVA. Chapter 13 discusses some of the statistical techniques commonly used after ANOVA.

ANOVA is a family of techniques. We will study two of these in this chapter: *one-way and two-way ANOVA*.

One-Way Analysis of Variance

One-way ANOVA is a statistical procedure that tests for differences between two or more means. With two samples, it is appropriate to compute either t or F.

Comparing two means with a t-test is a special case of one-way ANOVA. In fact, the outcome (not the actual value) of an analysis of variance done on two samples is identical to the outcome of a t-test done on those two samples.

Let's examine the logic of one-way ANOVA. Consider three groups of 10 subjects each. All the subjects were randomly selected from a population and independently assigned to groups. Each group was treated differently. Now imagine, for the moment, that the treatment (IV) had no effect on the DV. We might find the following kinds of results:

```
GROUP A    X XX    XXXXX X      X
                    X̄_a
GROUP B   XXXXX    XX           X XX
                    X̄_b
GROUP C    X X     XXXXX       X XX
                    X̄_c
```

Each X represents the score for a single subject. As you can see, within each group the individual scores vary around the group mean. The means of the three groups are similar but not identical.

Now, let's consider what kind of data we might have if the treatment did have an effect on the groups. We might see something like this.

```
GROUP A   X XX XX    XXXXX
           X̄_a
GROUP B              X XXX XXXX X X
                          X̄_b
GROUP C   XXX XXXX   X XX
              X̄_c
```

Within each group, the scores vary around the group mean. The group means are not as similar as when the treatment had no effect. However, we would not expect the means to be identical even if the treatment had no effect. They would vary somewhat because of sampling fluctuation. The question is "how different must the group means be before we conclude that the differences are probably not due to sampling variation alone?" In other words, "how much variation is expected when the groups come from populations with equal means?"

If there is no treatment effect, the populations from which the groups were drawn would have identical means and thus, we may treat the samples as if they came from the same population. Any variation in the sample means would be considered chance variation. If, however, the treatment did have an effect, the samples come from populations with different means and we would expect the variation between the sample means to be quite large.

Partitioning the Variance

Looking at the examples given in the previous section, we can identify three kinds of variation. The individual scores *vary around their subgroup means*. The subjects within each group are different and so their scores are different. This is variation inherent in the subjects themselves. **Inherent variation** or **error variance** is free of the effects of the treatment. It is the variation we see because of individual differences between our subjects.

> **Error variance:** Variability between subjects that is free of treatment effects.

The subgroup means are not the same. The *subgroup means vary around the combined mean*, the overall mean of the experiment. These group means are different for two reasons. First, the group means differ partly due to inherent variation of the subjects. Second, they differ due to the effect of the treatment, if indeed it had an effect. The variation between subgroup means is due to *inherent variation plus variation due to treatment*.

Finally, the individual scores vary around the combined mean of the entire distribution. Each score varies from the overall mean. This is the **total variation in the experiment**.

We have three kinds of variation:

1. the total variation as reflected in the difference between the scores and the combined mean;
2. the variation of the scores within each group from their own group mean; and
3. the variation of the group means from the combined mean.

The second kind of variation is due to inherent variability only. The third kind of variation is due to inherent variation and the effect of the treatment. If the treatment had no effect we would expect the second and third kinds of variation to be equal. In other words, if the treatment had no effect, then these two measures should be more or less the same, given some amount of sampling fluctuation. This is the logic of analysis of variance.

The **total variability** in an experiment may be partitioned thus:

1. the variability of subjects **within groups** and
2. the variability **between groups**.

Any individual score in any group can vary from the combined mean of all the groups ($X - \overline{X}_c$). Any score can vary from the mean of its own group ($X - \overline{X}$). Each group mean can vary from the combined mean ($\overline{X} - \overline{X}_c$). If we squared each of these deviation scores and summed the squares, we would have three measures of variability in "sum of squares" form. Analysis of Variance involves computing these various sums of squares (**SS**) and comparing them.

> **Total variability:** Variability of all the scores from the combined mean.
> **Within group variability:** Variability of scores within groups from the group mean.
> **Between group variability:** Variability of group means from combined mean.

Calculating the Sums of Squares

Since we have three measures of variability, we compute three separate sums of squares. The measure of total variability (called **SS$_{TOT}$**) is composed of two parts: (i) the variability within groups (called **SS$_{WG}$**) and (ii) the variability between groups (called **SS$_{BG}$**). The defining formula which partitions the total variability in an experiment into its two component parts is:

$$SS_{TOT} = SS_{BG} + SS_{WG}$$

$$\Sigma^k \Sigma^n (X_i - \overline{X}_c)^2 = \Sigma_n^k (\overline{X}_k - \overline{X}_c)^2 + \Sigma^k \Sigma^n (X_i - \overline{X}_k)^2$$

where $\overline{X}_c$ is the combined mean
$\overline{X}_k$ is the group mean
X_i is the raw score

Now, don't let this throw you! Examine the expression to the left of the equal sign. This tells us to subtract the combined mean from each score in the entire experiment, square these differences, and sum them. This is the total variability in the experiment. The first expression to the right of the equal sign tells us to subtract the combined mean from each group mean, square each difference, and sum these.

$$SS_{BG} = (\overline{X}_1 - \overline{X}_c)^2 + (\overline{X}_2 - \overline{X}_c)^2 + ... + (\overline{X}_k - \overline{X}_c)^2$$

This is the variability between groups.

The last expression tells us to subtract the group mean from each score in the group, square these differences, sum them, and to do this for all the groups.

$$SS_{WG} = \Sigma x_1^2 + \Sigma x_2^2 + ... + \Sigma x_k^2$$

This is the variability within groups.

In the past, we have found that the defining formulas are not usually used computationally. This is true here. There are simplified formulas to be used in the actual computation of the sums of squares.

The computational formula for the total sum of squares is:

$$SS_{TOT} = \Sigma X_{tot}^2 - \frac{(\Sigma X_{tot})^2}{n_{tot}} \quad \text{computational formula for } SS_{TOT}$$

X_{tot} refers to all the raw scores in the experiment.
n_{tot} refers to the total number of observations in the experiment.

This formula tells us to

1. square all the raw scores in the experiment.
2. sum the squared raw scores.
3. sum the raw scores; square the sum, and divide by the total number of observations in the experiment.
4. subtract the result of step 3 from that of step 2.

The computational formula for the between group sum of squares is

$$SS_{BG} = \frac{(\Sigma X_1)^2}{n_1} + \frac{(\Sigma X_2)^2}{n_2} + ... + \frac{(\Sigma X_k)^2}{n_k} - \frac{(\Sigma X_{tot})^2}{n_{tot}} \quad \text{computational formula for } SS_{BG}$$

This formula tells us to

1. sum the raw scores in each group.
2. square each group sum and divide each by is group size.
3. sum all the values obtained in Step 2.
4. sum all the scores in the entire experiment; square this sum and divide by the total number of observations.
5. subtract the result of step 4 from that of step 3.

Since the total sum of squares is composed of the SS_{BG} plus the SS_{WG}, we can obtain the sum of squares within groups by subtraction ($SS_{TOT} - SS_{BG}$). If we wished to calculate the SS_{WG} directly, we would determine the sum of squares within each of our groups using our usual formula for any sum of squares:

$$SS = \Sigma x^2 = \Sigma X^2 - (\Sigma X)^2/n$$

We would compute this value for each group and then sum the resulting values. The formula would look like this

---

$$SS_{WG} = [\Sigma X_1^2 - (\Sigma X_1)^2/n_1] + [\Sigma X_2^2 - (\Sigma X_2)^2/n_2] + \ldots + [\Sigma X_k^2 - (\Sigma X_k)^2/n_k]$$

computational formula for SS_{WG}

Calculating the Mean Squares

In the past, we have divided sums of squares by degrees of freedom to obtain unbiased estimates of the population variance. We will do the same here. Dividing each SS by its associated degrees of freedom produces unbiased estimates of the variance called **mean squares**.

> **Mean square:** Estimate of the population variance, found by dividing sum of squares by df.

When we compute the total sum of squares, we effectively ignore the groups and treat all the scores as one large group. We subtract each raw score from the overall or combined mean, square each difference, and sum the squared differences. Because we use the combined mean in our calculation, it is fixed, and we use up one degree of freedom. Therefore, $n_{tot} - 1$ scores are left free to vary. When computing SS_{TOT} then

$$df_{tot} = n_{tot} - 1 \quad \text{degrees of freedom for } SS_{TOT}$$

Computing the sum of squares between groups requires that we subtract the combined mean from each subgroup mean, square each difference, and sum the squared differences. Because we use the combined mean in our computations, it is fixed. We have as many difference values as we have groups (k), but we have used up one degree of freedom. When computing SS_{BG} then

$$df_{bg} = k - 1 \quad \text{degrees of freedom for } SS_{BG}$$

The sum of squares within groups is found by measuring the amount of variability of the group scores around their own means. We subtract the subgroup mean from all the scores in its group, square the differences, and sum them. We do this for each group in our experiment. Because we use the subgroup means in our calculation, each is fixed, and we use up one degree of freedom for each group mean used. When computing SS_{WG} then

$$df_{wg} = n_1 - 1 + n_2 - 1 + \ldots + n_k - 1$$
$$= n_{tot} - k \quad \text{degrees of freedom for } SS_{WG}$$

In an experiment, the total sum of squares can be partitioned into the sum of squares between, plus the sum of squares within, groups. The total number of degrees of freedom in the experiment can be partitioned into two parts as well: degrees of freedom between groups plus degrees of freedom within groups. Therefore

$$df_{tot} = df_{bg} + df_{wg}$$
$$n_{tot} - 1 = k - 1 + n_{tot} - k$$

The partitioning of the variability and degrees of freedom in a one-way ANOVA is illustrated in Figure 11-2.

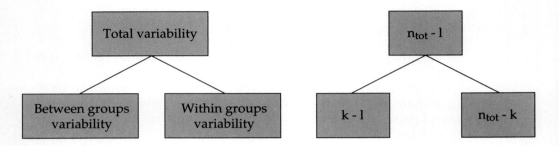

Figure 11-2 Partitioning the variability and degrees of freedom for a one-way ANOVA

Dividing each sum of squares by its associated degrees of freedom produces unbiased estimates of the population variance: mean squares. If the treatment in our experiment had no effect on the DV, we would expect the estimate of the variance between groups (MS_{BG}) to equal the estimate of the variance within groups (MS_{WG}). This is because the variance estimate between groups reflects inherent variation plus treatment; the variance estimate within groups reflects inherent variation only. If the treatment has no effect, these two measures are estimating the same thing: *inherent variation*. We are interested, then, in these two unbiased estimates: the mean square between, and the mean square within, groups. Each is found by dividing the sum of squares by degrees of freedom.

In summary

$$MS_{BG} = \frac{SS_{BG}}{df} = \frac{SS_{BG}}{k-1}$$
$$MS_{WG} = \frac{SS_{WG}}{df} = \frac{SS_{WG}}{n_{tot}-k}$$

mean squares

Now we can compare these two variance estimates to determine the effect of the treatment. If the treatment didn't work, each estimates the same population variance. If the treatment did work, then the MS_{BG} would be larger than the MS_{WG}, since it reflects not only inherent variation, but also treatment effects.

Calculating and Interpreting the F-Ratio

The F-ratio is the ratio between the between group variance estimate and the within groups variance estimate:

$$F = MS_{BG}/MS_{WG} \quad \text{F-ratio}$$

Clearly, if the treatment had no effect, we would expect this ratio to be 1, on the average. If the treatment did have an effect, we would expect this value to be greater than 1. Table B-3, in Appendix B near the back of the book, provides the critical values of F for the 5% and 1% level of significance. This table is read by locating the degrees of freedom associated with the numerator (MS_{BG}) along the top, and locating the degrees of freedom associated with the denominator (MS_{WG}) along the side. As usual, to reject the null hypothesis, the obtained F value must be equal to or larger than the critical value. If the null is rejected, we conclude that the treatment had a significant effect on the DV. In other words, the MS_{BG} is so much greater than the MS_{WG} that we claim that this is not due to chance, but is caused by the treatment variable.

Let's work our way through an example in detail to see how ANOVA is done.

Running a One-Way ANOVA

As a psychology instructor, I am always looking for ways to help students improve their study skills and test performance. Let's assume that I have randomly selected three groups of 15 students each, and I have given special training to two of the groups. In one group, I have concentrated their training on test-taking skills (Group T). Another group has been trained in study skills (Group S). The third group has received no special training. This is the control group (Group C). The trained groups have been instructed to use their new skills when studying and taking weekly tests for a period of one month. At the end of this time all the students take a common test to measure their knowledge about the preceding month's work. Here are the data:

	Group T	Group S	Group C	X_1^2	X_2^2	X_3^2
	64	56	45	4096	3136	2025
	78	76	60	6084	5776	3600
	68	55	65	4624	3025	4225
	57	53	67	3249	2809	4489
	76	76	54	5776	5776	2916
	75	75	53	5625	5625	2809
	73	51	58	5329	2601	3364
	66	62	59	4356	3844	3481
	87	69	49	7569	4761	2401
	89	63	72	7921	3969	5184
	68	52	63	4624	2704	3969
	59	53	69	3481	2809	4761
	72	81	61	5184	6561	3721
	83	90	53	6889	8100	2809
	61	84	58	3721	7056	3364
Sums	1076	996	886	78528	68552	53118
Means	71.73	66.40	59.07			

We have all the raw scores and their squares. Now let's go ahead and run a one-way ANOVA on these data.

Step 1. Compute the sums of squares

$$SS_{TOT} = \Sigma X_{tot}^2 - (\Sigma X_{tot})^2/n_{tot}$$

$$\Sigma X_{tot}^2 = 78528 + 68552 + 53118 = 200198$$

$$\Sigma X_{tot} = 1076 + 996 + 886 = 2958$$

$$(\Sigma X_{tot})^2/n_{tot} = 2958^2/45 = 194439.20$$

$$SS_{TOT} = 200198 - 194439.20 = 5758.80$$

$$SS_{BG} = \frac{(\Sigma X_1)^2}{n_1} + \frac{(\Sigma X_2)^2}{n_2} + \frac{(\Sigma X_3)^2}{n_3} - \frac{(\Sigma X_{tot})^2}{n_{tot}}$$

$$= \frac{1076^2}{15} + \frac{996^2}{15} + \frac{886^2}{15} - 194439.20$$

$$= 195652.53 - 194439.20 = 1213.33$$

$$SS_{WG} = SS_{TOT} - SS_{BG}$$

$$= 5758.80 - 1213.33 = 4545.47$$

We can verify the SS_{WG} by computing it directly.

SS within Group T = $\Sigma X_1^2 - (\Sigma X_1)^2/n_1$ = $78528 - 1076^2/15 = 1342.933$

SS within Group S $= \Sigma X_2^2 - (\Sigma X_2)^2/n_2 = 2417.60$

SS within Group C $= \Sigma X_3^2 - (\Sigma X_3)^2/n_3 = 784.933$

$SS_{WG} = 4545.47$

Step 2. Compute the mean squares

To calculate the F-ratio we use MS_{WG} and MS_{BG}. We have a total of $n_{tot} - 1$ degrees of freedom ($45 - 1 = 44$). Because we have three groups, the MS_{BG} has 2 degrees of freedom. The within group MS has 42 df (i.e., $n_{tot} - k$).

$MS_{BG} = SS_{BG}/df = 1213.33/2 = 606.67$

$MS_{WG} = SS_{WG}/df = 4545.47/42 = 108.23$

Step 3. Compute the F-ratio

$F = MS_{BG}/MS_{WG} = 606.67/108.23 = 5.61$

Step 4. Compare the obtained F value with the critical value and make a decision.

$F_{crit} = F_{(2, 42)} = 5.15$ at $\alpha = .01$

Since our obtained value is larger than the critical value, we reject the null hypothesis. We have evidence that there is a significant difference between the means of the populations from which our samples were drawn. We can say that training makes a difference in test performance. The next step would be to find out exactly where that difference lies. This requires that we follow our ANOVA with another statistical technique designed to compare individual means. The more common comparison procedures are discussed in Chapter 13.

The outcome of any ANOVA can be summarized in a table called an **ANOVA Summary Table**. The summary table for the analysis we just did would look like this.

ANOVA Summary Table

Source of Variance	Sum of Squares	df	Mean Squares	F	p
Between groups	1213.33	2	606.60	5.61	<.01
Within groups	4545.47	42	108.23		
Total	5758.80	44			

Summary of One-Way ANOVA

Hypotheses
H_o: $\mu_1 = \mu_2 = ... = \mu_k$
H_a: H_o is false

Assumptions
1. Subjects are randomly selected and independently assigned to groups.
2. Population distributions are normal.
3. Population variances are homogeneous.

Decision Rules
$df_{bg} = k - 1$
$df_{wg} = n_{tot} - k$
If $F_{obt} \geq F_{crit}$, reject the H_o
If $F_{obt} < F_{crit}$, do not reject H_o

Formula
$$F = \frac{MS_{BG}}{MS_{WG}}$$

Two-Way Analysis of Variance

One-way ANOVA is a method for comparing groups receiving different treatments or different levels of *one* independent variable. Another ANOVA technique allows us to simultaneously study the effects of *two* independent variables.

Two-way ANOVA simultaneously measures the effects of two treatment conditions or independent variables. Perhaps we are interested in determining the readability of four computer type styles under fluorescent, versus incandescent light. We could do two experiments: one to study the readability of the four styles under fluorescent light, and a second to study readability under incandescent light. This approach is not very efficient, however. Two-way ANOVA allows us to investigate the two independent variables (light and style) at the same time in a single experiment. This design is particularly important because it provides an analysis of the interaction between the two variables.

The Logic of Two-Way ANOVA

A two-way ANOVA provides three different F-tests to answer three different questions about the effects of the treatments. Using the previous example, let's consider the questions we can ask. First, does type style make a difference in readability, overall? Second, is there a difference, overall, in readability under incandescent versus fluorescent light? Third, whatever the difference in readability of the four styles, is this difference the same under both light conditions? The first two questions are asking about **main effects**. The third question asks whether or not there is an **interaction** between type style and lighting conditions.

> **Main effect:** In ANOVA, the effect of an independent variable on performance of groups.
>
> **Interaction:** In ANOVA, the effect of one independent variable on the other.

Main Effects

Main effect refers to the effect of each independent variable. If type style made a difference in readability, we would say there is a *main effect of style*. If light conditions also made a difference, we would say there is a *main effect of lighting*. The readability scores from our experiment are as follows:

Light	Chicago	Geneva	Monaco	Princeton	Sums	Means
Fluorescent	35	22	20	31	108	27
Incandescent	28	23	8	29	88	22
Sums	63	45	28	60		
Means	31.5	22.5	14.0	30.0		

Let's consider the main effect of type style: Does style make a difference overall? To determine the effect of style we examine the sums (or means) for each style, ignoring light conditions, for the moment. We can see that the readability score is highest for Chicago and lowest for Monaco. Let's graph the main effect of style. See Figure 11-3.

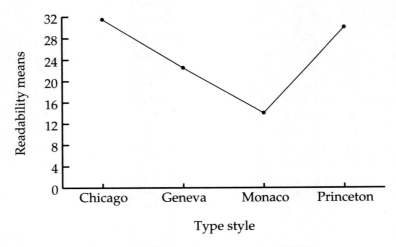

Figure 11-3 The main effect of type on readability

This graph indicates that readability is poorest for Monaco, best for Chicago and Princeton and intermediate for Geneva. If the line was flat, there would be no main effect due to type style.

The second independent variable was light condition. If we graphed the data on readability under the two kinds of lighting, we could examine the main effect of lighting. See Figure 11-4.

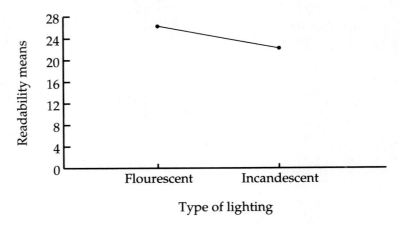

Figure 11-4 The main effect of lighting on readability

This graph indicates that readability was better under fluorescent lighting conditions. The third question we asked was "Whatever the effect of one of the independent variables, is it the same under the levels of the other IV?" In other words, "Is there an interaction between the two IV's?"

The Interaction

An interaction, in our example, means that the effect of type style on readability is different under fluorescent and incandescent lighting. To graph the interaction, we separate the scores under the two lighting conditions.

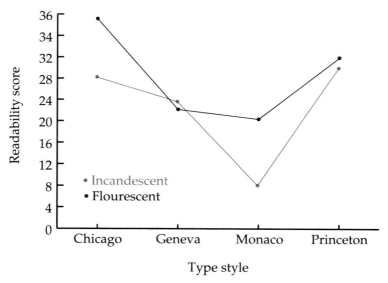

Figure 11-5 The interaction between lighting and type style

Figure 11-5 indicates that the Monaco type style was particularly hard to read under incandescent light. It appears to be the style most affected by the change in lighting conditions. If the effect of lighting was the same for all type styles, the two lines of our graph would be more or less parallel.

The F-test for the interaction measures the degree to which the lines are parallel. If it is significant, we conclude that the lack of parallelism is not due to chance alone. Of course, we would not expect the lines to be exactly parallel; we would expect some deviation. If the deviation is very large, however, we have a significant interaction.

Finding a significant interaction affects how we interpret our data. Consider an example where two teachers are interested in the effectiveness of two instructional methods on student performance. Professor A is very effective when she uses a small-group discussion approach. When she uses a straight lecture approach, however, her students do not do very well. Professor B, on the other hand, is a very effective lecturer and students do much better when he lectures than when he uses a small-group approach. If we obtained overall performance scores from the students under each teaching method, we might find the situation shown in Figure 11-6.

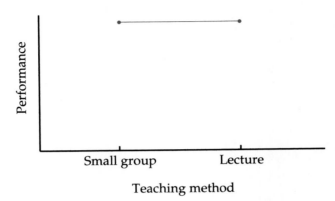

Figure 11-6 The main effect of teaching method on performance

This graph indicates that there is no difference in overall performance under the two teaching methods, that is, there is *no main effect of teaching method*. When we look at the two professors, ignoring method, the data might look like Figure 11-7.

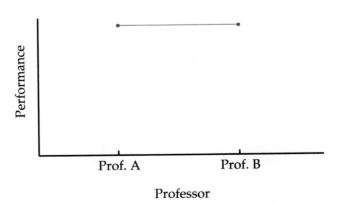

Figure 11-7 The main effect of professor on performance

This graph indicates that there is no difference in performance between Professor A's students and Professor B's students, that is, there is *no main effect of teacher*. If our interpretation of the data stopped here, it would be misleading. The lack of main effects does not necessarily mean that there are no differences. We must also examine the interaction between teacher and method. The graph of the interaction would look like Figure 11-8.

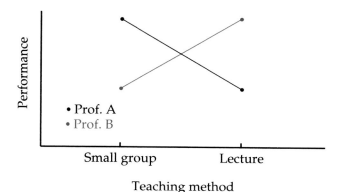

Figure 11-8 The interaction between professor and teaching method

Now we can see what really happened. Professor A was very effective with the small group approach and Professor B was very effective with the lecture approach. The teaching method interacted with the teacher using it. If we had looked only at the main effects we would have concluded, incorrectly, that neither teacher nor method made a difference in student performance. Two-way ANOVA allows us to examine the interaction between the two independent variables. It provides us with important information that we do not have with one-way ANOVA.

Partitioning the Variance

Let's consider an experiment with two independent variables (A and B), each having two levels (1 and 2). This design is called a **2X2 complete factorial**. We have two variables or factors, each of which has two levels. In total, we have four groups of subjects. Like one-way ANOVA, we can partition the total variance in the experiment into its component parts. The total sum of squares can be divided into the sum of squares between groups, (often called the treatment sum of squares) and the sum of squares within groups.

What is new with two-way ANOVA is that the *sum of squares between groups can be partitioned into three sums of squares* ($SS_{BG} = SS_A + SS_B + SS_{AXB}$):

1. the sum of squares associated with the first independent variable (SS_A),

2. the sum of squares associated with the second independent variable (SS_B), and
3. the sum of squares associated with the interaction (SS_{AXB}).

Each sum of squares, when divided by its associated degrees of freedom, gives us an unbiased estimate of the population variance. These variance estimates are called mean squares as before.

$$MS_A = SS_A/df$$
$$MS_B = SS_B/df \qquad \text{mean squares}$$
$$MS_{AXB} = SS_{AXB}/df$$

If neither A nor B had an effect, then these three mean squares estimate the same population variance as the within-group mean square. With a two-way ANOVA, we have three new tests of significance and three new F-ratios. The F-ratios are determined, as before, by dividing the between-group variance estimates by the within-group variance estimate. In summary

$$\text{F for the A Main Effect} = MS_A/MS_{WG}$$
$$\text{F for the B Main Effect} = MS_B/MS_{WG} \qquad \text{F-ratios}$$
$$\text{F for the Interaction} = MS_{AXB}/MS_{WG}$$

Each F-ratio is compared to the critical value in Table B-3 to determine its significance.

Let's look at an example to see how we would calculate the sums of squares for our three tests of significance.

Calculating the Sums of Squares

Below is an example of a 2X2 factorial design layout. Thirty-two subjects are randomly selected and independently assigned to four groups, with eight subjects in each.

	Groups			
	A_1		A_2	
Subject	B_1	B_2	B_1	B_2
1				
2				
3				
4				
5				
6				
7				
8				
Sums	A_1B_1	A_1B_2	A_2B_1	A_2B_2

Step 1. Calculate the total sum of squares.

This is done in the same way as before. Recall the formula for SS_{TOT}

$$SS_{TOT} = \Sigma X_{tot}^2 - (\Sigma X_{tot})^2/n_{tot}$$

Once again, we square all the raw scores, add them up and subtract from this value the square of the sum divided by the total number of scores in the experiment.

Step 2. Calculate the between-groups and the within-groups sum of squares.

We use the same procedure as we did with one-way ANOVA. We'll modify our earlier formula for the between sum of squares to avoid confusion.

The between-group sum of squares formula for a general two-way ANOVA is

$$SS_{BG} = \frac{(\Sigma A_1B_1)^2 + (\Sigma A_1B_2)^2 + \ldots + (\Sigma A_aB_b)^2}{n} - \frac{(\Sigma X_{tot})^2}{n_{tot}}$$

where n is the number of subjects in each group; a is the number of levels of the A independent variable; and b is the number of levels of the B independent variable.

And so, ΣA_aB_b is the sum of the scores in the last group. For the design presented above, $\Sigma A_aB_b = \Sigma A_2B_2$, the fourth group in the experiment. Obviously, for this design ab is the total number of groups in the experiment, which we often call k.

The within-group sum of squares is easily found by subtraction.

$$SS_{WG} = SS_{TOT} - SS_{BG}$$

Step 3. Calculate the sums of squares for the main effects and the interaction.

Recall that we have three between-group tests of significance because we partitioned the between-group sum of squares into three parts: the two main effects and the interaction. We must determine the sum of squares for the A main effect, for the B main effect, and for the AXB interaction. The general formula for computing the sum of squares for the A main effect is

$$SS_A = \frac{(\Sigma A_1)^2 + (\Sigma A_2)^2 + \ldots + (\Sigma A_a)^2}{bn} - \frac{(\Sigma X_{tot})^2}{n_{tot}}$$

SS for the A main effect

where bn is the total number of subjects in each level of the A independent variable.

For the A main effect, in our 2X2 design, we must sum over the two levels of B for A_1 and over the two levels of B for A_2, square each sum, and divide by the number of subjects contributing to that sum, i.e., bn. We ignore the B independent variable and look only at the difference between the levels of A. We then subtract the same term: the square of the sum of all the scores in the experiment divided by the total number of scores. Our formula is

$$SS_A = \frac{(\Sigma A_1)^2 + (\Sigma A_2)^2}{bn} - \frac{(\Sigma X_{tot})^2}{n_{tot}}$$

To calculate the B main-effect sum of squares, the general formula is

$$SS_B = \frac{(\Sigma B_1)^2 + (\Sigma B_2)^2 + \ldots + (\Sigma B_b)^2}{an} - \frac{(\Sigma X_{tot})^2}{n_{tot}}$$

SS for the B main effect

where an is the total number of subjects in each level of B.

For our design, this formula is simplified to

$$SS_B = \frac{(\Sigma B_1)^2 + (\Sigma B_2)^2}{an} - \frac{(\Sigma X_{tot})^2}{n_{tot}}$$

Here we ignore the A IV and look only at the difference between the two levels of B.

Remember that the between-groups sum of squares is composed of the sum of squares for A, the sum of squares for B and the sum of squares for the AXB interaction. The interaction sum of squares, then, can be found by subtraction.

$$SS_{AXB} = SS_{BG} - SS_A - SS_B \qquad \text{SS for the interaction}$$

Calculating the Mean Squares

Each sum of squares is divided by its degrees of freedom to provide mean squares. Recall that the total degrees of freedom in the experiment is $n_{tot} - 1$. The within-group sum of squares has $n_{tot} - k$ degrees of freedom, and the between-group sum of squares has $k - 1$ degrees of freedom. Recall that k for a two-way ANOVA is the product of a and b (i.e., the number of levels of A and the number of levels of B).

Since the between-group sum of squares is partitioned into three sums of squares, we might expect the degrees of freedom between groups to be partitioned as well; and this is so. The degrees of freedom for the A main effect are found by subtracting 1 from the number of levels of A. If there are two levels of A, we have 1 df for the A main effect. The same is true for the main effect of B. The degrees of freedom are the number of levels of B minus 1. The remaining degrees of freedom between groups are taken by the interaction. The interaction, then, has $k - 1 - df_a - df_b$. The degrees of freedom for the interaction can also be obtained by $(df_a)(df_b)$. A 2X2 experiment with four groups would have 3df between groups: 1df for the A main effect, 1df for the B main effect and 1df for the interaction. In summary:

$$df_{bg} = df_a + df_b + df_{axb}$$

The mean squares are now easy to obtain.

between-group means squares

$MS_A = \dfrac{SS_A}{df_a}$ df is $(a - 1)$, where a is the number of levels of A

$MS_B = \dfrac{SS_B}{df_b}$ df is $(b - 1)$, where b is the number of levels of B

$MS_{AXB} = \dfrac{SS_{AXB}}{df_{axb}}$ df is $(df_{bg} - df_a - df_b)$ or $(df_a)(df_b)$

Partitioning of the variability and degrees of freedom for a two-way ANOVA is illustrated in Figure 11-9.

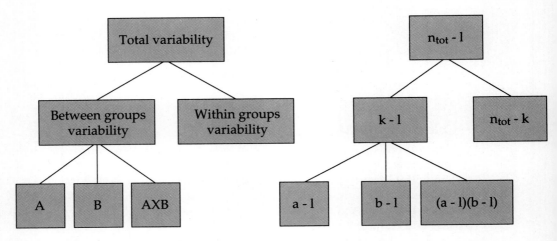

Figure 11-9 Partitioning the variability and degrees of freedom for a two-way ANOVA

Calculating and Interpreting the F-Ratios

Now we can test the three mean squares for significance.

$$F_A = MS_A/MS_{WG}$$
$$F_B = MS_B/MS_{WG}$$
$$F_{AXB} = MS_{AXB}/MS_{WG}$$

F-ratios

All three F-ratios use the MS within groups in the denominator. Each is tested for significance by locating the appropriate degrees of freedom in Table B-3. The between-group, or treatment mean square itself, may be tested for significance with the within-group mean square in the denominator. Lack of significance of the between-group mean square does not preclude a significant result in the other tests, however. Often, we don't test the between-group mean square in a two-way ANOVA, since our interest is in the main effects and the interaction rather than the overall treatment mean square.

As in one-way ANOVA, we would expect the F ratios to be close to 1, on the average, if the independent variables had no effect on performance. With a two-way ANOVA, however, we have three questions to ask.

1. Did our first independent variable have an overall effect?
2. Did our second independent variable have an overall effect?
3. Was the effect of the first independent variable the same under each level of the second independent variable?

If the F ratio for the A main effect was significant, then we know that A made a difference in performance. If the B main effect was also significant, we know that B affected performance. If the interaction is significant, we know that the A independent variable affected performance differently under the different levels of the B independent variable.

Running a Two-Way ANOVA

Let's do a two-way ANOVA. Once again we'll use a 2X2 factorial design. A researcher decides to investigate the effect of practice and corrective feedback on problem-solving performance in elementary school children. She randomly selects 32 children and divides them into four groups of 8 each. Two of the groups are given 25 practice problems to work on and the other two groups are given 5 practice problems. In addition, she provides corrective feedback to one of the high-practice groups and to one low-practice group. The remaining two groups receive no feedback. Here are her data.

	No Feedback A_1		Corrective Feedback A_2	
	High Practice	Low Practice	High Practice	Low Practice
	B_1	B_2	B_1	B_2
	6	6	12	9
	9	5	9	8
	6	7	9	8
	9	4	8	9
	8	6	7	7
	6	2	9	9
	8	4	8	5
	4	7	6	6
Sums	56	41	68	61
Means	7.00	5.13	8.50	7.63

$\Sigma X_{tot} = 56 + 41 + 68 + 61 = 226$

Step 1. Compute the total sum of squares.

$$SS_{TOT} = \Sigma X_{tot}^2 - (\Sigma X_{tot})^2/n_{tot}$$
$$= 6^2 + 9^2 + 6^2 + \ldots + 6^2 - 226^2/32$$
$$= 1726 - 1596.13 = 129.88$$

Step 2. Compute the between group sum of squares.

$$SS_{BG} = \frac{(\Sigma A_1B_1)^2 + (\Sigma A_1B_2)^2 + (\Sigma A_2B_1)^2 + (\Sigma A_2B_2)^2}{n} - \frac{(\Sigma X_{tot})^2}{n_{tot}}$$
$$= \frac{56^2 + 41^2 + 68^2 + 61^2}{8} - \frac{226^2}{32}$$
$$= 1645.25 - 1596.12 = 49.13$$

Step 3. Compute the within group sum of squares.

$$SS_{WG} = SS_{TOT} - SS_{BG}$$
$$= 129.88 - 49.13 = 80.75$$

Step 4. Compute the A, B and AXB sums of squares.

$$SS_A = \frac{(\Sigma A_1)^2 + (\Sigma A_2)^2}{bn} - \frac{(\Sigma X_{tot})^2}{n_{tot}}$$
$$= \frac{97^2 + 129^2}{16} - \frac{226^2}{32}$$
$$= 32$$

$$SS_B = \frac{(\Sigma B_1)^2 + (\Sigma B_2)^2}{an} - \frac{(\Sigma X_{tot})^2}{n_{tot}}$$
$$= \frac{124^2 + 102^2}{16} - \frac{226^2}{32}$$
$$= 15.13$$

$$SS_{AXB} = SS_{BG} - SS_A - SS_B$$
$$= 49.13 - 32 - 15.13 = 2$$

Step 5. Compute the mean squares.

$$MS_A = SS_A/df$$
$$= 32/1 = 32$$
$$MS_B = SS_B/df$$
$$= 15.13/1 = 15.13$$

$$MS_{AXB} = SS_{AXB}/df$$
$$= 2/1 = 2$$
$$MS_{WG} = SS_{WG}/df$$
$$= 80.75/28 = 2.88$$

Step 6. Compute the F-ratios.

$$F_A = MS_A/MS_{WG}$$
$$= 32/2.88 = 11.10$$
$$F_B = MS_B/MS_{WG}$$
$$= 15.13/2.88 = 5.25$$
$$F_{AXB} = MS_{AXB}/MS_{WG}$$
$$= 2/2.88 = 0.69$$

Step 7. Complete the ANOVA Table.

The outcome of any analysis of variance is presented in a summary table.

ANOVA Summary Table

Source	SS	df	MS	F	p
Between					
A	32.00	1	32.00	11.10	< .01
B	15.13	1	15.13	5.25	< .05
AXB	2.00	1	2.00	0.69	> .05
Within	80.75	28	2.88		
Total	129.88	31			

What does all this mean? Our researcher has two significant main effects, one at $\alpha = .05$ and one at $\alpha = .01$, and no significant interaction. The A main effect tells her that providing feedback made a significant difference in performance. The B main effect tells her that practice also made a difference. The lack of significance of the interaction means that the two variables, practice and feedback, did not interact. The effect of feedback was similar under high and low practice conditions. Let's graph both main effects and the interaction to verify this.

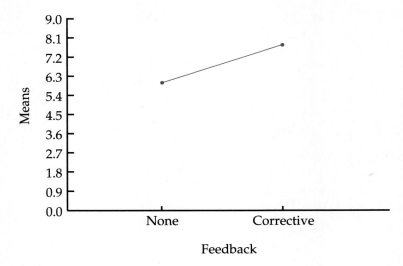

Figure 11-10   The main effect of feedback on problem-solving performance

We can see from Figure 11-10 that the groups given corrective feedback performed better than those not given feedback. Since the F-ratio was significant, we can claim that feedback improved performance.

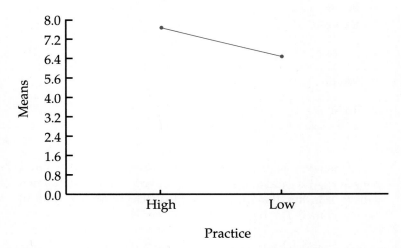

Figure 11-11   The main effect of practice on problem-solving performance

Let's look at the main effect of practice. We can from Figure 11-11 see that children given many practice problems did better than those given only a few; this is supported by a significant F-ratio.

Recall that the test of significance of the interaction involves testing whether the two lines depart significantly from parallelism. The interaction is not significant. As shown in Figure 11-12, the two lines do not depart from parallel more than expected by chance. They don't look exactly parallel but, nevertheless, they are not divergent enough for significance. There is no evidence that the effect of feedback was different under the two practice conditions.

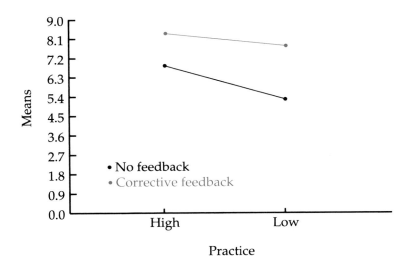

Figure 11-12 The interaction between practice and feedback

You may have noticed that all the examples of two-way ANOVA have used groups of equal sizes. This is not necessary; however, the calculations for a design with unequal group sizes is beyond the scope of this book.

Summary of Two-Way ANOVA

Hypotheses
  H_o: No main effects and no interaction.
  H_a: H_o is false.

Assumptions
  1. Subjects are randomly selected and independently assigned to groups.
  2. Population distributions are normal.
  3. Population variances are homogeneous.

Decision Rules
  $df_a = a - 1$
  $df_b = b - 1$
  $df_{axb} = (a - 1)(b - 1)$
  If $F_{obt} \geq F_{crit}$, reject the H_o
  If $F_{obt} < F_{crit}$, do not reject H_o

Formulas
$$F_A = \frac{MS_A}{MS_{WG}}$$
$$F_B = \frac{MS_B}{MS_{WG}}$$
$$F_{AXB} = \frac{MS_{AXB}}{MS_{WG}}$$

Assumptions Underlying Inference with the F-Distribution

The analysis of variance techniques we have studied assumes that the populations from which the samples were drawn are normally distributed. The Central Limit Theorem assures us that the assumption of normality won't be seriously violated as long as our samples are reasonably large and of the same size.

ANOVA also assumes that the populations from which the samples are drawn have equal variances. The F-test is quite robust, however, in that it is relatively insensitive to heterogeneity of variances as long as subjects have been randomly selected and independently assigned to groups.

Inferential Error

One of the important concerns in research is that of inferential error. You may recall the discussion, in Chapter 9, of Type I and Type II errors in statistical inference. A Type I error occurs when a true null hypothesis is rejected. The Type I error rate is set by alpha. Earlier in this chapter, I mentioned that one of the problems with using multiple t-tests was the increased probability of making an error. When many t-tests are run within a single experiment, the probability of rejecting at least one true null hypothesis is higher than alpha. The advantage of ANOVA is that the probability of a Type I error is maintained at alpha over the entire experiment. This is often referred to as the **experiment-wise error rate** (i.e., the probability of making at least one Type I error). In ANOVA, the experiment-wise error rate is $\leq \alpha$.

> **Experiment-wise error rate:** Probability of Type I error overall in an experiment.

Choosing the Appropriate Test of Significance

In this chapter we learned about two new tests of significance, one-way ANOVA and two-way ANOVA. Deciding which of these two analyses is appropriate for a given research study is a matter of determining how many independent variables are operating. We will assume that there are more than two groups of subjects in the experiment.

If you have a situation where there are two or more groups in the study, you must determine how many independent variables are involved. Do you have several groups of subjects under different levels of one independent variable, or do you have groups being treated with more than one independent variable?

With more than two groups of subjects, where each group is under a different level of a single independent variable, you will choose one-way ANOVA. If you determine that the experimental design involves two independent variables, where subjects have been randomly and independently assigned to all levels of both IV's, you choose a two-way ANOVA.

A biology student has three groups of randomly selected corpulent rats. This is a strain of rat that becomes obese quite naturally and are affectionately called "fat rats" by many researchers. The student is interested in the effects of a new drug on controlling weight gain. He uses three dosages of the drug, one dose level for each group. The subjects are weighed before and after the period of drug administration. The average weight gain of the groups are compared.

This study has one independent variable, dosage level, and a one-way ANOVA is the appropriate analysis.

Another biology student has three groups of corpulent rats and three groups of normal (thin) rats. He is interested in the differential effects of the new drug on controlling weight gain. He wonders if the drug may have different effects on the corpulent groups than on the thin groups. He uses three dosage levels, high, medium and low, on the fat rat groups and the same three levels on the thin rat groups. He compares weight gain after the drug administration period is over.

In this study there are two independent variables. The student is interested in the effects of the three levels of drug dose (first IV) and in the type of rat being tested (second IV). He will use a two-way ANOVA which will allow him to examine the overall effect of dosage, the overall effect of type of rat, and the interaction between the two. For example, he might find that the high dosage level has a greater effect on the fat rats than on the thin rats but that the low and medium dosage levels have similar effects on fat and thin rats.

This chapter has dealt with statistical techniques for research involving more than two groups of different subjects. The following chapter describes the use of analysis of variance in research where subjects serve in more than one group. We have called these "dependent groups designs." They are also known as **repeated measures** designs.

FOCUS ON RESEARCH

Benin and Edwards (1990)* were interested in the effects of family employment structure on adolescents' participation in family chores. Specifically, they wanted to know how family type affects the amount and kind of household chores adolescents perform.

The Data
The data were longitudinal and were collected by survey and from an earlier study. The sample included 176 children between the ages of 12 and 17 who had participated in an earlier study at the ages of 7–12.

The Variables
The major dependent variable was amount of time spent on several households tasks including traditional female tasks such as cooking and cleaning;

---

* Benin, M.H., and Edwards, D.A. (1990). Adolescents' Chores: The Difference between Dual- and Single-Earner Families, *Journal of Marriage and the Family*, 52, 361–73.

traditional male tasks such as car maintenance and household repairs; and neutral tasks such as pet care and running errands.

The independent variables included gender of child and family type. Three family types were identified: full-time dual-earner where both parents worked full-time outside the home, part-time dual-earner where the mother worked 20 hours or less per week, and traditional families where the mother was not employed outside the home.

The Analysis

The major dependent measure was total chore minutes per week and so a parametric analysis was used. Specifically a two-way ANOVA with gender (two categories) and family type (three categories) was used to assess the main effect and the interaction of gender by family type. Table 11-1 presents some of the results of this study.

Table 11-1 Total chore minutes per week

	Full-time	Part-time	Traditional	Sum
Male	164.98	144.21	435.21	744.4
Female	613.07	150	491.41	1254.48
Sum	778.05	294.21	926.62	

Source: Benin and Edwards (1990). Copyright 1990 by the National Council on Family Relations, 3989 Central Ave. N.E., Suite 550, Minneapolis, MN 55421. Reprinted by permission.

Inspection of the sums reveals that females seem to spend more time on chores than males and that adolescents from traditional families spend the most time on chores with adolescents from part-time families spending the least amount of time. Whether or not these are significant effects must be determined by the ANOVA. Closer inspection of all the table entries reveals that there may be an interaction between gender and family type. Let's look at some of the ANOVA results. See Table 11-2.

Table 11-2 ANOVA of reported data

Source	SS	df	MS	F	p
Main effects					
Gender	578 294	1	578 294	5.69	< .05
Family type	1 034 064	2	517 032	5.09	< .01
Gender X Family type	1 189 756	2	594 878	5.86	< .01

As expected from the first table, gender and family type make a significant difference in the amount of time spent on chores.

These effects, however, must be interpreted in light of the significant interaction of the two variables. Let's graph the time spent on chore measure for each gender and each family type to help interpret the results.

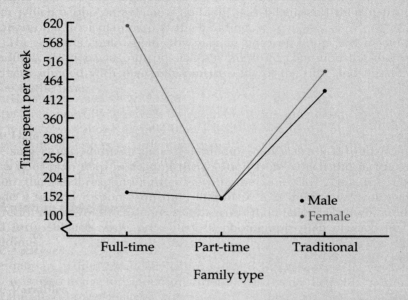

Figure 11–13   Time spent on chores by gender and family type

Source: Adapted from Benin and Edwards (1990).

From Figure 11-13 we can see the reason for the significant interaction. While boys contribute somewhat less help than girls in part-time and traditional families, this pattern does not hold in full-time families. Boys in full-time families contribute much less time doing chores than girls do.

You might wonder, as did the researchers, about the implications of this unfair division of labor in those households that we would have expected to be less susceptible to gender discrimination.

SUMMARY OF FORMULAS

One-Way ANOVA: Computational Formulas

Sums of Squares

Total $\quad SS_{TOT} = \Sigma X_{tot}^2 - \dfrac{(\Sigma X_{tot})^2}{n_{tot}}$

Between Groups $\quad SS_{BG} = \dfrac{(\Sigma X_1)^2}{n_1} + \dfrac{(\Sigma X_2)^2}{n_2} + ... + \dfrac{(\Sigma X_k)^2}{n_k} - \dfrac{(\Sigma X_{tot})^2}{n_{tot}}$

Within Groups $\quad SS_{WG} = SS_{TOT} - SS_{BG}$

Mean Squares

Between Groups $\quad MS_{BG} = \dfrac{SS_{BG}}{k-1}$

Within Groups $\quad MS_{WG} = \dfrac{SS_{WG}}{n_{tot}-k}$

F Ratio $\quad F = MS_{BG}/MS_{WG}$

Two-Way ANOVA: Computational Formulas

Sums of Squares

Total $\quad SS_{TOT} = \Sigma X_{tot}^2 - \dfrac{(\Sigma X_{tot})^2}{n_{tot}}$

Between Groups $\quad SS_{BG} = \dfrac{(\Sigma A_1 B_1)^2 + (\Sigma A_1 B_2)^2 + ... + (\Sigma A_a B_b)^2}{n} - \dfrac{(\Sigma X_{tot})^2}{n_{tot}}$

A $\quad SS_A = \dfrac{(\Sigma A_1)^2 + (\Sigma A_2)^2 + ... + (\Sigma A_a)^2}{bn} - \dfrac{(\Sigma X_{tot})^2}{n_{tot}}$

B $\quad SS_B = \dfrac{(\Sigma B_1)^2 + (\Sigma B_2)^2 + ... + (\Sigma B_b)^2}{an} - \dfrac{(\Sigma X_{tot})^2}{n_{tot}}$

AXB $\quad SS_{AXB} = SS_{BG} - SS_A - SS_B$

Within Groups $\quad SS_{WG} = SS_{TOT} - SS_{BG}$

Mean Squares

A $\qquad MS_A = \dfrac{SS_A}{a-1}$

B $\qquad MS_B = \dfrac{SS_B}{b-1}$

AXB $\qquad MS_{AXB} = \dfrac{SS_{AXB}}{(a-1)(b-1)}$

WG $\qquad MS_{WG} = \dfrac{SS_{WG}}{n_{tot}-k}$

F Ratios

$$F_A = MS_A/MS_{WG}$$
$$F_B = MS_B/MS_{WG}$$
$$F_{A\times B} = MS_{A\times B}/MS_{WG}$$

EXERCISES

1. The data below reflect the outcome of a one-way ANOVA.
   $SS_{BG} = 141.3$
   $SS_{WG} = 1278$
   $k = 4$
   $n_1 = n_2 = n_3 = n_4 = 25$
   a. Determine the MS_{BG}
   b. Determine the MS_{WG}
   c. Determine F
   d. What is the critical F value at $\alpha = .05$?
   e. What is your decision?

2. Complete the one-way analysis of variance for the following data.
   $SS_{TOT} = 540.30$
   $SS_{BG} = 433.20$
   $\alpha = .01$
   $n_1 = 5$
   $n_2 = 6$
   $n_3 = 4$

3. An investigator measures the running speed through a maze of two groups of cockroaches. One group had been pre-trained in the maze and the other group was a control group. Run a one-way ANOVA at $\alpha = .05$ on the data. (Note: With two groups a t-test or an ANOVA may be run).

Pre-trained roach speeds in seconds: 7, 9, 12, 10, 10, 9, 8, 8, 8, 4
Control roach speeds in seconds: 9, 11, 10, 10, 13, 14, 12, 12, 13, 14

4. Sketch a rough graph for each of the following outcomes of a two-way ANOVA:
   a. One main effect and no interaction
   b. Two main effects and no interaction
   c. One main effect and an interaction
   d. Two main effects and an interaction

5. The following data were obtained from a two-way ANOVA. Sketch each main effect and the interaction.

Mean Score

	B_1	B_2
A_1	22	3
A_2	14	8

6. A social psychologist was interested in the effects of televised violence on the aggressive behavior of children. She was also interested in the effects of the presence of an authority figure on their behavior. She decided to investigate the two variables simultaneously. She randomly selected four groups of 8 children each. Two of the groups were exposed to a violent cartoon show (V groups) and the other two groups were shown a neutral cartoon show (N groups). All the children were then allowed to play in a common area. Their behavior was monitored by a "blind" judge who counted the number of aggressive acts performed by each child. For one V group and one N group, an adult authority figure was present during the play period. For the other two groups no authority figure was present. Run a two-way ANOVA on the data at $\alpha = .05$.

Violent Groups		Neutral Groups	
Authority	No Authority	Authority	No Authority
2	6	0	0
1	3	1	2
3	7	2	3
2	5	0	1
3	4	1	1
1	6	2	3
2	4	1	1
1	5	3	4

7. Run an ANOVA on the following data with α = .05.

Group 1	Group 2	Group 3
7	1	7
3	3	9
1	6	10
4	8	8
4	5	7
8	5	5
2	5	9

a. SS_{TOT} =
b. SS_{BG} =
c. SS_{WG} =
   SS_{WG} (to check) = SS_{TOT} − SS_{BG} =
d. H_o:
   H_a:
e. $F_{.05}$ =
f. Complete the ANOVA summary table.
g. Put your decision in words.

8. Complete the ANOVA for the following data.

	Group 1	Group 2	Group 3	Group 4
ΣX	45	38	32	32
ΣX²	310	217	185	210
n	7	7	7	7

a. SS_{TOT} =
b. SS_{BG} =
c. SS_{WG} =
d. H_o:
   H_a:
e. $F_{.05}$ =
f. Complete the ANOVA summary table.
g. Put your decision in words.

9. Run a two-way ANOVA on the following data.

	A1		A2	
	B1	B2	B1	B2
	49	61	71	80
	64	72	72	47
	77	83	69	67
	52	77	75	56
	73	82	78	89
	70	65	58	43

a. $SS_{TOT} =$
b. $SS_{BG} =$
c. $SS_{WG} =$
d. $A_1 =$
   $A_2 =$
   $SS_A =$
e. $B_1 =$
   $B_2 =$
   $SS_B =$
f. $SS_{AXB} =$
g. Complete the ANOVA summary table.
h. Plot the interaction using the group means.

10. The Canadian military hired a consultant to conduct research on obedience to authority. The consultant was asked to determine the effects of perceived arbitrariness of a command and the effects of the authority figure on obedience to the command. Eighty randomly selected members of the armed forces were independently assigned to groups, such that there were twenty subjects in each of four groups. All subjects read a story describing a situation where military personnel issued a command to other military personnel. For two of the four groups (A) the story described commands that were arbitrarily based. In other words, no apparent rationale for the commanded behavior was provided. For the other two groups (R), the story included a rationale for the commanded behavior. In addition, for one group from each of the above, the command was issued to a subordinate by a superior ranking officer (S). For the remaining groups the command was issued by an equal ranked person (E). After the story was read, subjects were required to predict whether or not the individual being commanded would obey the command, using a rating scale where 1 = definitely would obey and 7 = definitely would not obey. The mean ratings of

each group are provided below. Run a two-way ANOVA to determine if authority figure and arbitrariness had an effect on the subjects predictions. Graph the interaction.

Arbitrary		Rationale	
S	E	S	E
6	4	7	6
6	3	6	6
6	4	6	5
5	1	5	5
5	3	6	7
7	2	7	3
1	2	2	7
7	4	6	6
6	3	5	5
2	4	5	4
5	3	3	7
5	2	3	1
5	2	6	5
5	1	5	7
6	3	5	5
1	4	2	6
6	2	5	6
6	3	1	2
7	4	6	5
5	2	6	6

Means

	S	E
A	5.10	2.80
R	4.85	5.20

CHAPTER 12

Analysis of Variance with Repeated Measures

LEARNING OBJECTIVES

After reading this chapter you should be able to:

1. Describe the partitioning of the variance for a one-way ANOVA with repeated measures and indicate the associated degrees of freedom.
2. Provide the F-ratio tested in one-way ANOVA with repeated measures.
3. Run a one-way ANOVA with repeated measures.
4. Describe the partitioning of the variance for a two-way ANOVA with repeated measures and indicate the associated degrees of freedom.
5. Provide the F-ratio tested in a two-way ANOVA with repeated measures.
6. Run a two-way ANOVA with repeated measures.
7. Complete an ANOVA summary table for a given analysis.
8. Determine the appropriate test of significance for a given research problem.

Researchers in psychology and related disciplines tend to study organisms that are quite variable in their behavior even under identical experimental conditions. People, for example, are generally more variable than are chemical compounds. People bring their different backgrounds and experiences into the experimental situation. In Chapter 10, we discussed the use of dependent groups designs to reduce the effects of individual differences as a source of variability.

Recall that ANOVA is a family of analyses; some of these are appropriate when the same subjects serve under more than one experimental condition.

Because these designs measure the same subjects' behavior under different conditions, these are called **repeated measures** designs. We will look at two repeated measures designs for analysis of variance.

One-Way ANOVA with Repeated Measures

In one-way ANOVA with repeated measures, all subjects serve under two or more levels (called treatments) of one independent variable. The order of treatment may not be the same for all subjects but, rather, is counterbalanced or randomized in some way. Because each subject is tested under all treatments, differences in performance between the subjects should not reflect treatment differences, but should represent individual differences. The repeated measures design allows us to remove the variability due to individual differences from the estimate of experimental error. Thus, it is a more powerful test of the treatment effect. We assume that the error variance based on repeated measures of the same subject, when the effects of the treatment are removed, will be less than the error variance based on different subjects under the same treatment.

Null and Alternative Hypotheses

The null and alternative hypotheses are the same as those for any one-way ANOVA. The null assumes no difference between population means and the alternative specifies that the null is false. As with other ANOVAs, specific differences between treatment means must be determined by a multiple comparison procedure.

Partitioning the Variance

The total variability in a one-way repeated measures experiment can be partitioned into two parts. The variability between subjects reflects individual differences. The variability within subjects reflects variation due to differences in treatments and to uncontrolled variation when the same subject is tested repeatedly.

The second component, variability within subjects, can be partitioned into 1) variability between treatments and 2) error variability (called subject by treatment or SXT). As you might expect, degrees of freedom can be partitioned similarly. Figure 12-1 illustrates the partitioning of variability and degrees of freedom for a one-way ANOVA with repeated measures, where k is the number of treatment groups and n is the number of subjects in the experiment.

ANOVA with Repeated Measures 261

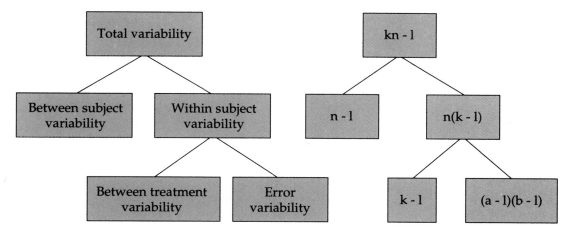

Figure 12-1 Partitioning the variability and degrees of freedom for a one-way ANOVA with repeated measures

Calculating the Sums of Squares

Below is an example of a one-way repeated measures design with three levels of the independent variable and five subjects tested under each level.

		Treatments		
Subjects	1	2	3	Sums
1				S_1
2				S_2
3				S_3
4				S_4
5				S_5
Sums	T_1	T_2	T_3	

Step 1. Calculate the total sum of squares.

This is done in the usual way. We square all the scores, sum them, and subtract from this value the square of the sum of all the scores divided by the total number of scores (kn) in the experiment.

$$SS_{TOT} = \Sigma X_{tot}^2 - \frac{(\Sigma X_{tot})^2}{kn}$$

Step 2. Calculate the between subject sum of squares.

For simplicity we'll call this the subject sum of squares. The general formula is

$$SS_S = \frac{(\Sigma S_1)^2 + (\Sigma S_2)^2 + ... + (\Sigma S_n)^2}{k} - \frac{(\Sigma X_{tot})^2}{kn} \quad \text{sum of squares subjects}$$

This formula tells us to 1) square each subject's sum, 2) sum the squares, 3) divide this sum by the number of treatments (k), and 4) subtract from the obtained value the square of the sum of all the scores divided by the total number of scores.

Step 3. Calculate the within subject sum of squares.

This can be done with the following formula:

$$SS_{WS} = \Sigma X_{tot}^2 - \frac{(\Sigma S_1)^2 + (\Sigma S_2)^2 + ... + (\Sigma S_n)^2}{k}$$

You can see that both parts of this formula have been calculated previously in determining the total and the subject sum of squares. Since the total sum of squares is composed of the within subject and the subject sum of squares, the within subject sum of squares can be easily obtained by subtraction.

$$SS_{WS} = SS_{TOT} - SS_S \quad \text{sum of squares within subjects}$$

Step 4. Partition the within subject sum of squares into the between treatment (or simply, treatment) sum of squares and the error (or SXT) sum of squares. The formula for the between treatment sum of squares is

$$SS_T = \frac{(\Sigma T_1)^2 + (\Sigma T_2)^2 + ... + (\Sigma T_k)^2}{n} - \frac{(\Sigma X_{tot})^2}{kn} \quad \text{sum of squares treatment}$$

This formula tells us to 1) square each treatment sum and sum the squares, 2) divide the value from 1) by the number of subjects (n), and

3) subtract from this sum the square of the sum of all the scores divided by the total number of scores. This is the source of variability we are interested in since it reflects the effect of the experimental treatment.

The error or SXT sum of squares is easily found by subtracting the treatment sum of squares from the within subject sum of squares.

$$SS_{SXT} = SS_{WS} - SS_T \quad \text{sum of squares subject by treatment}$$

This source of variability will be used in the denominator of the F-ratio to test for the significance of the treatment effect.

Calculating the Mean Squares

The two mean squares used in the F-ratio are obtained as always by dividing the sum of squares by the appropriate degrees of freedom.

The between treatment mean square is

$$MS_T = \frac{SS_T}{k - 1} \quad \text{mean square treatment}$$

The SXT or error mean square is

$$MS_{SXT} = \frac{SS_{SXT}}{(n - 1)(k - 1)} \quad \text{mean square error}$$

Notice that the degrees of freedom for the SXT sum of squares are the product of the degrees of freedom for the subject sum of squares (i.e., $n - 1$) and the treatment sum of squares (i.e., $k - 1$).

Calculating the F-Ratio

The F-ratio to test the significance of the experimental treatment is found in the usual way.

$$F = \frac{MS_T}{MS_{SXT}} \quad \text{F-ratio}$$

The obtained F value is evaluated for significance against the critical value of F from Table B-3 with $(k - 1)$ df in the numerator and $(n - 1)(k - 1)$ df in the denominator.

Running a One-Way ANOVA with Repeated Measures

The following data are the scores obtained by ten subjects under each of three treatment conditions. Subjects were tested for problem solving performance: alone, with one other person present, or with ten other people present. The researcher was interested in the effect of the presence of others (i.e., the treatment) on performance. The order of the three treatments was randomized for each subject.

		Treatment		
Subject	Alone 1	One Other Present 2	Ten Others Present 3	Sum
1	90	90	70	250
2	95	85	85	265
3	95	70	65	230
4	85	90	65	240
5	95	75	30	200
6	85	85	60	230
7	85	70	75	230
8	80	80	70	230
9	85	80	80	245
10	95	90	75	260
Sums	890	815	675	2380

Step 1. **Compute the total sum of squares.**

$$SS_{TOT} = \Sigma X_{tot}^2 - \frac{(\Sigma X_{tot})^2}{kn}$$

$$= 90^2 + 95^2 + \ldots + 75^2 - 2380^2/30$$

$$= 194100 - 188813.33$$

$$= 5286.67$$

Step 2. Compute the subject sum of squares.

$$SS_S = \frac{(\Sigma S_1)^2 + (\Sigma S_2)^2 + \ldots + (\Sigma S_{10})^2}{k} - \frac{(\Sigma X_{tot})^2}{kn}$$

$$= \frac{250^2 + 265^2 + \ldots + 260^2}{3} - \frac{2380^2}{30}$$

$$= 189850 - 188813.33$$

$$= 1036.67$$

Step 3. Compute the within subject sum of squares.

$$SS_{WS} = SS_{TOT} - SS_S$$

$$= 5286.67 - 1036.67 = 4250$$

Step 4. Compute the treatment and subject by treatment sum of squares.

$$SS_T = \frac{(\Sigma T_1)^2 + (\Sigma T_2)^2 + (\Sigma T_3)^2}{n} - \frac{(\Sigma X_{tot})^2}{kn}$$

$$= \frac{890^2 + 815^2 + 675^2}{10} - \frac{(2380)^2}{30}$$

$$= 191195 - 188813.33 = 2381.67$$

$$SS_{SXT} = SS_{WS} - SS_T$$

$$= 4250 - 2381.67 = 1868.33$$

Step 5. Compute the mean squares and F-ratio.

$$MS_T = \frac{SS_T}{k-1}$$

$$= 23.67/2 = 1190.83$$

$$MS_{SXT} = \frac{SS_{SXT}}{(n-1)(k-1)}$$

$$= 1868.33/18 = 103.80$$

$$F = MS_T/MS_{SXT}$$

$$= 11.47$$

With 2 and 18 degrees of freedom the obtained F value is larger than the critical value at the .01 level of significance, and so we reject the null hypothesis. We have statistical evidence that the presence of others affects problem solving performance. We would report our analysis in an ANOVA summary table.

ANOVA Summary Table

Source	SS	df	MS	F	p
Between Subjects	1036.67	9			
Within Subjects	4250.00	20			
Treatment	2381.67	2	1190.83	11.47	< .01
SXT	1868.33	18	103.80		
Total	5286.67	29			

Summary of One-Way ANOVA with Repeated Measures

Hypotheses
H_o: $\mu_1 = \mu_2 = ... = \mu_k$
H_a: H_o is false

Assumptions
1. Subjects are randomly selected.
2. Population distributions are normal.
3. Population variances are homogeneous.
4. Population covariances are equal.

Decision Rules
$df_t = k - 1$
$df_{sxt} = (n - 1)(k - 1)$
If $F_{obt} \geq F_{crit}$, reject the H_o
If $F_{obt} < F_{crit}$, do not reject H_o

Formula
$$F = \frac{MS_T}{MS_{SXT}}$$

Two-Way ANOVA with Repeated Measures on One Factor

In Chapter 11 we discussed two-way ANOVA as a useful design for simultaneously analyzing the effects of two independent variables with three tests of significance: two tests for main effects due to each independent variable, and the test for the interaction between the independent variables.

Two-way ANOVA can be used to analyze experiments where repeated measures are taken on one or both independent variables. We will concern ourselves with the case where one factor has repeated measures and the other does not. This is quite a common design in several areas of research. We may be interested in the effect of training on performance of groups of subjects who differ with respect to job experience. Perhaps we are investigating the effects of four drug dosages on visual acuity performance of three groups of subjects, each group having received different instructions about the task. If we randomly assigned subjects to instruction groups and tested each under all four dosage levels, we would have a 4X3 factorial design with repeated measures on one factor (drug dosage).

A 2X3 experiment with repeated measures on factor B may be represented as

```
        B₁  B₂  B₃
    A₁
    A₂
```

This repeated measures design reduces error variance for tests of the within subjects factors. Differences in performance found between the different levels of factor B under each level of A, for example, cannot be due to differences between subjects, since the same subjects serve under all levels of B. In other words, variability due to individual differences is removed from the analysis of the main effect of factor B. This is also true of the interaction effect. Statisticians say that the B treatment effect and the AXB interaction is *unconfounded* by between-subject differences. For this reason the test of significance for factor B and the AXB interaction is more sensitive than the test of significance for the A main effect. This design is particularly suitable for researchers who are more interested in the B factor than the A factor.

Null and Alternative Hypotheses

The null and alternative hypotheses are the same as those for any two-way ANOVA. The null assumes no main effects and no interaction.

Partitioning the Variance

The total variability in a two-way repeated measures experiment can be partitioned in a similar manner to that used for the one-way design. This is illustrated in Figure 12-2.

268 Chapter Twelve

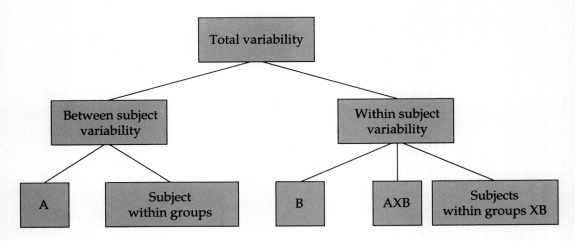

Figure 12-2 Partitioning the variability for a two-way ANOVA with repeated measures on factor B

The total degrees of freedom can be partitioned as shown in Figure 12-3; where a is the number of levels of factor A, b is the number of levels of factor B, and n is the number of subjects in each group.

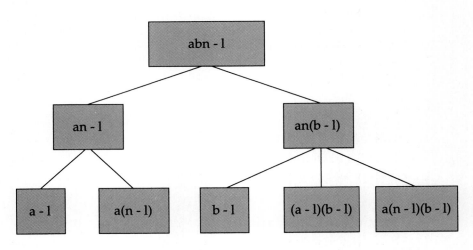

Figure 12-3 Partitioning the degrees of freedom for a two-way ANOVA with repeated measures on factor B

ANOVA with Repeated Measures

Calculating the Sums of Squares

Below is an example of a 2X3 repeated measures design, with two levels of the between subject factor (A), and three levels of the within subjects factor (B), and a total of ten subjects in the experiment.

	Subject	B_1	B_2	B_3	Sum	
A_1	1				S_1	
	2				S_2	
	3				S_3	
	4				S_4	
	5				S_5	
	Sum	A_1B_1	A_1B_2	A_1B_3		A_1
A_2	6				S_6	
	7				S_7	
	8				S_8	
	9				S_9	
	10				S_{10}	
	Sum	A_2B_1	A_2B_2	A_2B_3		A_2
	Sum	B_1	B_2	B_3		

Step 1. Calculate the total sum of squares.

$$SS_{TOT} = \Sigma X_{tot}^2 - \frac{(\Sigma X_{tot})^2}{abn} \quad \text{sum of squares total}$$

We square all the raw scores, sum them and subtract from this value the square of the sum of all the scores divided by the total number of scores in the experiment. For a two-way repeated measures design, there is a total of abn scores in the experiment.

Step 2. Calculate the subject sum of squares (SS_S) and its component parts, the sum of squares for A (SS_A) and the sum of squares for subjects within groups, $SS_{S(gps)}$.

$$SS_S = \frac{(\Sigma S_1)^2 + (\Sigma S_2)^2 + \ldots + (\Sigma S_{an})^2}{b} - \frac{(\Sigma X_{tot})^2}{abn} \quad \text{sum of squares subjects}$$

The subject sum of squares is found by 1) summing across all levels of B for each subject in the experiment, 2) squaring each sum, 3) adding all these squared sums, 4) dividing the value in 3 by the number of levels of B, and 5) subtracting from the value in 4, the same value we used to obtain the total sum of squares in Step 1 (i.e., the squared sum of all the scores in the experiment divided by the total number).

This subject sum of squares can now be partitioned into its component parts. We first find the sum of squares for factor A.

$$SS_A = \frac{(\Sigma A_1)^2 + (\Sigma A_2)^2 + \ldots + (\Sigma A_a)^2}{bn} - \frac{(\Sigma X_{tot})^2}{abn} \quad \text{sum of squares A}$$

This sum of squares is found by summing across all subjects and levels of factor B for each level of factor A, squaring each of these sums, summing the squares and dividing this value by the number of scores contributing to the sum (i.e., bn) and, finally, subtracting the same value as we used before.

The subjects within groups sum of squares can now be found by subtraction.

$$SS_{S(gps)} = SS_S - SS_A \quad \text{sum of squares S(groups)}$$

Step 3. Calculate the within subject sum of squares and its component parts, the B, AXB, and subjects within groups XB sums of squares.

The within subject sum of squares is easily obtained by subtracting the subject sum of squares from the total sum of squares.

$$SS_{WS} = SS_{TOT} - SS_S \quad \text{sum of squares within subjects}$$

Now we compute the sum of squares for factor B.

$$SS_B = \frac{(\Sigma B_1)^2 + (\Sigma B_2)^2 + \ldots + (\Sigma B_b)^2}{an} - \frac{(\Sigma X_{tot})^2}{abn} \quad \text{sum of squares B}$$

You can see that the procedure for calculating the sum of squares for factor B is much the same as that for factor A. We sum across all subjects and levels of A for each level of B, square each sum, add the squares and divide by the total number of subjects in each level of B (i.e., an).

Next, we compute the sum of squares for the AXB interaction.

$$SS_{AXB} = \frac{(\Sigma A_1 B_1)^2 + (\Sigma A_1 B_2)^2 + \ldots + (\Sigma A_a B_b)^2}{n} - \frac{(\Sigma X_{tot})^2}{abn} - SS_A - SS_B$$

sum of squares AXB

The interaction sum of squares is found first by computing the sum for each combination of A and B. For a 3x2 design, we would have six sums. Then we add up the squares of all the sums, divide by the number of subjects in each group (i.e., n) and subtract from this value the same value we have used before. Then we subtract the SS_A and the SS_B.

Finally, we find the third component of the within subject sum of squares, the subjects within groups X B sum of squares ($SS_{S(gps)XB}$), by subtraction.

$$SS_{S(gps)XB} = SS_{WS} - SS_B - SS_{AXB} \quad \text{sum of squares S(groups) XB}$$

Calculating the Mean Squares

As with any two-way ANOVA, we will have three tests of significance, one for each main effect and one for the interaction.

The between subjects main effect of interest will be the A main effect; the mean square for A will be tested for significance with the mean square for subjects within groups (i.e., the error mean square for between subject comparisons).

The within subjects tests will be for the main effect of B and for the interaction of A and B. Both mean squares will be compared with the mean square for subjects within groups X B (i.e., the error mean square for the within subjects comparisons).

All mean squares are found by dividing the sums of squares by the appropriate degrees of freedom.

---

between subjects mean squares

$$MS_A = \frac{SS_A}{a - 1} \quad \text{where a is the number of levels of factor A}$$

$$MS_{S(gps)} = \frac{SS_{S(gps)}}{a(n - 1)} \quad \text{where n is the number of subjects in each group}$$

---

within subjects mean squares

$$MS_B = \frac{SS_B}{b - 1} \quad \text{where b is the number of levels of factor B}$$

$$MS_{AXB} = \frac{SS_{AXB}}{(a - 1)(b - 1)}$$

$$MS_{S(gps)XB} = \frac{SS_{S(gps)XB}}{a(n - 1)(b - 1)}$$

Calculating and Interpreting the F-Ratios

Now the three mean squares can be tested for significance.

$$F_A = \frac{MS_A}{MS_{S(gps)}}$$

$$F_B = \frac{MS_B}{MS_{S(gps)XB}} \quad \text{F-ratios}$$

$$F_{AXB} = \frac{MS_{AXB}}{MS_{S(gps)XB}}$$

Each F-ratio is compared with the critical value from Table B-3, by entering the appropriate degrees of freedom. Interpretation of the outcome of a two-way ANOVA is discussed in Chapter 11. A repeated measures design is interpreted in much the same way. Recall, however, that because subjects serve under all levels of B, tests of the within subjects treatment effects will be more sensitive.

Running a Two-Way ANOVA with Repeated Measures

Carla has been hired by the Police Department to assess the performance of its officers in several areas related to their jobs. The Department is primarily interested in three areas of competence: 1) general knowledge of police procedure, 2) general knowledge about the law and justice system in the province and 3) decision making ability in "real life" situations. The Department has a secondary interest in whether "time on the force" is an important factor.

Carla decides to use standardized tests available from the Police Department. All the multiple-choice tests are scored out of a maximum of 40 points. She randomly selects ten officers from each of four categories of "time on the job": 1) one year, 2) two to four years, 3) five to ten years, and 4) more than ten years on the Force.

All officers are tested in each of the three areas of competence. Carla, being a well-trained researcher, is concerned about the effects of previous testing on later test performance so she randomizes the order of the three tests in such a way that an equal number of officers within each group receive each order. In this way, she feels confident that the effects of repeated testing will be balanced among her groups. Carla's design is a 3X4 factorial design with repeated measures on factor B, type of test. Table 12-1 shows her design.

Table 12-1 Design for Research Example

Factor A: Time on Force	Subject	Factor B: Type of Test		
		Procedure B_1	Law B_2	Decision Making B_3
A_1 one year	1			
	2			
	3			
	4			
	5			
	6			
	7			
	8			
	9			
	10			
A_2 2–4 years	11			
	12			
	13			
	14			
	15			
	16			
	17			
	18			
	19			
	20			
A_3 5–10 years	21			
	22			
	23			
	24			
	25			
	26			
	27			
	28			
	29			
	30			
A_4 >10 years	31			
	32			
	33			
	34			
	35			
	36			
	37			
	38			
	39			
	40			

And Table 12-2 shows her data.

Table 12-2 Data for Research Example

	B_1	B_2	B_3	Sum		B_1	B_2	B_3	Sum
	37	15	12	64		30	39	23	92
	28	20	11	59		22	33	27	82
	30	24	13	67		13	31	26	70
	22	25	12	59		15	25	15	55
A_1	33	21	14	68	A_3	17	30	18	65
	29	30	12	71		35	28	19	82
	27	35	13	75		33	22	18	73
	31	21	11	63		10	27	20	57
	36	22	11	69		18	32	24	74
	33	25	11	69		26	24	20	70
	25	28	13	66		26	22	23	71
	28	21	14	63		22	36	25	83
	30	30	17	77		21	33	28	82
	19	31	16	66		30	32	23	85
A_2	22	36	13	71		15	27	27	69
	29	22	13	64	A_4	18	25	27	70
	31	15	26	72		21	37	29	87
	13	20	13	46		27	20	26	73
	15	18	14	47		22	21	29	72
	20	30	15	65		16	17	27	60

Let's sum the scores for the subjects within each combination of A and B.

	B_1	B_2	B_3	Sum
A_1	306	238	120	664
A_2	232	251	154	637
A_3	219	291	210	720
A_4	218	270	264	752
Sum	975	1050	748	2773

Step 1. Calculate the total sum of squares.

$$SS_{TOT}^2 = \Sigma X_{tot}^2 - \frac{(\Sigma X_{tot})^2}{abn}$$

$$= 37^2 + 28^2 + \ldots + 27^2 - 2773^2/120$$

$$= 70349 - 64079.41$$

$$= 6269.59$$

Step 2. Calculate the SS_S and its component parts, SS_A and $SS_{S(gps)}$.

$$SS_S = \frac{(\Sigma S_1)^2 + (\Sigma S_2)^2 + \ldots + (\Sigma S_{40})^2}{b} - \frac{(\Sigma X_{tot})^2}{abn}$$

$$= \frac{64^2 + 59^2 + \ldots + 60^2}{3} - 64079.41$$

$$= 65349.00 - 64079.41 = 1269.59$$

$$SS_A = \frac{(\Sigma A_1)^2 + (\Sigma A_2)^2 + (\Sigma A_3)^2 + (\Sigma A_4)^2}{bn} - \frac{(\Sigma X_{tot})^2}{abn}$$

$$= \frac{664^2 + 637^2 + 720^2 + 752^2}{30} - 64079.41$$

$$= 64352.30 - 64079.41 = 272.89$$

$$SS_{S(gps)} = SS_S - SS_A = 996.70$$

Step 3. Calculate SS_{WS} and its component parts, the B, A×B, and subjects within groups ×B sums of squares.

$$SS_{WS} = SS_{TOT} - SS_S$$

$$= 5000.00$$

$$SS_B = \frac{(\Sigma B_1)^2 + (\Sigma B_2)^2 + (\Sigma B_3)^2}{an} - \frac{(\Sigma X_{tot})^2}{abn}$$

$$= \frac{975^2 + 1050^2 + 748^2}{40} - 64079.41$$

$$= 65315.73 - 64079.41 = 1236.32$$

$$SS_{AXB} = \frac{(\Sigma A_1B_1)^2 + (\Sigma A_1B_2)^2 + \ldots + (\Sigma A_4B_3)^2}{n} - \frac{(\Sigma X_{tot})^2}{abn} - SS_A - SS_B$$

$$= \frac{306^2 + 238^2 + \ldots + 264^2}{10} - 64079.41 - 272.89 - 1236.32$$

$$= 67208.30 - 64079.41 - 272.89 - 1236.32 = 1619.68$$

$$SS_{S(gps)XB} = SS_{WS} - SS_B - SS_{AXB}$$

$$= 2144.00$$

Step 4. Calculate the mean squares.

$$MS_A = \frac{SS_A}{a - 1}$$

$$= 272.89/3 = 90.96$$

$$MS_{S(gps)} = \frac{SS_{S(gps)}}{a(n-1)}$$
$$= 996.70/36 = 27.69$$

$$MS_B = \frac{SS_B}{b-1}$$
$$= 1236.32/2 = 618.16$$

$$MS_{AXB} = \frac{SS_{AXB}}{(a-1)(b-1)}$$
$$= 1619.68/6 = 269.95$$

$$MS_{S(gps)XB} = \frac{SS_{S(gps)XB}}{a(n-1)(b-1)}$$
$$= 2144.00/72 = 29.78$$

Step 5. Calculate the F-ratios.
$$F_A = \frac{MS_A}{MS_{S(gps)}} = \frac{90.96}{27.69} = 3.29$$

$$F_B = \frac{MS_B}{MS_{S(gps)XB}} = \frac{618.16}{29.78} = 20.76$$

$$F_{AXB} = \frac{MS_{AXB}}{MS_{S(gps)XB}} = \frac{269.95}{29.78} = 9.07$$

Step 6. Enter the results in an ANOVA summary table.

ANOVA Summary Table

Source	SS	df	MS	F	p
Between Subjects	1269.59	39			
A	272.89	3	90.96	3.29	< .05
S(gps)	996.70	36	27.69		
Within Subjects	5000.00	80			
B	1236.32	2	618.16	20.76	< .01
AXB	1619.68	6	269.95	9.07	< .01
S(gps)XB	2144.00	72	29.78		
Total	6269.59	119			

Now, of course, we need to interpret these results. Since both main effects are significant, we know that type of test made a difference in performance and that length of time on the force made a difference in performance. However, the presence of a significant interaction tells us that the test difference pattern is not identical for the four groups. The best way I know of determining what went on in a design as complicated as this one is to present the data graphically.

Interpreting a Two-Way ANOVA with Repeated Measures

First we will look at the main effect of time on force. See Figure 12-4.

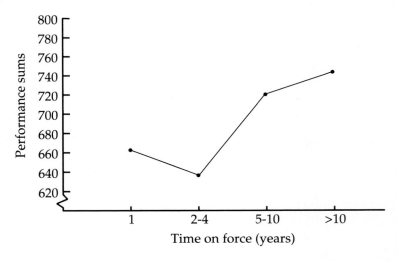

Figure 12-4   The main effect of time on force on performance

We can see that, overall, the more senior officers tended to do better; although the first year group did better than the 2–4 year group. In order to determine which groups are significantly different, this analysis would be followed by a multiple comparison technique as discussed in Chapter 13.

Let's look at the main effect of type of test as shown in Figure 12-5. Overall, we see that the officers performed best on the law test and worst on the decision-making test.

Both these main effects must be interpreted somewhat cautiously because of the existence of a significant interaction between the variables. Let's look at the interaction (Figure 12-6). Examination of this chart indicates that as experience (i.e., years on the force) increases, performance on the decision making test increases also. The new officers did particularly well on the procedure test. We might speculate that the years of experience in the field improved the scores of the senior officers in "real life" decision-making tests but that they tend to be a little complacent about matters involving procedure and law. We might also speculate that the new officers,

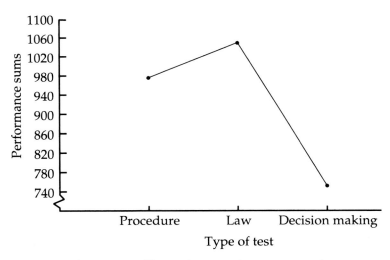

Figure 12-5 The main effect of type of test on performance

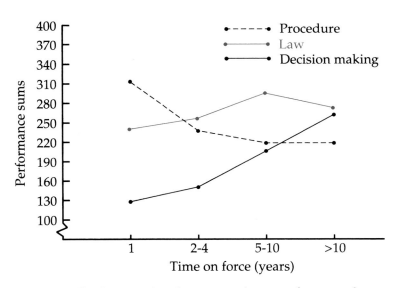

Figure 12-6 The interaction between time on force and type of test

on the other hand, lack real life experience but are keener about "book learning."

These speculative comments, however, should be supported by appropriate multiple comparison procedures.

Summary of Two-Way ANOVA with Repeated Measures

Hypotheses
   H_o: No main effects and no interaction
   H_a: H_o is false

Assumptions
   1. Subjects are randomly selected with repeated measures on factor B.
   2. Population distributions are normal.
   3. Population variances are homogeneous.
   4. Population covariances are equal.

Decision Rules
   $df_a = a - 1$
   $df_b = b - 1$
   $df_{axb} = (a - 1)(b - 1)$
   $df_{s(gps)} = a(n - 1)$
   $df_{s(gps)xb} = a(n - 1)(b - 1)$
   If $F_{obt} \geq F_{crit}$, reject the H_o
   If $F_{obt} < F_{crit}$, do not reject H_o

Formulas

$$F = \frac{MS_A}{MS_{S(gps)}}$$

$$F_B = \frac{MS_B}{MS_{S(gps)XB}}$$

$$F_{AXB} = \frac{MS_{AXB}}{MS_{S(gps)XB}}$$

Assumptions Underlying ANOVA with Repeated Measures

One of the assumptions of ANOVA is that the populations from which the samples are drawn are normally distributed with equal variances. We discussed this assumption of homogeneity of variance in Chapter 11, where we learned that the F-test is quite robust (i.e., insensitive to violations of this assumption) when the subjects have been randomly selected and independently assigned to groups, and when sample sizes are similar.

ANOVA with Repeated Measures

With repeated measures designs, subjects are not independently assigned to groups and so the assumption of homogeneity takes on added importance. Another assumption of ANOVA is that the population correlations (often called covariances) are constant. If subjects are independently assigned to groups, it is reasonable to assume that they are constant. When the same subjects participate in all treatment levels, however, this is unlikely to be true. When there is reason to believe that both assumptions (homogeneity of variances and covariances) have been violated, a more conservative test is recommended (e.g., Geisser & Greenhouse, 1958).[1] Discussions of the problems of homogeneity of variances and covariances can be found in most upper-level statistics textbooks.

Choosing the Appropriate Test of Significance

You have now learned about four F-tests of significance: one- and two-way ANOVA with repeated measures in this chapter, and one- and two-way ANOVA without repeated measures in Chapter 11. Let's go through the steps we need to decide which of these four analyses is appropriate. We will not include two-group studies in the present discussion.

Step 1. Determine the number of groups in the experiment.

If there is only one group of subjects, and each subject contributes several observations, then repeated measures have been taken and you will choose one-way ANOVA with repeated measures. If there are more than two groups, we go to Step 2.

Step 2. Determine the number of independent variables.

If you have a situation where there are more than two groups in the study, you must determine how many independent variables are involved. Do you have several groups of subjects under different levels of one independent variable, or do you have groups being treated with more than one independent variable? With more than two groups of subjects, where each group is under a different level of a single independent variable, you choose one-way ANOVA. If the experiment has two independent variables, we must go to Step 3.

Step 3. Determine whether repeated measures have been taken on one of the two independent variables.

If subjects have been randomly and independently assigned to all levels

---

[1] Geisser, S. and Greenhouse, S.W. (1958), An Extension of Box's Results on the Use of the F-Distribution in Multivariate Analysis. *Annals of Mathematical Statistics, 29,* 885–91.

of both IV's, you choose a two-way ANOVA. If one of the independent variables involves measures on the same subjects, i.e. a repeated measures design, then you will run a two-way ANOVA with repeated measures.

Let's go through the steps to decide which analysis to use in the following examples.

Example A   A researcher has randomly selected forty subjects to participate in a learning experiment. All subjects are required to learn three different lists of words. The lists differ in terms of the relationship between the items. For example, in List S, the items are semantically similar, they have similar meanings. In List R, the words rhyme. The last list (C) is a control condition where the words are not related to each other in any way. The number of trials it takes the subjects to learn each list is the dependent variable.

Step 1.   Determine the number of groups in the experiment.
There is only one group of subjects in this experiment, and each subject contributes three observations (the number of trials to learn each of the three lists). Repeated measures have been taken and the researcher will use a one-way ANOVA with repeated measures.

Example B   A Provincial Board of Health has decided to investigate three treatment programs for treating alcohol abuse. Three groups of abusers are randomly selected: one group of heavy abusers, a second of moderate abusers, and a third of light abusers of alcohol. Each group participates in a six-month treatment program. For the first two months, the subjects receive training in behavioral observation and monitoring of their drinking behavior. For the next two months, the subjects receive group therapy. For the final two months, subjects receive individual therapy. Measures of drinking behavior and attitude are taken after each treatment period.

Step 1.   Determine the number of groups in the experiment.
There are three groups of subjects in this study: a heavy abusing group, a moderate abusing group, and a light abusing group. We go to Step 2.

Step 2.   Determine the number of independent variables.
This experiment has two independent variables, level of abuse and treatment program, and so we must go to Step 3.

Step 3.   Determine whether repeated measures have been taken on one of the two independent variables.
The three levels of abuse groups were randomly selected and all subjects went through the three-treatment program. Repeated measures, therefore, were taken after each treatment period from all subjects. The appropriate analysis is a two-way ANOVA with repeated measures on type of treatment. The researcher will discover whether level of abuse overall makes a differ-

ence, whether treatment program overall makes a difference and whether the two variables interact in some way. For example, perhaps the heavy abusers benefit more from one-on-one individual therapy than do the other groups.

Example C   A Provincial Board of Health has decided to investigate three treatment programs for treating alcohol abuse. Six groups of abusers are randomly selected: two groups of heavy abusers, two groups of moderate abusers, and two groups of light abusers of alcohol. Each group participates in a two-month treatment program. One group of each pair is randomly assigned to one of three treatment programs: behavioral treatment, group therapy, or individual therapy. In other words, one group of heavy abusers, one group of moderate abusers, and one group of light abusers receive behavioral treatment for two months. A second set of abusers (i.e. heavy, moderate, and light) receive group therapy for two months. The third set receive individual therapy for two months. Following the therapy period, measures of drinking behavior and attitude are taken.

Step 1.   Determine the number of groups in the experiment.
    There are six groups of subjects in this study: two heavy abusing groups, two moderate, and two light abusing groups.

Step 2.   Determine the number of independent variables.
    This experiment has two independent variables, level of abuse and treatment program, and so we must go to Step 3.

Step 3.   Determine whether repeated measures have been taken on one of the two independent variables.
    Repeated measures have not been taken. Groups were randomly assigned to treatment condition. A two-way ANOVA is the appropriate analysis for this study.

FOCUS ON RESEARCH

Warren, Rossano, and Wear (1990)* were interested in the kinds of features people use in reading maps to find their way around. For example, to use a map effectively, we must be able to match the environment to the representations on the map. Although the environment around us is a three-dimensional detailed space, a map is only a two-dimensional simplified

---

* Warren, D.H., Rossano, M.J., and Wear, T.D. (1990), Perception of Map-Environment Correspondence: The Roles of Features and Alignment, *Ecological Psychology, 2*, 131–50.

diagram. An understanding of what features are important is necessary for construction of useful maps. Part of this study is discussed here.

One of the concerns addressed by this study was the relation between the orientation of a map and the orientation of the environment the map represents. They investigated this by having subjects decide the location from which a photograph of a building was taken, and then mark that location on a floor plan map of the building.

The subjects could rotate the map in one condition and in another condition rotation was not possible. In the fixed condition the map was correctly aligned with the environment some of the time and misaligned some of the time.

The Data
The subject was shown a slide of a building and was asked to mark a dot on a floor-plan map indicating the location from which the picture was taken (the initial response). After viewing the same slide again, the subject made a second response on the same map. A response was counted as correct if it fell within 15 degrees of the correct direction. The two hundred and forty subjects were presented 40 photographs, ten of each of four buildings.

The Variables
Half of the subjects were in the fixed condition and the other half in the rotation condition.

The Analysis
The data were the number of correct responses on the initial and the second response. Since each subject contributed two responses for each view, the data were analyzed with a two-way ANOVA with repeated measures. Some of the results were as follows. There was a main effect of first versus second response ($F_{(1,22)} = 31.49$, $p < .001$), indicating that performance improved on the second try. The opportunity to rotate the map improved performance ($F_{(1,22)} = 5.56$, $p < .05$) compared with the group not permitted to rotate the map. Within the fixed condition, subjects performed better when the map was aligned with the picture than they did when the map was misaligned ($F_{(1,11)} = 4.86$, $p < .05$). The researchers concluded that people attempt to spatially align maps with the environment when making location decisions and when they align incorrectly or are unable to align, they make more errors.

SUMMARY OF FORMULAS

One-Way ANOVA with Repeated Measures—Computational Formulas

Sums of Squares

Total
$$SS_{TOT} = \Sigma X_{tot}^2 - \frac{(\Sigma X_{tot})^2}{kn}$$

Between Subject
$$SS_S = \frac{(\Sigma S_1)^2 + (\Sigma S_2)^2 + ... + (\Sigma S_n)^2}{k} - \frac{(\Sigma X_{tot})^2}{kn}$$

Within Subject
$$SS_{WS} = SS_{TOT} - SS_S$$

Treatment
$$SS_T = \frac{(\Sigma T_1)^2 + (\Sigma T_2)^2 + ... + (\Sigma T_k)^2}{n} - \frac{(\Sigma X_{tot})^2}{kn}$$

Subject by Treatment
$$SS_{SXT} = SS_{WS} - SS_T$$

Mean Squares

Treatment
$$MS_T = \frac{SS_T}{k - 1}$$

Subject by Treatment
$$MS_{SXT} = \frac{SS_{SXT}}{(n - 1)(k - 1)}$$

F-Ratio

$$F = \frac{MS_T}{MS_{SXT}}$$

Two-Way ANOVA with Repeated Measures — Computational Formulas

Sums of Squares

Total
$$SS_{TOT} = \Sigma X_{tot}^2 - \frac{(\Sigma X_{tot})^2}{abn}$$

Between Subjects
$$SS_S = \frac{(\Sigma S_1)^2 + (\Sigma S_2)^2 + \ldots + (\Sigma S_{an})^2}{b} - \frac{(\Sigma X_{tot})^2}{abn}$$

A
$$SS_A = \frac{(\Sigma A_1)^2 + (\Sigma A_2)^2 + \ldots + (\Sigma A_a)^2}{bn} - \frac{(\Sigma X_{tot})^2}{abn}$$

Subjects within Groups
$$SS_{S(gps)} = SS_S - SS_A$$

B
$$SS_B = \frac{(\Sigma B_1)^2 + (\Sigma B_2)^2 + \ldots + (\Sigma B_b)^2}{an} - \frac{(\Sigma X_{tot})^2}{abn}$$

AXB
$$SS_{AXB} = \frac{(\Sigma A_1 B_1)^2 + (\Sigma A_1 B_2)^2 + \ldots + (\Sigma A_a B_b)^2}{n} - \frac{(\Sigma X_{tot})^2}{abn} - SS_A - SS_B$$

Subjects within Groups XB
$$SS_{S(gps)XB} = SS_{WS} - SS_B - SS_{AXB}$$

Mean Squares

A
$$MS_A = \frac{SS_A}{a - 1}$$

Subjects within Groups
$$MS_{S(gps)} = \frac{SS_{S(gps)}}{a(n - 1)}$$

B
$$MS_B = \frac{SS_B}{b - 1}$$

AXB
$$MS_{AXB} = \frac{SS_{AXB}}{(a - 1)(b - 1)}$$

Subjects within Groups XB
$$MS_{S(gps)XB} = \frac{SS_{S(gps)XB}}{a(n - 1)(b - 1)}$$

F-Ratios

$$F_A = \frac{MS_A}{MS_{S(gps)}}$$

$$F_B = \frac{MS_B}{MS_{S(gps)XB}}$$

$$F_{AXB} = \frac{MS_{AXB}}{MS_{S(gps)XB}}$$

EXERCISES

1. Below is a layout for a one-way ANOVA with repeated measures.

	Treatment				
Subject	1	2	3	4	5
1					
.					
.					
.					
20					

   Give the number of degrees of freedom for:
   a. Total SS
   b. Between subject SS
   c. Within subject SS
   d. Between treatment SS
   e. Subject by treatment SS

2. Run a one-way ANOVA at $\alpha = .05$ on the following data. All subjects served under each treatment condition.

	Treatment		
Subject	1	2	3
1	22	34	21
2	35	36	20
3	31	40	17
4	17	41	23
5	22	33	27
6	20	36	29
7	35	28	31
8	21	29	22
9	33	34	15
10	10	30	28

3. Twenty randomly selected students were given a standardized intelligence test that produced scores in each of three major areas: verbal fluency, mathematical ability, and spatial ability. Run an ANOVA on the data below to see if the students differed in performance in each of the three dimensions of intelligence.

Subject	Verbal	Mathematical	Spatial
1	87	65	35
2	77	55	45
3	45	48	55
4	68	69	67
5	90	45	50
6	86	76	60
7	86	80	40
8	80	78	55
9	63	77	45
10	59	68	60
11	85	65	50
12	64	63	53
13	70	57	50
14	60	60	48
15	63	56	55
16	58	55	47
17	63	65	69
18	59	60	55
19	68	45	43
20	60	50	49

4. Complete the ANOVA summary table for the following. There were 4 levels of A and 3 levels of B with 9 subjects under each level of A. Use $\alpha = .05$.

	SS
Total	3500
Subject	250
A	50
S(gs)	200
WS	3250
B	700
AXB	550
S(gps)XB	2000

5. A sociology professor was interested in the effects of socio-economic status on three different areas of marital satisfaction. She randomly selected 8 couples from each of two SES groups: upper/middle and lower SES. She wants to compare their perception as a couple on three areas of marital relationships: communication (C), domestic chore equity (DE), and personal self-esteem (SE). She uses a questionnaire that yields scores out of 100. Run a two-way ANOVA with repeated measures on the marital satisfaction category at $\alpha = .01$.

SES Upper/Middle	C	DE	SE
1	88	87	90
2	76	75	80
3	65	70	75
4	40	68	65
5	76	75	70
6	78	84	80
7	40	56	60
8	80	83	79
Lower			
1	75	75	80
2	72	78	80
3	56	63	70
4	69	74	70
5	63	76	75
6	71	70	72
7	73	69	69
8	64	69	78

6. Graph the two main effects and the interaction from Exercise 5. Use group means on your graphs.

7. Run a two-way ANOVA on the following data where repeated measures are taken on Factor B.

	Subjects	B1	B2	B3	B4
	1	2	4	5	7
	2	4	5	5	8
	3	7	6	2	6
A1	4	6	4	3	5
	5	5	3	4	4
	6	2	7	3	7
	7	9	8	2	9
	8	7	9	1	9
	9	8	2	6	6
	10	4	3	5	5
	11	6	6	3	7
A2	12	5	7	6	4
	13	7	6	7	6
	14	3	8	9	7
	15	9	9	5	3
	16	10	10	4	8

a. $SS_{TOT} =$
b. $SS_s =$
c. $SS_A =$
d. $SS_{A(gps)} =$
e. $SS_{WS} =$
f. $SS_B =$
g. $SS_{AXB} =$
h. $SS_{S(gps)XB} =$
i. Complete the ANOVA summary table.
j. Using the group sums, graph the interaction.

8. A clinical psychologist was interested in the influence of psychotherapeutic labels on people's judgements of mental health. She randomly assigned ten subjects to each of three groups. All the subjects read short stories about people with various psychological problems. After each story was read, subjects were required to rate the mental health of the person described in the story, where low ratings = poor mental health

and high ratings = good mental health. A third of the stories described people with anxiety disorders (AD), a third described people with personality disorders (PD), and a third described people with depressive disorders (DD). For one of the three groups, each story ended with a behavioral label diagnosing the disorder (BL). In another group, a psychiatric label from the Diagnostic and Statistical Manual of Mental Disorders was used (DSM3). In the last group, no label was given. Run the appropriate ANOVA on the mean rating data from this study.

	AD	PD	DD
No label	5.6	5.8	4.7
	4.3	6.1	4.3
	3.8	6.7	4.7
	5.9	6.1	2.7
	5.0	5.4	5.2
	5.1	5.8	6.0
	4.1	6.8	4.8
	3.7	1.8	2.5
	6.2	6.4	5.1
	4.8	5.3	5.3
DSM3	5.6	3.5	5.0
	5.1	3.7	3.0
	4.6	2.8	3.0
	5.8	1.6	6.0
	5.0	3.9	5.0
	6.1	4.0	5.0
	5.7	5.3	4.2
	4.9	4.6	3.6
	4.7	3.4	4.5
	4.0	4.2	5.1
BL	5.9	6.3	5.3
	4.8	5.7	5.4
	4.5	6.0	4.8
	6.0	5.6	6.1
	5.6	5.9	6.2
	6.7	6.2	5.7
	4.8	4.6	5.0
	6.2	6.3	6.1
	5.9	5.2	5.2
	3.7	4.9	5.0

9. The academic dean of a large university decided to do some research to see whether there was a difference in student performance in three different classes of a senior seminar in organic chemistry. He selected three senior classes, each taught by a different professor. All three professors used the same term-exams. The dean collected the term-exam scores of the students in each of the three classes. His primary interest was whether the professor had an influence on the scores. He expected that performance would improve over the term. Run the appropriate ANOVA on the data he collected.

	Student	Exam 1	Exam 2	Exam 3
Professor A	1	87.0	74.0	35.0
	2	77.0	58.0	45.0
	3	45.0	50.0	55.0
	4	68.0	50.0	67.0
	5	90.0	63.0	70.0
	6	86.0	76.0	45.0
	7	86.0	80.0	55.0
	8	80.0	78.0	65.0
	9	63.0	77.0	69.0
	10	59.0	68.0	62.0
Professor B	1	85.0	65.0	50.0
	2	75.0	55.0	65.0
	3	65.0	48.0	45.0
	4	58.0	69.0	50.0
	5	50.0	45.0	60.0
	6	60.0	55.0	40.0
	7	60.0	58.0	55.0
	8	59.0	65.0	45.0
	9	68.0	45.0	60.0
	10	60.0	50.0	52.0
Professor C	1	60.0	63.0	53.0
	2	67.0	57.0	50.0
	3	64.0	60.0	48.0
	4	70.0	56.0	55.0
	5	60.0	55.0	47.0
	6	63.0	65.0	69.0
	7	58.0	60.0	55.0
	8	63.0	55.0	43.0
	9	63.0	51.0	49.0
	10	54.0	49.0	50.0

CHAPTER 13

Multiple Comparison Procedures

LEARNING OBJECTIVES

After reading this chapter you should be able to:

1. Describe the difference between *a priori* and *post hoc* comparisons.
2. Use the planned comparison approach to test for differences between means.
3. Use the Scheffé method to test for differences between means.
4. Use the Tukey method to test for differences between means.
5. Describe the hypotheses, assumptions and decision rules for each multiple comparison technique.
6. Describe the appropriate conditions in which to use each multiple comparison technique.

In Chapters 11 and 12, we learned that the outcome of ANOVA tells us whether or not a significant difference exists. It does not tell us where that difference lies. ANOVA must be followed by additional statistical procedures to determine which means are different.

Controlling the Error Rate

One of the important concerns in doing inferential statistics is the possibility of making an error. A Type I error, you will recall, is made when we reject a null hypothesis that should not have been rejected. ANOVA keeps the Type I error rate at alpha over the entire experiment. If, on the other hand, we do multiple t-tests, rather than ANOVA, the Type I error rate is higher than alpha. Although the probability of a Type I error for each individual t-test is alpha, the probability of making at least one Type I error with many t-tests within one experiment is higher than alpha. The **experiment-wise**

error rate is higher than the error rate for each t-test comparison. The experiment-wise error rate will depend on the number of t-test comparisons that are made within a single experiment. Since researchers must control the overall experiment-wise error rate, other procedures are recommended for comparing group means following ANOVA. Some common multiple comparison procedures are discussed in the following sections.

A Priori or Planned Comparisons

A priori, as you know, means before the fact, and so *a priori* (or **planned**) **comparisons** are those planned in advance of the experiment, usually on the basis of some theory or previous research. It is not required that the ANOVA yield a significant result for planned comparisons to be made.

As is often the case in statistics there is some disagreement about the specifics of a planned comparison analysis and students should consult an upper level statistics text for clarification.*

Each planned comparison is evaluated for significance with a t-ratio. For our purposes we will assume that the means to be compared are based on equal sample sizes. In this case, the numerator of the t-ratio is simply the difference between the pair of means of interest and the denominator uses the error mean square from the ANOVA to compute the standard error of the comparison. The t formula for a planned comparison is

$$t = \frac{\overline{X}_1 - \overline{X}_2}{\sqrt{2MS_{error}/n}} \qquad \text{t-ratio for the planned comparison}$$

In Chapter 11 we ran an ANOVA to see if training students in study and test-taking skills made a difference in their performance. A control group received no training. There were 15 subjects in each group. The relevant data are presented below.

ANOVA Summary Table

Source	SS	df	MS	F	p
Between groups	1213.33	2	606.60	5.61	< .01
Within groups	4545.47	42	108.23		
Total	5758.80	44			

---

* For a discussion see Keppel, G. (1973) *Design and Analysis*. Englewood Cliffs, N.J.: Prentice-Hall, pp. 92–93. The present text assumes comparisons need not be orthogonal.

$\overline{X}_1$ (Control) = 59.07
$\overline{X}_2$ (Study) = 66.40
$\overline{X}_3$ (Test) = 71.73

Let's use a planned comparison technique to compare the control group with each of the treatment groups. We can first compute the standard error for the t-ratio. It will be the same for both comparisons.

$$\text{Standard error} = \sqrt{2MS_{error}/n}$$
$$= \sqrt{2(108.23)/15}$$
$$= \sqrt{14.43} = 3.80$$

The t-ratio for the planned comparison of the control group with the study group is

$$t = \frac{\overline{X}_2 - \overline{X}_1}{\text{standard error}}$$
$$= \frac{66.40 - 59.07}{3.80} = 1.93$$

The t-ratio for the planned comparison of the control group with the test group is

$$t = \frac{\overline{X}_3 - \overline{X}_1}{\text{standard error}}$$
$$= \frac{71.73 - 59.07}{3.80} = 3.33$$

To evaluate the comparisons for significance, let's use the .05 level of significance. We enter the the degrees of freedom associated with the error mean square (i.e. 42) into Table B-2 of Appendix B and we find the critical value of t for a two-tailed test is approximately ±2.02.

We will conclude that training in test-taking skills improved performance over no-training. And there was no evidence that training in study skills made a difference in performance.

Summary of Planned Comparisons

Hypotheses
  H_o: No difference between population means
  H_a: H_o is false

Assumptions
  The outcome of the ANOVA need not be significant.

Decision Rules
  If $t_{obt} \geq t_{crit}$, reject H_o
  If $t_{obt} < t_{crit}$, do not reject H_o

Formula
$$t = \frac{\overline{X}_1 - \overline{X}_2}{\sqrt{2MS_{error}/n}}$$

A Posteriori or *Post-Hoc* Comparisons

A posteriori (or *post-hoc*) means after the fact. **Post-hoc comparisons** are usually not planned until after the researcher has examined the data and noted trends. *Post-hoc* comparisons require that the ANOVA yielded a significant outcome.

The Scheffé Method

The **Scheffé method** is appropriate for making any and all comparisons on a set of means. This method is considered superior to some of the other techniques when complex comparisons are of interest and/or when sample sizes are not equal. When samples are the same size and when simple comparisons are of interest, the Scheffé method is more conservative (less powerful) than some of the other techniques.

Constructing the Comparison

The Scheffé method allows comparisons between any and all means. In any comparison, two quantities are contrasted. These quantities may both be sample means or averages of means. For example, a researcher who used a control group and two experimental groups may wish to compare the control group mean with the average of the experimental group means. This could be expressed as

$$\overline{X}_c \text{ compared with } \frac{\overline{X}_1 + \overline{X}_2}{2}$$

Or, he may wish to compare the two experimental group means with each other: $\overline{X}_1$ compared with $\overline{X}_2$.

To construct a comparison, each quantity is multiplied by a coefficient. In the first example, $+1$ is the coefficient for the control mean and $-1/2$ is the coefficient for each experimental group mean. Since the null hypothesis is at the population level for this example, it is

$$H_o: 1\mu_c - \frac{1}{2}\mu_1 - \frac{1}{2}\mu_2 = 0$$

For the second example, the coefficients are $+1$ and -1 and the null hypothesis is

$$H_o: 1\mu_1 - 1\mu_2 = 0$$

Alternative hypotheses are always non-directional.

In general, any comparison (C) may be expressed by the following, where c is the coefficient for each mean and k is the number of groups.

$$C = c_1\overline{X}_1 + c_2\overline{X}_2 + \ldots + c_k\overline{X}_k \qquad \text{comparison}$$

Note that the sum of the coefficients must be zero, i.e., $(c_1 + c_2 + \ldots + c_k = 0)$. Group means not included in the comparison are assigned coefficients of zero.

The Standard Error of the Comparison

To test the significance of a comparison, we need to determine the standard error (s_c). The general formula is as follows, where MS_{error} is the appropriate error variance estimate from the ANOVA, c is the coefficient for the group mean, and n is the sample size.

$$s_c = \sqrt{MS_{error}\left(\frac{c_1^2}{n_1} + \frac{c_2^2}{n_2} + \ldots + \frac{c_k^2}{n_k}\right)} \qquad \text{standard error}$$

Evaluating the Comparison for Significance

To evaluate a comparison for significance, we first must calculate F_s, the critical value of F used for a Scheffé comparison.

$$F_s = \sqrt{(k-1)F_{crit}} \quad \text{Scheffé's critical F}$$

In this equation, k is the number of groups. F_{crit} is the tabled value of F with $(k-1)df$ in the numerator and the degrees of freedom associated with the MS_{error} from the analysis of variance in the denominator.

Now we can go ahead and test our comparison for significance. The formula is

$$F' = C/s_c \quad \text{Scheffé F' statistic}$$

As usual, if the obtained F value for any comparison (i.e., F') is equal to or larger than the critical value (i.e., F_s), we reject the null hypothesis.

Running a Scheffé Test

Let's use the same example we analyzed with a planned comparison approach in the preceding section to see how the Scheffé method differs. The data were

ANOVA Summary Table

Source	SS	df	MS	F	p
Between groups	1213.33	2	606.60	5.61	< .01
Within groups	4545.47	42	108.23		
Total	5758.80	44			

$\overline{X}_1$ (Control) = 59.07
$\overline{X}_2$ (Study) = 66.40
$\overline{X}_3$ (Test) = 71.73

The ANOVA told us that there was a significant difference between the three kinds of students: those trained in study skills, those trained in test-taking skills and those receiving no training. Six comparisons can be examined: S vs T, S vs C, T vs C, ST vs C, TC vs S, SC vs T. Let's run a Scheffé test to determine whether the training made a difference. In other words we will compare the control group with the two trained groups. The null hypothesis will be: H_o: $1/2\ \mu_2 + 1/2\ \mu_3 - 1\ \mu_1 = 0$.

Step 1. Construct the comparison.

$$C = c_1\overline{X}_1 + c_2\overline{X}_2 + c_3\overline{X}_3$$
$$= \left(\frac{1}{2}\right)(66.40) + \left(\frac{1}{2}\right)(71.73) + (-1)(59.07)$$
$$= 69.07 - 59.07 = 10$$

Step 2. Determine the standard error.

$$s_c = \sqrt{MS_{WG}\left(\frac{c_1^2}{n_1} + \frac{c_2^2}{n_2} + \frac{c_3^2}{n_3}\right)}$$

$$= \sqrt{108.23\left(\frac{\left(\frac{1}{2}\right)^2}{15} + \frac{\left(\frac{1}{2}\right)^2}{15} + \frac{(-1)^2}{15}\right)}$$

$$= 3.29$$

Step 3. Determine Scheffé's critical F.

$$F_s = \sqrt{(k-1)F_{crit}}$$

F_{crit} is the tabled value with $(k-1)$df in the numerator and the df associated with the MS_{WG} (i.e., the error mean square from ANOVA) in the denominator.

$$F_{(2, 42)} \text{ at } \alpha \text{ equals } .05 = 3.22$$
$$F_s = \sqrt{2(3.22)} = 2.54$$

Step 4. Test the comparison for significance.

$$F' = C/s_c$$
$$= 10/3.29 = 3.04$$

Step 5. Make a decision.
Since the obtained F value is larger than the critical value, we reject the null and claim that the training significantly improved performance.

The Scheffé method is particularly appropriate when complex combinations of sample means are being compared.

Summary of the Scheffé Test

Hypotheses
H_o: No difference between population means
H_a: H_o is false

Assumptions
The outcome of the ANOVA was significant.

Decision Rules
If $F' \geq F_s$, reject the H_o
If $F' < F_s$, do not reject H_o

Formulas
$F' = C/s_c$
$F_s = \sqrt{(k-1)F_{crit}}$

The Tukey Method

The **Tukey method** is more powerful than Scheffé's for comparing pairs of means. However, it is less powerful for comparing combinations of means. The Tukey method compares the difference between each pair of means with a value called the **honestly significant difference (HSD)**. The value of HSD is found by

$$\text{HSD} = q(\alpha, df_{error}, k) \sqrt{MS_{error}/n} \quad \text{Tukey's honestly significant difference}$$

where q is the value from Table B-5 in Appendix B; df_{error} is the degrees of freedom associated with the MS_{error} from ANOVA; k is the number of groups; and n is the number of subjects within a group.

The value of q is found by entering Table B-5 with the α level, the df associated with the MS_{error} from the ANOVA, and the number of groups involved in the analysis. The differences between pairs of means can then be compared with the value of HSD. If any difference is greater than or equal to the value of HSD, the two means are significantly different or "honestly significantly different."

As with the Scheffé test the null hypotheses specify no difference between the population means, and the alternative hypotheses are nondirectional.

Running a Tukey Test

Let's use the same example we used earlier to run a Tukey test at $\alpha = .05$ on each pair of means. The three samples had 15 observations each and the outcome of the ANOVA was as follows:

ANOVA Summary Table

Source of Variance	Sum of Squares	df	Mean Squares	F	p
Between groups	1213.33	2	606.60	5.61	< .01
Within groups	4545.47	42	108.23		
Total	5758.80	44			

$\overline{X}_1$ (Control) = 59.07
$\overline{X}_2$ (Study) = 66.40
$\overline{X}_3$ (Test) = 71.73

Step 1. Determine the difference between each pair of group means.

$$\text{Study} - \text{Control} = 66.40 - 59.07 = 7.33$$
$$\text{Test} - \text{Control} = 71.73 - 59.07 = 12.66$$
$$\text{Test} - \text{Study} = 71.73 - 66.40 = 5.33$$

Step 2. Compute the value of HSD.

$$\text{HSD} = q(\alpha, df_{wg}, k)\sqrt{MS_{WG}/n}$$
$$= q(.05, 42, 3) \sqrt{108.23/15}$$
$$= 3.44(2.69) = 9.25$$

Step 3. Compare differences with the value of HSD and make a decision.

Since the only mean difference larger than HSD is that between the Test group and the Control group, we conclude that test training had a significant effect on performance compared to no training.

Several other techniques for *post-hoc* multiple comparisons have been developed but the Scheffé and Tukey methods are probably the most commonly used because of their generality and utility. Those of you wishing to learn more about multiple comparison techniques will find useful descriptions in Winer (1971) and Kirk (1968).*

---

* Winer, B.J. (1971). *Statistical Principles in Experimental Design*. New York: McGraw-Hill.
Kirk, R.E. (1968). *Experimental Design: Procedures for the Behavioral Sciences*. Belmont, Cal.: Brooks/Cole.

Summary of the Tukey Test

Hypotheses
H_o: no difference between population means.
H_a: H_o is false.

Assumptions
The outcome of the ANOVA was significant.

Decision Rules
Any mean difference $\geq$ HSD, reject the H_o

Formula
$$HSD = q(\alpha, df_{error}, k) \sqrt{MS_{error}/n}$$

FOCUS ON RESEARCH

Wahler and Gendreau (1990)* used the Correctional Personnel Rating Scale (CPRS) to assess effective characteristics of correctional officers in three correctional settings.

The CPRS is a scale that purports to measure correctional officer behaviors deemed important by correctional personnel. The researchers were interested in the views of other groups, especially supervisors of correctional officers and inmates, on what makes an effective correctional officer. A second interest involved comparing different correctional settings in terms of ratings of effectiveness.

The Data
The CPRS is a 4-point rating scale of 69 behaviors identified as contributing to the effectiveness of a correctional officer's job. The rating scale data and demographic data were collected by questionnaire.

The Variables
Three types of correctional facility were included: minimum/medium facility, maximum security facility, and small jail type facility.

Three samples from each facility were surveyed: correctional officers, supervisors, and inmates. Attempts to randomly sample were made although this was not always possible.

---

* Wahler, C. and Gendreau, P. (1990). Perceived Characteristics of Effective Correctional Officers by Officers, Supervisors, and Inmates across Three Different Types of Institutions, *Canadian Journal of Criminology, 32*, 265–77.

The Analyses

A correlational type analysis, called factor analysis, was performed on all the rating scale data to determine major dimensions of effectiveness/ineffectiveness. The researchers identified three dimensions: 1) Responsibility/Leadership skills such as report writing, enforcement of rules etc; 2) Behavior Skill Deficits such as failure to meet deadlines, poor communication with co-workers etc.; and 3) Inmate-Relationship skills such as compassion for inmates' feelings, interaction with inmates etc.

Mean scores on these three dimensions were then used in further analyses. Because mean scores were the data, an initial analysis of variance was performed and followed by the Tukey multiple comparison procedure to assess differences between samples and institutions. The initial ANOVA found no significant differences between ratings from the three types of facilities. Some of the additional findings are as follows.

Table 13-1 Analysis of data

Rating differences	Mean differences
Responsibility/Leadership skills	
Correctional officers – inmates	5.58
Supervisors – inmates	4.89
Inmate-Relationship skills	
Inmates – correctional officers	2.00
Inmates – supervisors	2.13

Source: Wahler and Gendreau (1990).

Correctional officers and supervisors attributed more importance to Responsibility/Leadership skills than did the inmates (both differences are larger than Tukey's HSD). Inmates attributed significantly greater importance to Inmate-Relationship skills than did either of the other two groups (both differences are larger than Tukey's HSD).

The sampling difficulties encountered by the researchers as well as other problems with this kind of research limit the generality of the findings. Nevertheless, the study suggests that supervisors, inmates, and fellow correctional officers may have some differences of opinion about what makes an effective correctional officer.

SUMMARY OF TERMS AND FORMULAS

Planned comparisons are made *a priori* and do not require a significant outcome from the ANOVA. Common *post-hoc* comparisons include the Scheffé and Tukey tests, which require a significant outcome from the ANOVA.

The **Scheffé method** is suitable for comparing any or all pairs of means as well as complex combinations of means. combinations of means. Samples need not be the same size. The Scheffé test requires computation of the **F'** statistic for each comparison of interest. Each F' statistic is then compared to **Scheffé's critical F value** for significance.

The **Tukey method** is used for comparing pairs of means and requires samples to be the same size. For simple comparisons, the Tukey method is considered to be more powerful than the Scheffé method. The Tukey test compares the mean difference between each pair of sample means with the value of the **honestly significant difference (HSD)**. Any mean differences equal or larger than the HSD are considered to be significant.

Test	Formulas
Planned comparisons	$t = \dfrac{\overline{X}_1 - \overline{X}_2}{\sqrt{2MS_{error}/n}}$
Scheffé	
F'	$F' = C/s_c$
Critical F	$F_s = \sqrt{(k-1)F_{crit}}$
Comparison	$C = c_1\overline{X}_1 + c_2\overline{X}_2 + \ldots + c_k\overline{X}_k$
Standard error	$s_c = \sqrt{MS_{error}\left(\dfrac{c_1^2}{n_1} + \dfrac{c_2^2}{n_2} + \ldots + \dfrac{c_k^2}{n_k}\right)}$
Tukey	
Honestly significant difference	$HSD = q(\alpha, df_{error}, k)\sqrt{MS_{error}/n}$

EXERCISES

1. Below is the outcome of a two-way ANOVA. Use a planned comparisons approach to test the six possible comparisons for significance at the .05 level. There were six subjects in each group.

Source	SS	df	MS	F	p
A	16.67	1	16.67	0.11	>.05
B	8.17	1	8.17	0.05	>.05
A×B	383.99	1	383.99	2.58	>.05
WS	2981.00	20	149.05		
Total	3389.83	23			

$\overline{X}_{A_1B_1} = 64.17$
$\overline{X}_{A_1B_2} = 73.33$
$\overline{X}_{A_2B_1} = 70.50$
$\overline{X}_{A_2B_2} = 63.67$

2. Below is the outcome of an ANOVA. Use the planned comparisons approach to see if Group 2 is significantly different from each of the other groups at the .01 level of significance. There were twenty subjects in each group.

Source	SS	df	MS	F	p
A	23.11	1	23.11	9.41	<.01
B	19.01	1	19.01	7.74	<.01
AXB	35.11	1	35.11	14.29	<.01
WG	186.75	76	2.46		

Means:
Group 1   5.10
Group 2   2.80
Group 3   4.85
Group 4   5.20

3. The outcome of a one-way ANOVA is provided below. Run a Scheffé test at $\alpha = .05$ for the following null hypotheses.
   a. $1\mu_1 - 1\mu_2 = 0$
   b. $1\mu_3 - 1/2\mu_1 - 1/2\mu_2 = 0$
   c. $1\mu_2 - 1\mu_3 = 0$

Source	df	MS	F	p
Between Groups	2	32.6	7.36	<.05
Within Groups	12	4.43		

Means: Group 1 = 4.60
        Group 2 = 3.00
        Group 3 = 8.00
$n_1 = n_2 = n_3 = 5$

4. Run a Tukey test on the following data for all possible comparisons at $\alpha = .05$.

Subject	Control	Group A	Group B
1	6	1	4
2	4	3	4
3	9	3	5
4	10	2	6

5. For the following data, complete the ANOVA summary table and run Scheffé's test for all possible comparisons ($\alpha = .05$).

Source	SS	df	MS	F
Between	28.40	2		
Within	9.20	6		

$\bar{X}_1 = 6.30$
$\bar{X}_2 = 1.70$
$\bar{X}_3 = 2.40$
$n_1 = n_2 = n_3 = 3$

6. A kayak manufacturer measured the time to complete a race course by professional racers in 4 different types of kayaks for 6 trials each. Here are the data.

Eclipse	Mirage	Dancer	Mark IV
1.4	1.7	2.0	3.0
1.2	1.8	2.1	3.1
1.0	1.9	2.0	2.9
1.6	2.2	2.4	2.8
1.8	2.4	2.6	3.4
1.0	2.7	2.8	3.5

   a. Run a one-way ANOVA on the data above at $\alpha = .05$.
   b. Compare the Eclipse with the Mirage using Scheffé's test ($\alpha = .05$). Do they differ?
   c. Compare the Eclipse with the average of the other three boats using Scheffé's test ($\alpha = .05$). What is your conclusion?
   d. Compare all possible means with Tukey's test ($\alpha = .05$). What are your conclusions?

7. The following data are from a two-way ANOVA found in Chapter 11 of the text. Compare the means with a Tukey test at $\alpha = .05$.

No Feedback		Corrective Feedback	
High Practice	Low Practice	High Practice	Low Practice
7.00	5.13	8.50	7.63

$MS_{error} = 2.88$ with 28 df
$n = 8$ for each group

a. HSD =
   b. NH-NL =
      CH-NH =
      CL-NH =
      CH-NL =
      CL-NL =
      CH-CL =
   c. Which means are significantly different?
8. Using the data below, compare the average of means 1 and 2 with the average of means 3 and 4 using the Scheffé test at $\alpha = .05$.

   Means: Group 1 = 6.43
          Group 2 = 5.43
          Group 3 = 4.57
          Group 4 = 4.57
   $MS_{error} = 5.58$
   n = 7

   a. C =
   b. s_c =
   c. F_s =
   d. F' =
   e. What is your decision?

CHAPTER 14

Inference with the Chi-Square Distribution

LEARNING OBJECTIVES

After reading this chapter you should be able to:

1. Describe the difference between a parametric technique and a non-parametric technique.
2. List the steps for constructing the chi-square distribution.
3. Provide the formula for chi-square.
4. Describe the shape of the chi-square distribution.
5. List the rule for determining degrees of freedom for a chi-square test for goodness of fit.
6. Run a chi-square test for goodness of fit for a given set of data.
7. Describe the null and alternative hypotheses for a chi-square test for independence.
8. Provide the formula for determining expected values for a chi-square test for independence.
9. List the rule for determining degrees of freedom for a chi-square test for independence.
10. Run a chi-square test for independence for a given set of data.
11. Determine the appropriate test of significance for a given research problem.

When we make inferences about the mean of a population or the difference between means of two or more populations, for example, we are using parametric techniques. We are inferring the values of population parameters. Some research questions do not involve specific parameters of a distribution but, rather, the entire frequency distribution. An automobile dealer might be interested in the relative popularity of six of her car models, for example. If her data showed that one model was more popular with her customers than the others, she might use this information when ordering new cars from the manufacturer. In this example, the data are not mean scores; rather, they are the number of cars sold of each type that interests the dealer.

If we are interested in the nature of the entire population, we may find a **non-parametric** technique to be appropriate. The **chi-square test** (symbolized by χ^2) is a non-parametric test that allows us to make inferences about population frequencies from sample frequencies. Non-parametric tests are useful for analyzing data measured on nominal and ordinal scales, since they do not make as many assumptions as parametric tests.

Chi-square tests compare obtained sample frequencies with those expected according to the null hypothesis. Chi-square can be used with frequency data or with proportion data, since proportions can always be converted into frequencies. Chi-square can be used for discrete variables or for continuous variables which have been categorized into discrete intervals.

The chi-square test compares the frequencies obtained in a sample with those expected if the null hypothesis were true. The null hypothesis states the expected frequencies of sample data based on certain assumptions about the population from which the sample was drawn. Of course, we would not expect sample frequencies to be *exactly* equal to expected frequencies, even if the null were true. Sample frequencies will vary somewhat from their hypothesized values because of sampling fluctuation. The question is "How much variation between obtained sample frequencies and their expected values would likely occur if the null were true?" To answer this question, we need a sampling distribution.

Non-parametric techniques: Used to compare population distributions rather than parameters.

Chi-square test: A non-parametric analysis used to test hypotheses about frequencies of categorical or discrete variables.

The Chi-Square Distribution

Like the t- and F-distributions, the chi-square distribution is a family of distributions; the shape of each is determined by degrees of freedom. The chi-square distribution is a relative frequency distribution based on discrepancies between obtained frequencies and their expected values. The value of chi-square will be smaller when the obtained and expected frequencies are similar, and the value will be larger when they are not. If the hypothesized frequencies are not the true population frequencies, the discrepancies between obtained and expected values will be large and so will the value of chi-square. We need to discover what values of chi-square would occur with random sampling when the null is true. We can then compare our obtained chi-square value with this distribution of values and determine whether our outcome is a likely one or not according to the null hypothesis.

Constructing the Sampling Distribution of Chi-Square

The random sampling distribution of chi-square is constructed in the following manner:

Step 1. Randomly select a sample from a population of a discrete variable whose expected frequencies are known and record the frequency for each category.

Step 2. Subtract the expected frequency (E) for each category from the observed frequency (O). Square each difference and divide it by the associated expected frequency i.e., $(O - E)^2/E$. Sum these values for all categories of the variable. This is the chi-square statistic.

Step 3. Return the sample to the population.

Step 4. Repeat the first three steps until all possible samples have been drawn from the population.

Step 5. Place the chi-square values in a relative frequency distribution. This relative frequency distribution is the random sampling distribution of the chi-square statistic.

Characteristics of the Chi-Square Distribution

Because the chi-square value is computed by squaring the differences between the observed and expected values, it can never be negative.

The null hypothesis states that the category frequencies in the population equal a set of values. A sample selected from that population should reflect that set of values. When the obtained frequencies are larger or smaller than those expected, the value of chi-square increases. For this reason, the region of rejection always appears in the upper tail of the distribution, as illustrated in Figure 14-1.

Although the critical region lies in one tail, the chi-square test is nondirectional. A very low chi-square value simply means that the obtained frequencies are closer to the expected values than chance would predict.

The chi-square distribution changes shape depending on degrees of freedom. In the other distributions we have looked at, degrees of freedom

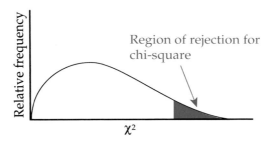

Figure 14-1 An example of a chi-square distribution

have been determined in relation to sample size. Degrees of freedom for the chi-square test are not related to sample size but rather are related to the number of discrepancies, (O − E)'s, that are independent and free to vary. In a chi-square test, we assume the total number of observations for total frequency is fixed and determine how many discrepancies are free to vary.

Using the Chi-Square Distribution

We will discuss the two chi-square tests: the **chi-square test for goodness of fit** and the **chi-square test for independence**. The first is used when we have one variable. The second test is used when we wish to discover whether two variables are related.

The Chi-Square Test for Goodness of Fit

This test is used when we have two or more categories or levels of one variable. We are interested in whether the frequencies we obtain for each category in our sample match the expected frequencies specified by the null hypothesis.

Null and Alternative Hypotheses

The null and alternative hypotheses for a chi-square test of goodness of fit are determined before data collection; that is *a priori*. How the null and alternative are stated depends upon the research question. For example, a tavern owner may be interested in customer preference for four types of beer. He may decide to have 100 customers taste each beer and indicate their preference. If the population from which his customers came had no preference for any of the four types, he would expect 25 people to choose each one. These would be the expected frequencies. The null hypothesis would specify "no difference in preference" and the expected value for each brand would be 25. The alternative hypothesis would state "preference differs" and that the true frequencies in the population were different than those hypothesized in the null.

> H_o: No difference in preference for types of beer.
> H_a: Preference for types of beer differs.

Calculating Chi-Square

Let's run a chi-square test for goodness of fit to answer the tavern owner's question. Suppose he finds, after 100 customers choose which of the four types of beer they prefer, the following frequencies.

	Types				
	Ale	Beer	Lager	Porter	Total
Observed Frequencies	10	20	55	15	100
Expected Frequencies	25	25	25	25	100

We find the value of chi-square as follows:

$$\chi^2 = \Sigma \frac{(O - E)^2}{E} \qquad \text{chi-square}$$

$$\chi^2 = \frac{(10 - 25)^2}{25} + \frac{(20 - 25)^2}{25} + \frac{(55 - 25)^2}{25} + \frac{(15 - 25)^2}{25}$$
$$= 50$$

Now he needs to compare the obtained χ^2 value with the critical value. The critical values for chi-square are found in Table B-4, in Appendix B, for various degrees of freedom. As usual, if the obtained value is equal to or larger than the critical value, the null hypothesis is rejected.

Recall that degrees of freedom for chi-square are determined by the number of comparisons between observed and expected frequencies that are free to vary. The total frequency is fixed. Looking at our example, we can see that three frequencies can vary but the fourth must be fixed to keep the sum at 100. Three discrepancies can vary, but the fourth cannot. One degree of freedom is used so the total can stay at 100. This problem, then, has three degrees of freedom.

The critical value of chi-square for 3 df is 11.34 at $\alpha = .01$. Since the obtained value of 50 is greater than the critical value, the null is rejected. The tavern owner has statistical evidence of a significant difference in population preference for his four types of beer.

In this example the expected frequencies for each category were equal. This is not always the case. Remember Mendel? Imagine a botanist has determined that seedlings should show four particular characteristics in the ratio of 4:3:2:1, according to Mendel's Law. The first characteristic should appear in 4/10 of the seedlings, the second in 3/10, and so on. If the botanist collected a random sample of 200 seedlings, the expected frequencies for each characteristic would be 80, 60, 40, and 20. The obtained values could then be compared with these expected values.

Both of these examples have four categories and three degrees of freedom. A special situation exists when there are two categories and one degree of freedom. With only two categories of frequencies, either a chi-square test for goodness of fit or a Z-test for a proportion may be used, as long as the assumptions of Z have been met. The outcome will be the same. For example, suppose a researcher counts the number of gerbils who prefer a pink running wheel and the number who prefer a turquoise running wheel when given a choice between the two in their daily exercise period. Of the 50 gerbils in the experiment, 33 chose the pink wheel and 17 chose the turquoise wheel. The investigator wants to know if the color of the wheel affected their choice. If color makes no difference, we would expect equal numbers of gerbils to select each wheel. This experiment has two categories (pink and turquoise) and 1 degree of freedom; we may run a chi-square test or a Z-test for a proportion since our frequencies can be easily converted to proportion. Let's do both at $\alpha = .01$. The null and alternative hypotheses for a chi-square test are

H_o: Equal preference for pink and turquoise wheels
H_a: Preference differs

$$\chi^2 = \frac{(33-25)^2}{25} + \frac{(17-25)^2}{25} = 5.12$$

With 1 df, the critical value of $\chi^2 = 6.64$ at $\alpha = .01$; we would not reject the null hypothesis. Gerbils, evidently, have no preference for the color of their running wheels.

With a Z-test for a proportion we hypothesize that the proportion of gerbils in the population who prefer pink running wheels is 0.50. In our sample, the proportion who chose the pink wheel was 33/50 = 0.66. Our hypotheses are as follows:

H_o: P = 0.50
H_a: P ≠ 0.50

Then we conduct a Z-test for a proportion.

$$Z = \frac{p - P_p}{\sqrt{PQ/n}}$$
$$= \frac{0.66 - 0.50}{\sqrt{(0.5)(0.5)/50}} = \frac{0.20}{0.07} = 2.29$$

The critical value of Z is ±2.58 at α = .01, so we cannot reject the null. There is no evidence that the proportion of gerbils preferring pink running wheels is different than 0.50.

Interpreting Chi-Square

The tavern owner interested in customer preference chose to test four types of beer. What if he had decided to test ten types? The degrees of freedom would be 9, not 3. The computed chi-square value would be larger because there were six more discrepancies in its calculation.

We found in the t- and F-distribution that as degrees of freedom increase, the critical value decreases. Perhaps, you are wondering why we don't just add more categories, increasing the value of our obtained chi-square, and making it easier to reject the null. A good point. If you examine the chi-square table, you will notice that as degrees of freedom increase, the critical value of chi-square *gets larger, not smaller*. Adding more categories does not make it easier to reject the null. The table takes the number of degrees of freedom into account when it determines the critical value. With more degrees of freedom in your experiment, you must obtain a larger chi-square value to reject the null.

The chi-square test for goodness of fit compares obtained frequencies with *a priori* expected values stated by the null hypothesis. As we will see in the next section, the chi-square test for independence makes a different comparison.

Summary of the Chi-Square Test for Goodness of Fit

Hypotheses
H_o: O's = E's
H_a: O's ≠ E's

Assumptions
1. Subjects are randomly selected.
2. Categories are mutually exclusive.

Decision Rules
df = number of categories − 1
If $\chi^2_{obt} \geq \chi^2_{crit}$, reject H_o
If $\chi^2_{obt} < \chi^2_{crit}$, do not reject H_o

Formula
$$\chi^2 = \Sigma \frac{(O - E)^2}{E}$$

The Chi-Square Test for Independence

The chi-square test for independence is used to measure the association between two variables. This is often called the "two variable case." The question asked is "Are the two variables independent?" Suppose the tavern owner, discussed earlier, wished to know if preference for his four types of beer depended on whether the customer was female or male. His research question in this case would be "Are gender and beer preference independent?" Similarly, the gerbil researcher may wonder if preference for pink and turquoise running wheels depends on the previous experience of the gerbils in such wheels. His research question would be "Are preference for wheel color and previous experience independent?"

Null and Alternative Hypotheses

In the chi-square test for independence, the null hypothesis always states that the two variables are independent, and the alternative hypothesis states that they are dependent.

In the one-variable case (goodness of fit) expected frequencies were determined *a priori* by some theoretical assumption. In the two-variable case, the expected values are determined after data collection, or *post hoc*, from the values of the obtained or observed frequencies.

Determining Expected Frequencies

Let's call on our tavern owner again to illustrate how expected frequencies are determined in a chi-square test for independence. Suppose he randomly selected 150 men and 100 women and asked each to declare his or her preference for the four types of beer. Here are his data.

	\multicolumn{4}{c}{Observed Frequencies}			
	Ale	Beer	Lager	Porter	Total
Women	35	25	15	25	100
Men	20	30	70	30	150
Total	55	55	85	55	250

To find the expected frequencies for this problem, we must determine the frequencies we would expect in each category if gender made no difference to preference. If we examine the column totals we see that, overall, lager is the "preferred type" and the other three are ranked equally. If gender and preference are independent, then that pattern of results would be expected for both genders. In other words, if gender didn't matter, how many women would prefer each type and how many men would, considering the size of our two samples? The formula for determining these expected values is

$$E = \frac{(\text{row sum})(\text{column sum})}{\text{total}} \quad \begin{array}{l}\text{expected values for the}\\ \text{chi-square test for}\\ \text{independence}\end{array}$$

Using this formula, our expected frequencies for each group would be

Expected Frequencies

	Ale	Beer	Lager	Porter	Total
Women	22	22	34	22	100
Men	33	33	51	33	150
Total	55	55	85	55	250

Notice that the row and column totals are the same as those of the observed frequencies. This is always true. Now we are ready to compute our chi-square.

Calculating Chi-Square

$$\chi^2 = \Sigma \frac{(O - E)^2}{E}$$

$$= \frac{(35 - 22)^2}{22} + \frac{(25 - 22)^2}{22} + \frac{(15 - 34)^2}{34} + \frac{(25 - 22)^2}{22} +$$

$$\frac{(20 - 33)^2}{33} + \frac{(30 - 33)^2}{33} + \frac{(70 - 51)^2}{51} + \frac{(30 - 33)^2}{33}$$

$$= 31.75$$

Now, we need to look up the critical value of chi-square and compare it to our obtained value. However, we need to know the degrees of freedom. Degrees of freedom are determined by the number of discrepancies that are free to vary. In a chi-square test for independence, we assume that the row and column sums are fixed. Degrees of freedom are equal to the number of cells in the table of expected values that are independent and, therefore, free to vary. One way to determine degrees of freedom is to ask how many expected values must be calculated before we can obtain the rest by subtraction. Let's look at our table of expected values, for a moment.

Expected Frequencies

	Ale	Beer	Lager	Porter	Total
Women	*				100
Men					150
Total	55	55	85	55	250

Let's calculate the expected frequency for the box marked with an asterisk.

$$E = \frac{(\text{Row Sum})(\text{Column Sum})}{\text{Total}}$$

$$= \frac{(100)(55)}{250} = 22$$

We can find the expected value for men choosing ale by subtraction. It must be 55 − 22 = 33. This value, then, is not free to vary. How many more values must we compute before we can obtain the rest by subtraction? Clearly, we need to calculate only two more values. Three expected values, altogether, must be calculated before the rest are fixed. Our problem, then, has 3 df.

For any chi-square test of independence, degrees of freedom are calculated by:

$$df = (\text{number of rows} - 1)(\text{number of columns} - 1)$$

Returning to our problem:

$$df = (2 - 1)(4 - 1) = 3$$

The critical value of χ^2 is 7.82 at $\alpha = .05$. Our obtained value is larger than the critical value and so we reject the null hypothesis. We have evidence that gender and preference for four types of beer are dependent. In other words, women and men do not prefer the same types of beer.

Interpreting Chi-Square

Like the goodness of fit test, as categories are added to one or both variables, the χ^2 value will increase. The table takes this into account; the critical values increase with larger degrees of freedom.

A significant value of χ^2 means that the two variables are related in some systematic way. When two variables are related, we often say they are **correlated**. Correlation, as a statistical technique, is discussed in detail in Chapter 15. A significant value of chi-square, then, tell us that the variables depend on each other or are correlated. But how dependent or correlated are they? A statistic that has been developed to measure the strength of this relationship is called **Cramer's measure of association** (ϕ'). This statistic is appropriate for computing the strength of the relationship when the chi-square test for independence produces a significant result. This statistic ranges from 0 (when the two variables are not related) to 1 (when the variables are perfectly related). Students should consult an upper level statistics text for detailed information on this measure.

Summary of the Chi-Square Test for Independence

Hypotheses
  H_o: The variables are independent.
  H_a: The variables are dependent.

Assumptions
  1. Subjects are randomly selected.
  2. Observations have been classified simultaneously on two independent categories.

Decision Rules
  df = (number of rows − 1)(number of columns − 1)
  If $\chi^2_{obt} \geq \chi^2_{crit}$, reject H_o
  If $\chi^2_{obt} < \chi^2_{crit}$, do not reject H_o

Formula
  $$\chi^2 = \Sigma \frac{(O - E)^2}{E}$$

Assumptions Underlying Inference with the Chi-Square Distribution

Chi-square assumes that the sample was randomly selected from the population, the observations are independent, and the variable discrete. Each particular observation can only be recorded in one cell. In other words, the categories are mutually exclusive.

In repeated experiments, chi-square requires that observed frequencies are normally distributed around their expected frequencies. This makes sense, because if we have an expected frequency of 15, occasionally we would observe a much higher or lower frequency, but most of the time we would see frequencies close to the expected value, given the null is true. This assumption may cause problems when expected frequencies are very small. With an expected frequency of 3, for example, the observed frequencies would be positively skewed around 3 since their distribution is limited at zero. Some statisticians recommend that all expected frequencies should be 5 or greater.

Choosing the Appropriate Test of Significance

This chapter has dealt with two non-parametric tests of significance: chi-square test for goodness of fit and chi-square test for independence.

Deciding which of these two tests should be used is not difficult for most students. What many students have trouble with is deciding whether the data in a particular research study lend themselves to a parametric or a nonparametric approach. This decision is made by examining the kinds of data collected in the study.

In this section we will go through the steps involved in deciding whether ANOVA or chi-square is the appropriate analysis. We will not include ANOVA designs where repeated measures have been taken.

Step 1. Determine the kind of data collected in the experiment.

The first step in deciding between chi-square and ANOVA is to examine the dependent variable data to see if measures of performance or categories of frequencies have been collected. If measures were taken from subjects that will be used to compute means, then ANOVA is the likely analysis. On the other hand, if subjects have been categorized into frequency groups then chi-square is the likely approach.

Step 2. Determine the number of independent variables.

If you have a situation where there are two or more groups in the study, you must determine how many independent variables are involved. With two or more groups or categories of subjects, each group under a different level of a single independent variable, you will choose one-way ANOVA if the data are measures and you will choose chi-square test for goodness of fit if the data are frequency counts. If you determine that the experimental design involves two independent variables, then you know you will run a two-way ANOVA if the data are measures and you will run a chi-square test for independence if the data are frequency counts.

Let's use the steps to decide which analysis is appropriate for the following research studies.

Example A An investigator has classified 400 randomly selected business executives according to their profiles from a standardized personality test, into high-anxious, medium-anxious, and low-anxious. He wonders if the proportions of each type are similar.

Step 1. Determine the kind of data collected in the experiment.

This is an easy one. The term "classified" and the term "proportions" are clues that these data are frequency counts. Although measures have been taken, they have not been used directly in any computation of average; they have been used to categorize the subjects.

Step 2. Determine the number of independent variables.

There is only one variable in this example: level of anxiety. A chi-square test for goodness of fit will be used to determine if there is a difference in proportion between the three levels.

Example B The music department at a large college classifies a randomly selected group of music students into expert, intermediate, and novice pianists. Half of the students in each group are given intensive piano training using an innovative approach to teaching. The other half is given standard training for the same length of time. Following the training period all students are required to give a piano recital and the number of errors made by each student is recorded. The average number of errors made by each group is compared.

Step 1. Determine the kind of data collected in the experiment.

Although the use of the term "classifies" might have led you to think the data are frequency data, you can see that this is not the case. "Number of errors made" was the measure and averages for each group were computed.

Step 2. Determine the number of independent variables.

There are two variables in this study: level of expertise and type of training. The investigator will run a two-way ANOVA to see if expertise overall made a difference in performance, to see if training overall made a difference, and to see if the two variables interact. For example, perhaps the innovative training was particularly helpful to the novice students.

Example C The music department at a large college is hosting a recital by its piano students. Each performance at the recital is categorized, by an impartial member of the department, as excellent, fair, or poor. Some of the students had received intensive piano training using an innovative teaching approach for several weeks before the recital. Others had been given standard training for the same length of time. A researcher tallies the students in terms of what kind of training they had received, innovative or standard, and what rating they were given for their recital, excellent, fair, or poor.

Step 1. Determine the kind of data collected in the experiment.

In this version the data are clearly frequency counts. The researcher has counted the number of students in each category.

Step 2. Determine the number of independent variables.

Two variables are involved: training type and performance category. Students have been simultaneously categorized by type of training and recital rating. A chi-square test for independence will tell the music department whether recital performance and type of training are independent or dependent. If type of training wasn't important we'd expect the same number of excellent, fair, and poor performances from each group.

Example D The Dolphin Show manager at Sea World has become concerned about the influence of the trainer on the dolphins' performance. He has noticed that some of the dolphins seem to perform differently with different trainers. He randomly assigned 20 dolphins to each of three trainers. The dolphins are signaled by their trainers, one at a time, to perform a high leap out of the water. Impartial judges are on hand to determine if each jump was successful (reached a certain height) or was not successful.

The number of dolphins succeeding and the number failing are counted for each of the three trainers.

Step 1. Determine the kind of data collected in the experiment.

These data are frequency data. The manager is interested in how many dolphins peform successfully with each trainer.

Step 2. Determine the number of independent variables.

There are two independent variables. The dolphins have been categorized into two groups based on whether they succeeded or not in their jumps and simultaneously on a second variable, which trainer was present. A chi-square test for independence will help the manager determine if success or failure is dependent upon the trainer involved.

Example E The Dolphin Show manager at Sea World has become concerned about the influence of the trainer on the dolphins' performance. He has noticed that some of the dolphins seem to perform differently with different trainers. He randomly assigned 20 dolphins to each of three trainers. The dolphins are signaled by their trainers, one at a time, to perform a high leap out of the water. Impartial judges are on hand to measure the height of the jump against a backdrop ruler. The average jump height of the dolphins assigned to each trainer is compared.

Step 1. Determine the kind of data collected in the experiment.

In this example, a measure for each subject is collected (i.e., height of jump) and a mean will be computed for each group (i.e., mean height under each trainer).

Step 2. Determine the number of independent variables.

There is only one independent variable in this study, the trainer. The analysis will compare the mean performance of the animals under three different trainers. A one-way ANOVA is the appropriate test of significance. The dolphins were randomly assigned to a trainer and so if Trainer 1's dolphins jumped significantly higher than the rest, the manager might have reason to believe that Trainer 1 is a more effective trainer than the others.

FOCUS ON RESEARCH

Skiing Louise ski resort installed new snow making equipment on several runs in the Lake Louise ski area in 1989. Any construction in a Canadian National Park is of concern to a variety of groups, in particular environmental groups. Consultants are routinely hired to assess the effects of development on the alpine terrain. I was involved as a research and statistical consultant on this project. I worked with an environmental scientist* who was responsible for determining the extent of the damage to the terrain as a result of the construction. From this analysis he would make recommenda-

---

* David Walker & Assoc., Consultants to the Lake Louise ski area, 1989.

tions to Skiing Louise as to what kind of repair to the terrain was required to meet his criterion. He had established the criterion based on previous work. If at least 90% of the area was adequate in terms of vegetation, then restorative planting would not be necessary. If significantly less than 90% was adequate, then he would recommend various methods for restoring the terrain. My job was to recommend how the terrain should be sampled and how the data should be analyzed. No standard scientific procedures had been set up for this kind of research and so we were breaking new ground. We had to develop a procedure for randomly sampling the disturbed alpine area in order to assess the damage and make inferences about the condition of the entire area. Two ski runs where snow-making equipment had been installed were to be assessed, the Wiwaxi ski run and the Juniper run.

The Data
Based on typical research in biology and botany, a sample element was defined as one-square meter of terrain (called a site). Each site was rated as adequate or inadequate for coverage, where "adequate" = vegetation covers 90% or more of site and "inadequate" = vegetation covers less than 90% of site. The same criterion was used to evaluate density. Each site, then, provided two measures and the data were dichotomous, i.e. Yes/No.

Sample selection
For various practical reasons, true random selection was not possible. Site locations were selected according to a pre-determined "random" scheme with the following restrictions:
1. vertical distance from site to site was not less than 5 meters and not more than 350 meters and
2. the horizontal span was from 8 to 18 meters. The horizontal span was determined by the nature of the disturbance.

Sample size
Determining an adequate sample size was constrained by a variety of factors. Sixty sites on the Wiwaxi snowmaking right of way and 31 sites on the Juniper run were examined for a total of 91 in the sample.

Procedure
The site location was determined by two randomly generated numbers with the restrictions discussed above. For example, if Site 1 = 45:7L, the site evaluator paced off 45 meters vertical distance down the mountain and 7 meters to the left of the centre of the disturbed area. A one-square meter grid was dropped at that point and the vegetation within the grid was rated for coverage and density as described above. This procedure was continued to the end of the critical area.

The Analyses
The data were proportion data in that we counted the number of sites meeting the agreed on criteria. Chi-square analyses were used to assess the impact of the development on the critical terrain. Since the *a priori* criterion

was that at least 90% of the area be adequate, this was used as the expected value in the chi-square analysis test for goodness of fit. We were testing for significantly less than 90% and so chi-square was used only in cases where less than 90% of the sites met criterion.

Table 14-1 presents the results for the entire sampled area.

Table 14-1   Sites meeting criterion

	Density		Coverage	
	Yes	No	Yes	No
O's	82	9	43	48
E's	81.9	9.1	81.9	9.1

Overall the critical area was adequate for density but did not approach the criterion for coverage ($\chi^2_{(1)} = 184.76, p < .01$).

Separate analyses were conducted on various sub-areas. Coverage on part of the Wiwaxi run, called the Olympic Cattrack, seemed to be particularly poor. The data are presented in Table 14-2.

Table 14-2   Sites meeting criterion on the Olympic Cattrack

	Density		Coverage	
	Yes	No	Yes	No
O's	31	0	6	25
E's	27.9	3.1	27.9	3.1

Chi-square analyses determined that the coverage on the Olympic Cattrack was significantly lower than the criterion of 90% ($\chi^2_{(1)} = 34.38, p < .01$).

The lower part of the Wiwaxi run and the Sunny T areas were adequate for density ($\chi^2_{(1)} = 0.46, p > .05$) but inadequate for coverage ($\chi^2_{(1)} = 9.44, p < .01$). The data are presented in Table 14-3.

Table 14-3   Sites meeting criterion on lower Wiwaxi and Sunny T

	Density		Coverage	
	Yes	No	Yes	No
O's	25	4	15	14
E's	26.1	2.9	26.1	2.9

The condition of the Juniper run was much like the lower Wiwaxi area with adequate density ($\chi^2_{(1)}$ = 1.29, p > .05) and inadequate coverage ($\chi^2_{(1)}$ = 12.48, p < .01). The Juniper results are presented in Table 14-4.

Table 14-4 Sites meeting criterion on Juniper run

	Density		Coverage	
	Yes	No	Yes	No
O's	26	5	22	9
E's	27.9	2.1	27.9	2.1

We presented the results of our analyses to Skiing Louise with recommendations that they replant the entire disturbed area to improve the vegetation coverage.

SUMMARY OF TERMS AND FORMULAS

The **chi-squares tests** are **non-parametric** analyses used to test hypotheses about frequencies of categorical or discrete variables.

The test for **goodness of fit** is used to evaluate the discrepancy between observed and expected frequencies for categories of a single variable.

The test for **independence** evaluates the relationship between two variables with a null hypothesis that the variables are unrelated.

Degrees of freedom for chi-square tests are determined by the number of discrepancies, used in the computation, that are independent and free to vary.

Chi-Square Formula

$$\chi^2 = \Sigma \frac{(O - E)^2}{E}$$

Degrees of Freedom

Test for Goodness of Fit number of categories − 1

Test for Independence (number of rows − 1)(number of columns − 1)

EXERCISES

1. For each of the following, determine the degrees of freedom and the critical value of chi-square.
   a. Test for goodness of fit, 6 categories, $\alpha = .05$
   b. Test for goodness of fit, 2 categories, $\alpha = .01$
   c. Test for independence, 4 categories for one variable and 5 categories for the second variable, $\alpha = .05$
   d. Test for independence, 2 categories for each variable, $\alpha = .01$

2. A local brewer observes that in a random sample of 100 women, 35 prefer light ale, 20 prefer pilsner, and 45 prefer a heavier malt brew. Test the hypothesis that women's preference is equal for the three types of beer.
   a. H_o:
      H_a:
   b. df =
   c. $\chi^2_{.05}$ =
   d. χ^2 =
   e. Decision:
   Put your decision in words:

3. A biologist wants to determine if a rare strain of rat will perform better on a problem-solving task than the more common strain. The results showed that 24 of the 30 rare rats succeeded in solving the problem and the remaining 6 failed. Twelve of the common strain solved the problem and the remaining 15 failed. With $\alpha = .05$, run a test for independence.

	Observed Frequencies	
	Success	Failure
Rare	24	6
Common	12	15

   a. H_o:
      H_a:
   b. df =
   c. $\chi^2_{.05}$ =
   d. χ^2 =
   e. Decision:
   Put your decision in words:

4. A psychologist administers a test assessing strength of religious values to 120 randomly selected churchgoers. He then administers a second questionnaire assessing their attitude toward censorship of rock videos. Use a χ^2 test to see if "piety" and attitude toward censorship are related at $\alpha = .01$.

	Observed Frequencies		
Censorship	Piety		
Attitude	High	Medium	Low
Pro	23	7	5
Neutral	20	20	20
Anti	8	22	25

    a. H_o:
       H_a:
    b. df =
    c. $\chi^2_{.05}$ =
    d. χ^2 =
    e. Decision:
Put your decision in words:

5. A breakfast cereal manufacturer observed that in a random sample of 60 children, 27 preferred a cornflakes product, 19 preferred a shredded wheat product, and 14 preferred a high-fibre product. Use chi-square to test the hypothesis that there is no difference in children's preference for the three cereals. Use α = .05.

6. A census determined that 60% of Canadians are Protestant, 30% are Catholic, and 10% have no religious affiliation. A small religious college of 500 students has 300 Protestants, 190 Catholics, and 10 students with no religious affiliation. Test the hypothesis at α = .05, that the college students are a random sample of the general Canadian population.

7. When offered a choice between popsicles and ice cream, 35 children chose popsicles and 15 chose ice cream. At α = .01, test the hypothesis that children's preference does not differ between the two treats.

8. A sporting goods manufacturer wants to determine if there is a relationship between gender and the riskiness of the sport each engages in. Over a six-month period, he records whether the equipment purchased is for a high-risk sport (kayaking, downhill skiing, skydiving) or a low-risk sport (cross-country skiing, skating, windsurfing) and whether the purchaser was male or female. He finds the following:

	High-Risk	Low-Risk
Men	22	37
Women	18	28

Test at α = .05 whether riskiness and gender are independent.

9. A psychologist administers a test to 120 randomly selected churchgoers to assess the strength of their religious values. A second test is then administered to the same group to assess attitude toward legalization of marijuana. Use a chi-square test to see if the two variables are related at $\alpha = .01$. The data are as follows:

Marijuana Attitude	High	Piety Medium	Low	Total
In Favor	5	10	20	35
Neutral	15	20	10	45
Against	20	10	10	40
Total	40	40	40	

10. A sociologist wonders if "Blondes have more fun." She selects a random sample of 50 blondes, 40 brunettes, and 35 redheads. She records the number of dates each girl has over a six-month period and classifies them into three categories. Test the hypothesis that hair colour and "popularity" are independent, at $\alpha = .05$. The data are as follows:

Number of Dates	Blondes	Brunettes	Redheads	Total
>50	39	15	13	67
25–50	8	20	10	38
<25	3	5	12	20
Total	50	40	35	

11. A scientist has been experimenting with black gerbils. He claims that as a result of certain injections, when two black gerbils are mated, the offspring will be black, white, and gray in the proportion 5:4:3. Many gerbils were mated after being injected with the chemical. Of 170 newborn gerbils, 61 were black, 69 were white, and 40 were gray. Test the scientist's claim at $\alpha = .01$.

12. Two kayaking buddies, Dan and Peter, enjoy racing each other down river. Over several years, they have been very evenly matched. Each has won about half the races. Last season, Peter read a book called "How to Win in Kayak Racing." Since then, Peter has lost 18 out of 20 races against Dan. Use chi-square, at $\alpha = .05$, to test the hypothesis that the book had no effect on Peter's performance.

13. A faculty-member and his wife are getting ready to attend a garden party given by his university. He wants to dress casually, but his wife thinks he should wear a suit. He explains to her that while most of the

administrative staff attending the party will be in suits, most of the faculty will not. He lost the argument, but when they arrived at the party he made a careful tally of who (administrators vs faculty) were wearing what (suit or no-suit). At α = .01, test the hypothesis that position and style of dress are independent. The data are as follows:

	Position at University		
	Administrator	Faculty	Total
Suit	45	8	53
No-Suit	10	32	42
Total	55	40	

14. A criminologist categorizes 315 randomly selected inmates, incarcerated in prisons across Canada, by type of offense and family structure of parental home. Are the variables independent? Use α = .05.

Family structure	Crimes of violence	Theft	Drug trafficking
Two-parent	2	87	60
Single-parent	4	93	40
Other	8	12	9

15. A political scientist randomly selects 200 people from each of three occupational categories and determines their political affiliation. Are the variables independent? Use α = .01.

	Cons	Lib	NDP	Total
Professional	30	85	85	200
Skilled	80	80	40	200
Unskilled	72	85	43	200
Total	182	250	168	600

CHAPTER 15

Additional Non-Parametric Techniques

LEARNING OBJECTIVES

After reading this chapter you should be able to:

1. Describe the relationship between the Mann-Whitney U test and the t-test for independent groups.
2. Run the Mann-Whitney U test for a given set of data.
3. Provide the Z-ratio for the U statistic.
4. Describe the relationship between the Wilcoxon test and the t-test for dependent groups.
5. Run the Wilcoxon test for a given set of data.
6. Provide the Z-ratio for the T statistic.
7. Describe the relationship between the one-way ANOVA and the Kruskal-Wallis test.
8. Run the Kruskal-Wallis test for a given set of data.
9. Describe the kind of research problem suitable for the rank-order correlation test.
10. Run the rank-order correlation test for a given set of data.
11. Determine the appropriate test of significance for a given research problem.

Many research studies involve rank order, rating scale, or frequency count data. These kinds of data are usually not interval or ratio in scale, and so inferences about means, for example, are inappropriate because the underlying assumptions of parametric analyses cannot be met. When we have nominal or ordinal data, we must use procedures specifically developed for them. Chapter 13 presented the chi-square test, a non-parametric technique appropriate for frequency data. This chapter presents some additional non-parametric analyses.

The Mann-Whitney U Test

The **Mann-Whitney U test** is used to make inferences about the difference between two populations. The test is sensitive to the entire distributions from which the samples were drawn as well as their central tendencies.

This test, used for ordinal data, is the non-parametric alternative to the t-test for the difference between independent groups.

Null and Alternative Hypotheses

The null hypothesis states that the populations from which the samples were drawn are identical. The alternative hypothesis states they are different.

H_o: The populations are identical.
H_a: The populations are not identical.

If the population distributions are similar in shape, the test compares their central tendencies. If the central tendencies are similar the test compares the entire distributions in general. As you can see, these hypotheses are slightly different from those used in inference with the t-distribution.

The Mann-Whitney U test requires that subjects are randomly selected and independently assigned to groups and that the scores are ranked in order.

The U Statistic

The Mann-Whitney test computes the **U** statistic which follows the U-distribution. The obtained U value is evaluated in terms of the sampling distribution of the U statistic. The U statistic which is tested for significance is the smaller of the following two values:

$$U_1 = n_1 n_2 + \frac{n_1(n_1 + 1)}{2} - \Sigma R_1$$

$$U_2 = n_1 n_2 + \frac{n_2(n_2 + 1)}{2} - \Sigma R_2$$

Mann-Whitney U statistic

where n_1 is the sample size of group 1; n_2 is the sample size of group 2; ΣR_1 is the sum of the ranks for group 1; and ΣR_2 is the sum of the ranks for group 2.

The critical values of U are found in Table B-6 (in Appendix B) for one- and two-tailed tests of significance. Enter the sample size for the first group along the top of the table, and the sample size of the second group along the side of the table. Unlike our previous tests, the obtained U value must be *smaller* than the critical value to be significant.

Running the Mann-Whitney U test

Step 1. Assign ranks to the scores in the groups.

This is done by combining and arranging the scores from both groups in order from the smallest to the largest and assigning a rank where 1 is the smallest score. For example, if a subject in Group 1 had the smallest score then that subject's rank would be 1. If the next smallest score was obtained by a subject in Group 2, then that subject would be assigned a rank of 2.

Step 2. Calculate the U statistic.

Step 3. Compare the obtained value with the critical value. The obtained value (U_{obt}) is the smaller of U_1 and U_2. If the obtained U value is smaller than the critical value, reject the null hypothesis; otherwise, do not reject the null hypothesis.

Ready for an example? Ten psychology professors and ten biology professors were given a questionnaire designed to measure their attitudes toward various controversial issues about the influence of heredity and environment on human behavior. Here are the data arranged in order for each group:

Scores on Questionnaire	
Biology Professors	**Psychology Professors**
2	6
3	8
11	16
13	17
15	23
25	24
27	26
33	37
39	38
45	49

First we need to assign ranks to all the scores. The smallest score, 2, appears in the biology professors' group and that score is assigned a rank of 1. Here are the rank order data:

| Ranks |
Biology Professors	Psychology Professors
1	3
2	4
5	8
6	9
7	10
12	11
14	13
15	16
18	17
19	20
Total = 99	Total = 111

Now we can use the formulas to compute each U value.

$$U_1 = n_1 n_2 + \frac{n_1(n_1 + 1)}{2} - \Sigma R_1$$

$$= 10(10) + \frac{10(11)}{2} - 99$$

$$= 100 + 55 - 99 = 56$$

$$U_2 = n_1 n_2 + \frac{n_2(n_2 + 1)}{2} - \Sigma R_2$$

$$= 10(10) + \frac{10(11)}{2} - 111$$

$$= 100 + 55 - 111 = 44$$

The second U value is smaller, so we compare it to the critical value. At $\alpha = .05$, the critical value is 23 for a two-tailed test (as listed in Table B-6). Since the smaller obtained U value is larger than the critical value, the null hypothesis is not rejected. We have no evidence that biology and psychology professors differ in terms of their attitudes toward the effect of heredity and environment on behavior. Remember that for this test the obtained U must be smaller than the critical value before we can reject the null.

Running the Mann-Whitney U Test for Large Sample Sizes

The sampling distribution of the U statistic approaches the normal distribution when both samples have 20 or more observations. In such cases, we can compute a Z value and use the normal curve tables in our test of significance.

After ranks have been assigned to the scores we can run the Mann-Whitney U in the following way:

Step 1. Determine the mean and standard deviation of the U statistic.
The sampling distribution of the U statistic has a mean of

$$\mu_u = n_1 n_2 / 2$$

and a standard deviation of

$$\sigma_u = \sqrt{\frac{n_1 n_2 (n_1 + n_2 + 1)}{12}}$$

Step 2. Compute the Z statistic.

Subtract the mean of the sampling distribution of our statistic (μ_u) from the obtained sample outcome (U) and divide by the standard error of the sampling distribution (σ_u). In notation:

$$Z = \frac{U - \mu_u}{\sigma_u} \quad \text{Z formula for the U statistic}$$

Step 3. Compare the obtained Z value with the critical value. If the obtained value is equal to or larger than the critical value, reject the null hypothesis; otherwise, do not reject the null hypothesis.

Ready for an example? Twenty randomly selected women and twenty randomly selected men are given a questionnaire designed to assess their feelings about the status of women in the work place. The data are considered ordinal. Arranged from lowest to highest, here are the scores and ranks.

Scores		Ranks	
Women	Men	Women	Men
3	5	1	3.5
4	7	2	6
5	9	3.5	8.5
6	10	5	10
8	11	7	11
9	18	8.5	17
12	19	12	18
14	20	13.5	19.5
14	21	13.5	21
16	23	15	23
17	24	16	24
20	29	19.5	27
22	31	22	28
27	34	25	30
28	37	26	33
32	39	29	35
35	41	31	36
36	46	32	38
38	48	34	39
43	52	37	40
		352.5	467.5

You will notice that some of the scores are equal. For example, two scores of 5 occurred, one in the women's group, the other in the men's. A common way to deal with tied scores is to assign the average of the ranks whose positions they take. Look at the two 5's that occurred. If these two scores were different, they would take positions 3 and 4. Because they are the same, they are assigned the average of those two rank positions, that is 3.5. If three 5's had occurred, each would be given the rank of 4, the average of positions 3, 4 and 5.

We can now go ahead and run our test. We first need to compute U_1 and U_2.

$$U_1 = n_1 n_2 + \frac{n_1(n_1 + 1)}{2} - \Sigma R_1$$

$$= 20(20) + \frac{20(21)}{2} - 352.5$$

$$= 257.5$$

$$U_2 = n_1 n_2 + \frac{n_2(n_2 + 1)}{2} - \Sigma R_2$$

$$= 20(20) + \frac{20(21)}{2} - 467.5$$

$$= 142.5$$

Since U_2 is the smaller value, we use 142.5 as the U value in our Z-test.

$$Z = \frac{U - \mu_u}{\sigma_u}$$

$$= \frac{U - n_1 n_2/2}{\sqrt{\frac{n_1 n_2 (n_1 + n_2 + 1)}{12}}}$$

$$= \frac{142.5 - (20)(20)/2}{\sqrt{(20)(20)(41)/12}}$$

$$= \frac{-57.5}{36.97}$$

$$= -1.56$$

The critical value for a Z-test is ± 1.96 for a two-tailed test at the .05 level of significance (as we discussed in Chapter 9). Since our obtained Z value was less than the critical value, we do not reject the null hypothesis. In other words, we have no evidence that men and women feel differently about the status of women in the workplace.

The Mann-Whitney test is the non-parametric alternative to the t-test for independent groups. It requires that the two samples be independent.

Additional Non-Parametric Techniques   335

If the two groups are dependent (for instance, the subjects are matched on certain characteristics or the groups contain the same subjects), then a different non-parametric test is required.

Summary of the Mann-Whitney U Test

Hypotheses
  H_o: Populations are identical.
  H_a: Populations are not identical.

Assumptions
  1. Subjects are randomly selected and independently assigned to groups.
  2. Measurement scale is at least ordinal.

Decision Rules
  If $U_{obt} \leq U_{crit}$, reject the H_o
  If $U_{obt} > U_{crit}$, do not reject the H_o

Formula
$$U_1 = n_1 n_2 + \frac{n_1(n_1 + 1)}{2} - \Sigma R_1$$
$$U_2 = n_1 n_2 + \frac{n_2(n_2 + 1)}{2} - \Sigma R_2$$
U_{obt} is the smaller of U_1 and U_2

The Wilcoxon Signed-Ranks Test

The **Wilcoxon signed-ranks test** is used for ordinal data obtained on the same or matched subjects.

Null and Alternative Hypotheses

The null and alternative hypotheses for the Wilcoxon test are identical to those in the Mann-Whitney test.

  H_o: The populations are identical.
  H_a: The populations are not identical.

The T Statistic

The Wilcoxon test computes the **T** statistic. (Note: This is not the same as the t-statistic). The T statistic follows the sampling distribution of T.
  The following procedure is used to conduct the Wilcoxon test.

Step 1. Calculate the difference between the two scores for each subject.

Step 2. Rank the absolute values (i.e., ignore the + or − sign of each value) of the difference scores from lowest to highest. Place the appropriate sign (+ or −) next to each rank.

Step 3. Sum the ranks with the less frequent sign. In other words, if there are fewer positive ranks than negative ranks, sum the values of the positive ranks. This is the T statistic.

Step 4. Compare the obtained value with the critical value.
Table B-7 (in Appendix B) provides the critical values of T for one- and two-tailed tests at various levels of significance. As with the Mann-Whitney test, the obtained T value must be *less* than the critical value for rejection of the null hypothesis.

Running the Wilcoxon Signed-Ranks Test

Let's work through an example. A French professor rated the pronunciation accuracy of 10 randomly selected students based on a pre-test. Scores could range from 0 to 15, with 15 representing excellent pronunciation. He provided these students with instruction in French pronunciation and then re-rated their accuracy on a post-test. Let's run a two-tailed test at $\alpha = .05$.

Student	Pre-test	Post-test	Difference	Rank
1	10	10	0	dropped
2	4	7	−3	−3.5
3	11	8	3	3.5
4	9	10	−1	−1
5	2	6	−4	−5
6	6	1	5	6
7	8	2	6	7
8	12	5	7	8
9	3	12	−9	−9
10	4	2	2	2

Like the Mann-Whitney test, tied difference scores are assigned shared ranks. Notice that when the two scores are equal and the difference is 0, the pair of scores is dropped from the analysis and n, the number of paired scores, is reduced accordingly.

There are fewer negatives than positives, so we sum all the ranks with negative signs. Our T value is 18.5.

To determine the critical value, we enter Table B-7 with the number of pairs of scores used in the final analysis. In our example, we dropped one pair of scores and so n = 9. We find that the critical value of T for a two-tailed test at α = .05 is 5. Since our obtained T value is greater than the critical value, we do not reject the null. Remember that, for this test, the obtained value must be smaller than the critical value to reject the null. There is no evidence that the professor's instruction affected the students' pronunciation accuracy.

Running the Wilcoxon Signed-Ranks Test for Large Sample Sizes

Like the Mann-Whitney test, when the samples are reasonably large (>20), the sampling distribution of T approaches the normal distribution and the Z statistic is used in the test for significance.

Step 1. Determine the mean and standard deviation of the T statistic.
The mean of the sampling distribution of T is

$$\mu_T = \frac{n(n+1)}{4}$$

and the standard deviation is

$$\sigma_T = \sqrt{\frac{n(n+1)(2n+1)}{24}}$$

Step 2. Compute the Z statistic.
The formula for converting T to Z is the following.

$$Z = \frac{T - \mu_T}{\sigma_T} \quad \text{Z formula for the T statistic}$$

Step 3. Compare the obtained Z value with the critical value. If the obtained Z value is equal to or larger than the critical value, reject the null hypothesis; otherwise, do not reject the null.

Let's look at an example. In a dog show, 20 Golden Retrievers were rated, by impartial judges, before and after receiving obedience training. Ratings were based on a scale from 0 to 5 with 5 representing excellent performance. Let's test the null hypothesis that training had no effect on the dog's behavior. Here are the total points received by each dog:

	Rating Before	Rating After	Difference	Rank
Spot	34	40	−6	−9.5
Fido	23	30	−7	−12
Breeze	56	55	1	1.5
Sydney	46	50	−4	−4.5
Amber	33	40	−7	−12
Dudley	38	39	−1	−1.5
Murphy	13	25	−12	−16
Karma	26	30	−4	−4.5
Shuba	22	25	−3	−3
Beast	37	43	−6	−9.5
Boga	19	36	−17	−20
Debit	27	34	−7	−12
Queenie	45	50	−5	−7
Bear	33	47	−14	−18
Murgatroyd	29	38	−9	−15
Fifi	30	25	5	7
Gemini	20	15	5	7
Phoenix	25	38	−13	−17
Luckenbach	15	31	−16	−19
Alfonse	50	42	8	14

In this example there are fewer positively signed ranks than negative ranks, so we sum the positive ranks. Our obtained T value is 29.5, the sum of the four positive ranks.

To compute the Z value:

$$Z = \frac{T - \mu_T}{\sigma_T}$$

$$= \frac{T - (n)(n+1)/4}{\sqrt{\frac{n(n+1)(2n+1)}{24}}}$$

$$= \frac{29.5 - 20(21)/4}{\sqrt{20(21)(41)/24}}$$

$$= \frac{-75.5}{26.79}$$

$$= -2.82$$

The critical Z at $\alpha = .01$ is ± 2.58; our obtained Z value is larger numerically than the critical value so we reject the null hypothesis and accept the alternative. Training had a significant effect on the ratings.

The Mann-Whitney and Wilcoxon tests are alternative analyses to t-tests. When the assumptions underlying inference with the t-distribution have not been met (for example, the data are ordinal in scale), then these tests are appropriate for testing hypotheses about the difference between two population distributions.

Summary of the Wilcoxon signed-ranks test

Hypotheses
H_o: Populations are identical
H_a: Populations are not identical

Assumptions
1. Subjects are randomly selected.
2. Same or matched subjects.
3. Measurement scale is at least ordinal.

Decision Rules
If $T_{obt} \leq T_{crit}$, reject the H_o
If $T_{obt} > T_{crit}$, do not reject the H_o

Formula
n = number of pairs with non-zero differences.
T is the sum of the absolute ranks with the less frequently appearing sign.

The Kruskal-Wallis Test

In Chapter 11, you learned how to use the F-distribution to test hypotheses about several population means. When the assumptions underlying ANOVA have not been met an alternative analysis is appropriate. The non-parametric analog to the one-way ANOVA is the Kruskal-Wallis test.

The **Kruskal-Wallis test** is used for ordinal data when subjects have been randomly selected and independently assigned to groups. The calculations for this test are similar to those used in the Mann-Whitney test.

Null and Alternative Hypotheses

The null hypothesis of the Kruskal-Wallis test states that all populations have identical distributions. The alternative is that the populations are not identical.

H_o: Populations are identical.
H_a: Populations are not identical.

The H Statistic

The statistic computed in the Kruskal-Wallis test is the **H** statistic. The sampling distribution of the H statistic follows the chi-square distribution with (k − 1) degrees of freedom, where k is the number of samples or groups in the experiment.

The computational formula for the H statistic is

$$H = \frac{12}{n_{tot}(n_{tot} + 1)}\left[\frac{(\Sigma R_1)^2}{n_1} + \frac{(\Sigma R_2)^2}{n_2} + \ldots + \frac{(\Sigma R_k)^2}{n_k}\right] - 3(n_{tot} + 1)$$

Kruskal-Wallis H statistic

where n_{tot} is the total number of observations; ΣR is the sum of the ranks of the scores in the group; and k is the number of groups.

Running the Kruskal-Wallis Test

The following lists the steps for running the Kruskal-Wallis test.

Step 1. Assign ranks to the scores in the groups.

All the scores are rank ordered from the smallest to the largest regardless of group membership. Ties are treated in the usual way.

Step 2. Calculate the H statistic.

Step 3. Compare the obtained H value with the critical value of χ^2. If the obtained value is equal to or larger than the critical value, reject the null hypothesis; otherwise, do not reject the null.

Let's look at an example. The President of a small junior college has obtained teaching evaluation ratings of eight professors in each of three faculties, Arts, Science, and Education. We compute the Kruskal-Wallis H to test the hypothesis that the ratings for Arts, Science, and Education professors don't differ. Here are the data.

Arts professors	Science professors	Education professors
13	23	17
12	30	10
16	29	28
27	14	20
19	11	22
18	9	21
15	24	8
31	32	26

These evaluation scores must be combined and then ranked from smallest to largest. The smallest score was obtained by the seventh Education professor, so this score is assigned the rank of 1. Here are the rank data.

Arts professors	Science professors	Education professors
6	16	10
5	22	3
9	21	20
19	7	13
12	4	15
11	2	14
8	17	1
23	24	18
93	113	94

Using our formula for the H statistic:

$$H = \frac{12}{n_{tot}(n_{tot}+1)} \left[\frac{(\Sigma R_1)^2}{n_1} + \frac{(\Sigma R_2)^2}{n_2} + ... + \frac{(\Sigma R_3)^2}{n_3} \right] - 3(n_{tot}+1)$$

$$= \frac{12}{24(24+1)} \left(\frac{93^2}{8} + \frac{113^2}{8} + \frac{94^2}{8} \right) - 3(24+1)$$

$$= 0.02(3781.75) - 75 = 0.63$$

The obtained H value is compared with the critical value of χ^2 with $(k-1)$ degrees of freedom. In our example, $k = 3$, and the critical value of χ^2 for 2 degrees of freedom, at $\alpha = .05$, is 5.99 (as listed in Table B-4). The obtained value is smaller than the critical value, so we do not reject the null hypothesis. We have no evidence that student evaluations of professors in Arts, Science, and Education are different.

Summary of the Kruskal-Wallis Test

Hypotheses
  H_o: Populations are identical
  H_a: Populations are not identical

Assumptions
  1. Subjects are randomly selected and independently assigned to groups.
  2. Measurement scale is at least ordinal.

Decision Rules
  df = k − 1
  If $H_{obt} \geq \chi^2_{crit}$, reject the H_o
  If $H_{obt} < \chi^2_{crit}$, do not reject the H_o

Formula
$$H = \frac{12}{n_{tot}(n_{tot} + 1)} \left[\frac{(\Sigma R_1)^2}{n_1} + \frac{(\Sigma R_2)^2}{n_2} + \ldots + \frac{(\Sigma R_k)^2}{n_k} \right] - 3(n_{tot} + 1)$$

The Spearman Rank-Order Correlation Test

The tests we have been studying are the non-parametric alternatives to some of the inferential techniques discussed in previous chapters. These are used for testing hypotheses about the equality of populations when the assumptions of parametric analysis have not been met.

Many research questions ask about the relationship between variables. In the next chapter, you will learn about Pearson's correlation test, a procedure for determining the strength of association between two variables. An adaptation of this test, the **rank-order correlation test**, is used for ordinal variables which have been rank-ordered.

When ordinal variables have been ranked and you wish to determine the relationship between the ranks, the **Spearman rank-order correlation test**, often called **Spearman's Rho**, is appropriate.

Null and Alternative Hypotheses

The null hypothesizes no correlation between the ranks. The alternative hypothesis may be non-directional (i.e., the correlation is not zero) or directional (i.e., the correlation is greater or less than zero).

H_o: Rho = 0
H_a: Rho ≠ 0, or Rho > 0, or Rho < 0

The rho Statistic

To be consistent, we will differentiate between the correlation in the population (Rho) and the sample statistic (rho).

The correlation rho is calculated on rank data with the following formula.

$$rho = 1 - \frac{6\Sigma d^2}{n(n^2 - 1)} \quad \text{Spearman rank-order correlation formula}$$

where n is the number of paired ranks; and d is the difference between the paired ranks.

Running the Spearman Rank-Order Correlation Test

The following describes the steps for running the rank-order correlation test.

Step 1. Determine the difference between the ranks for each subject.

Step 2. Square each difference and sum them.

Step 3. Calculate the rho statistic.

Step 4. Compare the obtained rho value with the critical value.
If the obtained value is equal to or larger than the critical value, reject the null hypothesis; otherwise, do not reject the null. Table B-8 (in Appendix B) provides the critical values of rho for various sample sizes and levels of significance. Remember that the sample size is the number of *pairs* of ranks.

Ready for an example? The Free Women's Coalition wishes to investigate the relationship between judges' rankings of entrants in the bathing suit competition and the talent competition in the Miss Canada Pageant. Here are the data:

	Rank-Orders			
Miss	Bathing Suit	Talent	d	d²
Edmonton	1	1	0	0
Vancouver	2	2	0	0
Regina	3	3	0	0
Winnipeg	4	4	0	0
Montreal	5	7	−2	4
Quebec	6	6	0	0
P.E.I.	7	5	2	4
Ottawa	8	9	−1	1
Toronto	9	8	1	1
Calgary	10	10	0	0
				10

Using our formula:

$$\text{rho} = 1 - \frac{6\Sigma d^2}{n(n^2 - 1)}$$

$$= 1 - \frac{6(10)}{10(100 - 1)}$$

$$= 1 - \frac{60}{990}$$

$$= 1 - 0.06 = 0.94$$

The critical value of rho is 0.65, at $\alpha = 0.05$ for a two-tailed test, when there are ten subjects (see Table B-8). The obtained value is larger than the critical value and the null hypothesis is rejected. There is a significant correlation between judges' rankings of the women in the bathing suit and talent competition.

The rank-order correlation test is very useful for ranked data. If the original data are not in rank order form, they must be converted to use the rho formula.

Summary of the Spearman Rank-Order Correlation Test

Hypotheses
  H_o: Rho = 0
  H_a: Rho ≠ 0 or Rho < 0 or Rho > 0

Assumptions
  1. Subjects are randomly selected.
  2. Observations are rank-ordered.

Decision Rules
  n = number of pairs of ranks
  If $rho_{obt} \geq rho_{crit}$, reject H_o
  If $rho_{obt} < rho_{crit}$, do not reject H_o

Formula
$$rho = 1 - \frac{6\Sigma d^2}{n(n^2 - 1)}$$

Choosing the Appropriate Test of Significance

In this chapter you learned about four non-parametric tests of significance, three of which are the non-parametric equivalents to parametric tests. The Mann-Whitney U test is the non-parametric equivalent to the t-test for independent means. The Wilcoxon Signed-Ranks test is the alternative to the t-test for dependent means. The Kruskal-Wallis test is the non-parametric equivalent to the one-way ANOVA. The more difficult aspects of making decisions between parametric and non-parametric approaches will be addressed elsewhere in this book but serious students should consult upper-level textbooks for clarification on issues concerning violation of parametric assumptions.

Let's go through the steps required to decide if the analysis should be a parametric or a non-parametric approach. Only the Mann-Whitney, the Wilcoxon, and the Kruskal-Wallis tests and their parametric equivalents will be considered in this section.

Step 1. Determine the number of groups in the experiment.
  If more than two groups are involved in the experiment, determine whether the data are measures from subjects in all groups or if the data are ranks of subjects in all groups. If subjects have been ranked, the appropriate analysis is the Kruskal-Wallis procedure. If measures have been taken and means will be computed, the appropriate analysis is the one-way ANOVA. If there are two groups or less in the experiment, we go to Step 2.

Step 2. Determine if repeated measures have been taken or if subjects have been matched in some way.

If subjects have contributed more than one observation, or if subjects have been matched on some variable, determine whether the data are measures from subjects in all groups or if the data are ranks of subjects in all groups. For data that are measures from subjects that will be used to compute means, a t-test for dependent means should be used. If the data are ranks, then the Wilcoxon test is appropriate. If there are two independent groups, we go to Step 3.

Step 3. Determine the kind of data involved.

If repeated measures have not been taken and groups have not been matched you have an independent groups design. With rank data you will run a Mann-Whitney U test and with measurement data you will run a t-test for independent groups.

Example A Six groups of randomly assigned laboratory rats have received different reinforcement experiences for running a maze. The amount of reinforcement varied from one pellet (Group 1) to six pellets (Group 6) of rat treats for each trial. After two weeks of experience, all the rats were placed in a maze they had not experienced previously. Each rat was given thirty trials in the new maze and the number of trials that the rat completed the maze within a given period of time was recorded. After all rats had been tested they were rank ordered according to the number of trials where completion occurred so that a rat who completed all thirty trials under the time limit was ranked number one and so on.

Step 1. Determine the number of groups in the experiment.

There are six groups in this experiment, each group receiving different amounts of reinforcement. Because the investigator rank ordered the animals, he will use the Kruskal-Wallis test to analyze the difference between the six groups.

Example B Six groups of randomly assigned laboratory rats have received different reinforcement experiences for running a maze. The amount of reinforcement varied from one pellet (Group 1) to six pellets (Group 6) of rat treats for each trial. After two weeks of experience, all the rats were placed in a maze they had not experienced previously. Each rat was given thirty trials in the new maze and the time to complete the maze was recorded. After all rats had been tested the average time to complete the maze was computed for each group.

Step 1. Determine the number of groups in the experiment.

There are six groups of animals in this experiment. The data consisted of mean time to complete the maze. The group performance will be compared using a one-way ANOVA.

Example C An industrial psychologist was hired by a large company to investigate employee morale. The company was interested in whether morale would improve if its employees could share in the profits of the company. The psychologist measured morale of twenty company employees with a rating scale. Six months after a profit-sharing scheme was introduced morale was measured again.

Step 1. Determine the number of groups in the experiment.
There is only one group in this experiment, the twenty employees, so we go to Step 2.

Step 2. Determine if repeated measures have been taken or if subjects have been matched in some way.
The twenty employees provided two observations: morale rating before and after the introduction of the profit-sharing program. Rating scale data are usually considered ordinal and the preferable analysis for this study is likely a Wilcoxon test.

Example D A sociologist measured the psychosocial well-being of thirty randomly selected single mothers and thirty randomly selected married mothers using an ordinal scale with several subscales. She wanted to compare the two groups.

Step 1. Determine the number of groups in the experiment.
There are two groups in the study, so we go to Step 2.

Step 2. Determine if repeated measures have been taken or if subjects have been matched in some way.
There are two independent groups, so we go to Step 3.

Step 3. Determine the kind of data involved.
The ordinal scale data involved in this study would most likely be analyzed using a Mann-Whitney U test.

Example E A criminologist compared the number of crimes committed per year in ten western cities with ten eastern cities all of approximately the same population. He was interested in determining whether average yearly crime rate differed between the east and the west.

Step 1. Determine the number of groups in the experiment.
There are two groups, so we go to Step 2.

Step 2. Determine if repeated measures have been taken or if subjects have been matched in some way.
The subjects in this study are cities. The groups are independent and so we go to Step 3.

Step 3. Determine the kind of data involved.
The data are mean crime rates and the appropriate analysis is a t-test for independent groups.

FOCUS ON RESEARCH

McKaye, Louda, and Stauffer, Jr., (1990) were interested in the effects of nest (bower) size on the female cichlid fish's choice of a mate (and therefore, male reproductive success).* Part of their study is discussed here. In the cichlid species the male builds the bower, which resembles a sand-castle, and defends it. It is a courtship and spawning site. The female enters the bower to deposit eggs. The researchers expected that male reproductive success improves as bower size increases. Specifically they expected that males above large bowers would attract more females and would defend the bower more aggressively than males above small bowers.

The Data
Forty-three pairs of males were observed for 10-minute periods. One of each pair of fish was above a "tall" bower and the other was above a "short" bower. The observers recorded courtship bouts and attacks on other fish. Reproductive success was estimated in part by counting the number of times a female entered the bower.

The Variables
The independent variable was bower size and the dependent variables included courtship and attack.

The Analyses
The data are paired frequency counts and so the Wilcoxon Signed-Ranks Test was used to test for significant difference between the tall-bower males and the short-bower males.

The expectations regarding courtship were confirmed. Males above tall bowers had more courtship opportunities ($p<.01$) and attracted more females into their bowers ($p<.01$) than the males above short bowers.

Their hypothesis that males would defend tall bowers more aggressively than short bowers was also confirmed with the Wilcoxon Test. Males spent more time and energy defending their bower from other breeding and non-breeding males of the same species ($p<.01$).

The authors concluded that the height of the bower is an important factor in the attraction of females to a bower and mate.

SUMMARY OF TERMS AND FORMULAS

When the underlying assumptions of parametric analyses have not been met, a **non-parametric** approach may be appropriate.

The **Mann-Whitney U test** is analogous to the t-test for the difference between independent means.

---

* McKaye, K.R., Louda, S.M., and Stauffer, Jr., J.R. (1990). Bower Size and Male Reproductive Success in a Cichlid Fish Lek. *The American Naturalist, 135,* 597–613.

For samples which are correlated or dependent, the **Wilcoxon signed-ranks test** is appropriate and is the non-parametric equivalent to the t-test for dependent means.

When the assumptions of ANOVA have not been met, the **Kruskal-Wallis test** may be used.

Spearman's rank-order correlation test is used to determine the relationship between two sets of rank-ordered data.

Test	Computational Formula
Mann-Whitney	$U_1 = n_1 n_2 + \dfrac{n_1(n_1 + 1)}{2} - \Sigma R_1$ $U_2 = n_1 n_2 + \dfrac{n_2(n_2 + 1)}{2} - \Sigma R_2$
Z Formula	$Z = \dfrac{U - n_1 n_2 / 2}{\sqrt{n_1 n_2 (n_1 + n_2 + 1)/12}}$
Wilcoxon Z formula	$Z = \dfrac{T - n(n+1)/4}{\sqrt{n(n+1)(2n+1)/24}}$
Kruskal-Wallis	$H = \dfrac{12}{n_{tot}(n_{tot} + 1)} \left[\dfrac{(\Sigma R_1)^2}{n_1} + \dfrac{(\Sigma R_2)^2}{n_2} + \ldots + \dfrac{(\Sigma R_k)^2}{n_k} \right] - 3(n_{tot} + 1)$
Spearman Rank-Order Correlation	$\text{rho} = 1 - \dfrac{6 \Sigma d^2}{n(n^2 - 1)}$

EXERCISES

1. A random sample of students from a Liberal Arts College and another random sample from a Church Work Training College are given a questionnaire designed to measure their attitude toward capital punishment. The scores are given below. A high score reflects pro capital punishment.

Liberal Arts Students	Church Work Students
10	6
11	5
12	3
14	7
18	6
8	2
9	4
7	10

   Run a Mann-Whitney U test on these data with $\alpha = .01$. What are your conclusions?

2. A social psychologist used an Aggression Scale to rate the aggressiveness of children before and after they viewed a violent cartoon show. Run a Wilcoxon test on the data below at $\alpha = .05$. What are your conclusions?

Aggressiveness Rating	
Before	After
2.0	2.5
3.5	2.5
1.5	2.0
2.5	2.5
3.0	1.5
4.0	4.5
1.0	2.5
3.0	2.5
1.5	3.0

3. Kayakers have been asked to rate the quality of 3 different boats. Run a Kruskal-Wallis test to see if the ratings differ ($\alpha = .05$). Do they?

	Ratings	
Eclipse	Mirage	Dancer
6.0	5.3	3.5
6.5	5.4	3.3
5.2	4.7	3.6
4.8	3.1	2.9
6.1	3.9	4.0

4. The ten Canadian provinces have been rank ordered according to crime rate in 1980 and in 1990. Run the rank-order correlation test to see if the rankings are related ($\alpha = .05$).

City	1980	1990
B.C.	1	3
Alta.	2	1
Man.	3	5
Sask.	4	4
Ont.	5	2
Que.	6	8
P.E.I.	7	6
N.S.	8	7
N.B.	9	9
N.F.	10	10

5. Plot the data from Exercise 4 on a scattergraph.

6. An ecologist has assessed pollution and crime rate for nine Canadian cities, using a standard index. Calculate Spearman's rho for the following raw score data. Remember you must rank the data first.

	Pollution	Crime rate
Toronto	20	3
Vancouver	17	9
Montreal	15	2
Ottawa	14	4
Regina	12	10
Calgary	12	1
Winnipeg	11	5
Edmonton	9	11
St. John's	6	8

7. Compute Spearman's rho for the following data.

Var 1	Var 2
51	62
53	69
55	63
56	52
57	53
59	81
61	90
64	84
66	45
68	60
68	65
72	67
73	54
75	53
75	58
76	59
76	49
76	72
78	63
83	69
87	61
89	53

8. Run a Mann-Whitney U test on the following data. Since there are more than 20 observations in each group you will run the test for large sample sizes.

Group 1	Group 2
64	62
78	69
68	63
57	52
76	53
75	81
73	90
66	84
87	45
89	60
68	65
59	67
72	54
83	53
61	58
56	59
76	49
55	72
53	63
76	69
75	61
51	53

a. $\Sigma R_1 =$
   $\Sigma R_2 =$
b. $U_1 =$
   $U_2 =$
c. $Z_{obt} =$
d. $Z_{.05} =$
e. Decision:

9. Run a Kruskal-Wallis test on the data given below.

Group 1	Group 2	Group 3
45	59	72
49	60	72
51	61	73
52	61	75
53	62	75
53	63	76
53	63	76
53	64	76
54	65	78
55	66	81
56	67	83
57	68	84
58	68	87
58	69	89
59	69	90

a. $\Sigma R_1 =$
 $\Sigma R_2 =$
 $\Sigma R_3 =$
b. $H =$
c. $\chi^2_{.05} =$
d. Decision:

CHAPTER 16

Pearson's Correlational Technique

LEARNING OBJECTIVES

After reading this chapter you should be able to:
1. Describe the difference between a positive and a negative correlation.
2. Compute Pearson's coefficient using a raw score, a deviation score, and a Z-score formula.
3. Describe the difference between linear and non-linear relationships.
4. Describe the term "homoscedasticity" as it refers to bivariate distributions.
5. Describe the effect of discontinuity on the coefficient of correlation.
6. Define and provide a formula for the coefficient of determination.
7. Provide the t-ratio for the correlation coefficient.
8. Run a correlation test of significance for a given set of data.

Correlational techniques are used to determine if two variables are related. In Chapter 2 you learned how to construct a scattergraph of a bivariate frequency distribution. A scattergraph shows the relationship between two variables. By examining a scattergraph, you can see whether or not two variables appear to be related. This relationship can be quantified by a *coefficient of correlation*, a value which indicates the strength of the relationship between two variables.

Correlation is a valuable statistical technique used in a great deal of research, particularly in medical research. For example, the general health of pregnant women is correlated with the birth weight of their babies. Stress is correlated with heart problems in men. Did you know that men's hair loss is correlated with their educational level? As number of years of education increase, so does the amount of hair lost in male adults. This latter example illustrates a very important rule: **correlation** *does not imply causation!* The correlation between two variables does not tell us that one variable caused the other, or vice versa. A correlation, no matter how strong, does not provide any information about cause. A strong correlation only tells us that two variables tend to vary together. Why they do this is a question that only a well-controlled *experiment* can answer.

When we say that two variables are positively correlated, we mean that the values of these variables tend to increase and decrease together. For example, studying is positively correlated with grades. In other words, if you increase your study time your grade point average will tend to increase as well.

When two variables are negatively correlated, the values of the first variable tend to increase as the values of the second variable decrease. Age and visual acuity are negatively correlated. As people get older, their vision tends to get poorer.

The correlation between high school grades and post-secondary performance may be of interest to you. After many years of collecting data, most colleges and universities have found that their students with higher high school grades tend to do better than those with poorer grades. In other words, there is a positive correlation between high school grades and college grades. Colleges and universities use this correlation for screening applicants to their programs. We will look at how correlational information is used to predict future events from current events in the next chapter.

Correlational techniques can be used not only to *describe* the relationship between two variables, but also to make inferences about the correlation between two variables in a population from a sample drawn from that population. We will start by discussing correlation as a descriptive technique. We will then discuss correlation as an inferential technique.

Correlation as a Descriptive Technique

When two variables are correlated, the values of the first variable tend to increase or decrease in a regular fashion with the values of the second variable. When high values of one variable are associated with high values of another, and low values of the first are associated with low values of the second, the two variables are *positively* correlated. On the other hand, when high values of one variable are associated with low values of another, the two variables are *negatively* correlated.

The **correlation coefficient** tells us how strongly the two variables are related and in what fashion. All correlation coefficients range from $+1$ to -1. A correlation coefficient of 1 is a perfect correlation and means that values of one variable are exactly related to values of another variable. A correlation coefficient of 0 indicates that the values of the first variable are unrelated to the values of the second variable.

Several ways of computing correlation coefficients have been developed. The choice of one over another depends upon the variables of interest. When both variables are continuous, Pearson's product-moment coefficient of correlation is used.

Pearson's Product-Moment Coefficient of Correlation (ρ)

Pearon's product-moment correlation coefficient is used to determine the extent of relationship between two variables. Pearson developed this coefficient by fitting a straight line to a bivariate frequency distribution. The line is called the **straight line of best fit**. The next chapter describes how Pearson fit this line to the data.

Basically, the coefficient of correlation (ρ, pronounced "rho") is a number describing how close the points in a bivariate frequency distribution fit a straight line. If all the points fall on the line, the correlation is 1: a perfect correlation. If all the points do not fall on the line, the correlation coefficient will be less than 1.

Calculating the Coefficient of Correlation (ρ)

The formula for calculating Pearson's coefficient of correlation varies depending on the data. We will look at versions of the formula for three types of data: raw scores, deviation scores, and Z-scores.

Data in Raw Score Form

For raw data, the formula for Pearson's ρ is

$$\rho = \frac{\Sigma XY - (\Sigma X)(\Sigma Y)/N}{\sqrt{[\Sigma X^2 - (\Sigma X)^2/N][\Sigma Y^2 - (\Sigma Y)^2/N]}} \quad \text{Pearson's } \rho \text{ for raw data}$$

In the numerator ΣXY is the sum of the *cross-products* of the values for each variable; $(\Sigma X)(\Sigma Y)$ is the product of the sum of X and the sum of Y; and N is the number of pairs of scores. In the denominator, the square root is taken of the product of the sum of squares in X and the sum of squares in Y.

Ready for an example? Suppose I gathered data about the television habits of ten children in my son's kindergarten class. I asked their teachers to rate the aggressiveness of each child, on a scale from 1 to 10, during each recess period for one month. Variable X is the mean rating per week for each child. I also asked the parents of these children to determine the amount of violent T.V. their children watch each week. The mean number of hours watched by each chi'd per week is my Y variable. I am interested in determining whether those children who are rated as most aggressive are also the children who watch a lot of violent television programs. Let's determine whether these two variables, aggressiveness (X) and T.V. habits (Y), are related.

Child	X	Y	X²	Y²	XY
Ben	8.5	5.8	72.3	33.6	49.30
Gabor	4.3	3.6	18.5	13.0	15.48
Linda	5.6	4.0	31.4	16.0	22.40
Luke	2.2	1.5	4.8	2.3	3.30
Hiro	6.5	6.3	42.3	39.7	40.95
Matthew	8.2	7.5	67.2	56.3	61.50
Mia	9.7	8.0	94.1	64.0	77.60
Ashley	1.0	2.2	1.0	4.8	2.20
Serge	3.5	3.1	12.3	9.6	10.85
Padraic	5.0	3.0	25.0	9.0	15.00
Totals	54.5	45.0	368.8	248.2	298.58

$$\rho = \frac{\Sigma XY - (\Sigma X)(\Sigma Y)/N}{\sqrt{[\Sigma X^2 - (\Sigma X)^2/N][\Sigma Y^2 - (\Sigma Y)^2/N]}}$$

$$= \frac{298.58 - (54.5)(45)/10}{\sqrt{[368.8 - (54.5)^2/10][248.2 - (45)^2/10]}}$$

$$= \frac{53.33}{(8.47)(6.76)} = 0.93$$

The correlation between teachers' ratings of the children's aggressiveness and number of hours watching violent TV, recorded by the parents, is 0.93. This suggests that the children who are rated most aggressive watch a lot of violent television programs, according to their parents.

Data in Deviation Score Form

When the data are in deviation score form, the formula for Pearson's coefficient is

$$\rho = \frac{\Sigma xy}{\sqrt{(\Sigma x^2)(\Sigma y^2)}} \qquad \text{Pearson's } \rho \text{ for deviation data}$$

Here Σxy is the sum of the cross-products of the deviation scores for each variable; (Σx^2) is the sum of the squared deviations in X; and (Σy^2) is the sum of the squared deviations in Y.

Let's use the previous example to verify our formula. Here are the data in deviation score form.

	x	y	x^2	y^2	xy
Ben	3.0	1.3	9.0	1.7	3.9
Gabor	−1.2	−0.9	1.4	0.8	1.1
Linda	0.1	−0.5	0.0	0.3	−0.1
Luke	−3.3	−3.0	10.9	9.0	9.9
Hiro	1.0	1.8	1.0	3.2	1.8
Matthew	2.7	3.0	7.3	9.0	8.1
Mia	4.2	3.5	17.6	12.3	14.7
Ashley	−4.5	−2.3	20.3	5.3	10.3
Serge	−2.0	−1.4	4.0	2.0	2.8
Padraic	−0.5	−1.5	0.3	2.3	0.8
Totals			71.77	45.74	53.33

Using the deviation score formula:

$$\rho = \frac{\Sigma xy}{\sqrt{(\Sigma x^2)(\Sigma y^2)}}$$

$$= \frac{53.33}{\sqrt{(71.77)(45.74)}} = \frac{53.33}{57.3} = 0.93$$

As you can see, the result is the same as that for the raw score data.

Data in Z-Score Form

When the data are in Z-score form, the formula for Pearson's correlation is

$$\rho = \frac{\Sigma(Z_x Z_y)}{N} \quad \text{Pearson's } \rho \text{ for Z-score data}$$

The cross-products of the Z-scores are summed and divided by the number of scores.

To show how this formula works, we will use the same data we used before. Now the scores have been converted to Z-scores.

	Z_x	Z_y	$Z_x Z_y$
Ben	1.12	0.61	0.68
Gabor	−0.45	−0.42	0.19
Linda	0.04	−0.23	−0.01
Luke	−1.23	−1.40	1.73
Hiro	0.37	0.84	0.31
Matthew	1.01	1.40	1.41
Mia	1.57	−1.64	2.56
Ashley	−1.68	−1.07	1.80
Serge	−0.75	−0.65	0.49
Padraic	−0.19	−0.70	0.13
Total			9.30

$$\rho = \frac{\Sigma(Z_x Z_y)}{N}$$

$$= \frac{9.30}{10} = 0.93$$

Once again, the result is the same because this formula is algebraically equivalent to the others.

Factors Influencing the Correlation Coefficient

I am sure every statistics student and most introductory psychology students have been told over and over that *correlation does not imply causation.* You know that the coefficient of correlation measures the degree to which two variables are related. It does not tell you anything about the reason for the relationship. If variable A is correlated with variable B, then we know that values of A tend to be associated with values of B. We do not know if A causes B, if B causes A, or if some other variable is responsible for the relationship. Earlier the correlation between hair loss and educational level of males was mentioned. It appeared that as men become more educated, they tend to lose more hair. Now if we were naive, we might think that education *causes* hair loss; perhaps studying causes stress which causes hair loss. Or perhaps hair loss *causes* men to seek more education; bald men do not date much, so they have more time to fill, so they take more courses. Clearly this is ridiculous. What we are actually seeing is a relationship between two variables, hair loss and education, which is caused by a third variable, age. Older men tend to have more years of education. Similarly, because they are older, they have less hair! Consider the following statements:

"People who brush with 'Brand X' toothpaste have fewer cavities."
"People who use 'Brand X' detergent have whiter clothes."

These statements imply that the use of a product will cause certain wonderful things to happen. This is not necessarily the case.

Linearity of Regression

The strength of the correlation depends on how closely the points hug the straight line of best fit. In a particular set of data, however, a straight line may or may not describe the relationship between the variables. A straight line is appropriate for variables that are linearly related. But what if X and Y are not linearly related?

Figure 16-1 presents are scattergraphs of two bivariate frequency distributions.

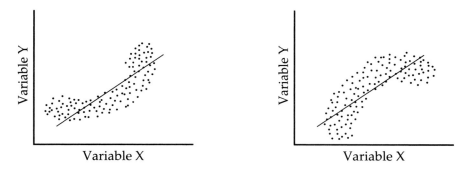

Figure 16-1   Examples of curvilinear relationships

If we calculated the correlation coefficient, ρ, for either of these distributions, it would be quite low; the points do not fit a straight line very well. In both cases, a curvilinear function best describes the relationship between the variables. Whenever the relationship between two variables is not linear, ρ will *underestimate* the strength of the relationship.

Homoscedasticity

When the amount of scatter is the same throughout a bivariate distribution, it is said to have the property of homoscedasticity or equal variability.

Examine the two scattergraphs in Figure 16-2. The scattergraph on the left shows homoscedasticity. No matter which value of X is chosen, the corresponding Y values are equally scattered around the straight line of best fit. In the scattergraph on the right, however, this is not the case. If X is low, Y does not vary much around the line; for higher values of X, the corresponding Y values vary a great deal. The second distribution does not have homoscedasticity.

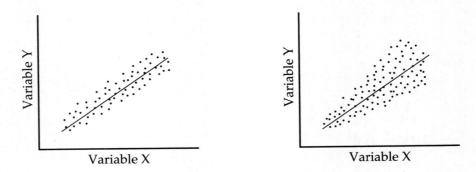

Figure 16-2 Bivariate distributions differing in homoscedasticity

Pearson's ρ reflects the "average" degree to which the scores hug the line of best fit. For the scattergraph on the right, ρ will underestimate the strength of the relationship for low values of X and overestimate it for high values of X.

Discontinuous Distributions

Whenever the range of one or both variables is restricted in some way, ρ will be affected. For example, if the middle of a distribution is excluded, the ρ will be higher than if the middle had been included. This might occur if we were to correlate the high and low scores without including the middle scores. Suppose the Dean of Arts wished to know if the grade point average of his 1st year Arts students correlated with their high school grades. He has data for students who failed and for those who received honors in their first year. He has no data for the middle students. If he calculates Pearson's ρ for this *discontinuous* distribution, the ρ value will be somewhat higher than if he had all the data available. Similarly, if the extreme scores were omitted from the calculation, ρ will tend to be lower.

Interpreting the Coefficient of Correlation

Unless ρ is 1, the coefficient of correlation does not directly indicate the association between Y and X. For example, a ρ value of 0.50 does not mean that there is a 50% association between the two variables. However, the square of ρ does indicate the degree of the association.

The coefficient of determination, ρ^2, reflects the degree of association between Y and X. For a correlation coefficient of 0.50, the coefficient of determination (ρ^2) is 0.25. This indicates the strength of the association. Specifically, 0.25 or 1/4 of the total Y variance is due to the correlation of Y with X. The coefficient of determination will be discussed in detail in the next chapter. For now, remember that ρ^2 reflects the amount of association between the two variables.

> **Coefficient of determination:** Indicates the strength of relationship between two variables.

Correlation as an Inferential Technique

When we draw samples from a population, determine the correlation between two variables, and make inferences about the value of the correlation in the population, we are using correlation as an inferential technique. Like any inferential technique, we do this when we can't obtain all the observations in a population.

We will examine one test involving correlation — testing the hypothesis that the population correlation is zero. As you will see, the formulas and notation change when we use correlation in inference.

Null and Alternative Hypotheses

The null hypothesis states that, in the bivariate population from which the sample was selected, the correlation is zero.

$$H_o: \rho = 0$$

The alternative hypothesis may be directional or non-directional.

$$H_a: \rho \neq 0$$
$$H_a: \rho > 0$$
$$H_a: \rho < 0$$

You will recall that whenever we sample from a population, the sample statistics vary from sample to sample. This is called sampling fluctuation. Even if the correlation in a population was truly zero, we would not expect a sample correlation of exactly zero. We would expect some variability. Our question here, as with any inferential technique, is "How far from zero would our sample correlation be expected to vary if the true population correlation is indeed zero?"

To answer this question, we need a distribution of correlations based on samples drawn from a population with a correlation of zero; the **random sampling distribution of the correlation coefficient**. The mean of this sampling distribution will be zero. The coefficient of correlation computed on a sample is called "r." The estimate of the standard deviation or standard error of this sampling distribution is denoted as s_r. When the null hypothesis is true, the sampling distribution of the correlation coefficient is close to the normal distribution for reasonably large samples.

Testing the Significance of the Correlation

To test the significance of a correlation, we need to compute r from the sample data. The formula is

$$r = \frac{\Sigma XY - (\Sigma X)(\Sigma Y)/n}{\sqrt{[\Sigma X^2 - (\Sigma X)^2/n][\Sigma Y^2 - (\Sigma Y)^2/n]}} \quad \text{coefficient of correlation for a sample}$$

The obtained r value may be compared with the critical value of r by entering the degrees of freedom into Table B-9 of Appendix B. The degrees of freedom for testing the correlation are number of pairs minus two (n − 2).

The significance of the correlation can also be determined with a t-test when n is large and r is small. However, if n is small and r is reasonably large it is easier and probably more accurate to use Table B-9 in Appendix B.

To use a t-test to determine the significance of a correlation we must convert our sample statistic, r, to a standard score. As you recall, this is done by subtracting the hypothesized parameter from the sample statistic and dividing the difference by the standard error of the sampling distribution of the statistic.

$$t = \frac{r - \rho}{s_r} \quad \text{t formula for the r statistic}$$

The estimate of the standard deviation, the standard error, is found by the following formula:

$$s_r = \sqrt{\frac{1 - r^2}{n - 2}} \quad \text{standard error for the r statistic}$$

When we do this for r, we obtain standard scores which follow the t-distribution with (n − 2) degrees of freedom, where n refers to the number of pairs of scores.

After computing the t value, we test our coefficient for significance by looking up the critical value of t for (n − 2) degrees of freedom.

Let's do an example. A researcher randomly selects ten students and administers a test of creativity and a test of mathematical competence. He discovers that the correlation between the scores on the two tests is 0.80. He wants to test the hypothesis that creativity is significantly correlated to mathematical competence.

$H_o: \rho = 0$
$H_a: \rho \neq 0$

$$s_r = \sqrt{\frac{1 - r^2}{n - 2}} = \sqrt{\frac{1 - 0.80^2}{8}} = 0.21$$

$$t = \frac{r - \rho}{s_r}$$

$$= \frac{0.80 - 0}{0.21} = 3.81$$

The critical value of t is ±2.31 with 8 df at $\alpha = .05$ (as listed in Table B-2). Since the obtained t falls in the region of rejection, the null hypothesis is rejected. The researcher has evidence that creativity and mathematical competence are significantly correlated.

Assumptions Underlying Inference about Correlations

The assumptions underlying tests of significance of correlation coefficients are similar to those of several parametric analyses we have discussed previously. First, the subjects are assumed to be randomly selected from the population. Second, normal population distributions of both X and Y are assumed. When the sample is reasonably large (30 or more), this assumption will not be badly violated because the sampling distribution of r tends to be normal, regardless of population shape.

Summary of the Pearson Correlation Test

Hypotheses
$H_o: \rho = 0$
$H_a: \rho \neq 0, \rho < 0, \rho > 0$

Assumptions
1. Subjects are randomly selected.
2. Both populations are normally distributed.

Decision Rules
If $t_{obt} \geq t_{crit}$, reject H_o
If $t_{obt} < t_{crit}$, do not reject H_o

Formula
$$t = \frac{r - \rho}{\sqrt{\frac{1 - r^2}{n - 2}}}$$

Other Correlation Coefficients

Several other correlation coefficients have been developed that are suitable for a variety of types of variables. Recall in Chapter 15 the rank-order correlation test which is appropriate when both variables are ranks. In Chapter 14, we referred to a correlation coefficient used to determine the strength of the relationship between variables following a chi-square test for independence. Although it is beyond the scope of this book to discuss additional coefficients in detail, mention of some of the available techniques might be in order. The Pearson coefficient, you will recall, measures the degree to which the points in a scattergraph hug the line of best fit. The line of best fit is a straight line. In others words, Pearson's coefficient measures only linear relationships. We have seen that when the relationship between two variables is non-linear, Pearson's coefficient will be inappropriate. A correlation coefficient that measures non-linear relationships is called the **correlation ratio** or **eta squared** (η^2). This coefficient is found by fitting the data points in a scattergraph to whatever line is appropriate. If the line is curved, for example, the coefficient fits the points to that curved line. Although there are statistical tests to determine whether the relationship is linear or non-linear, it's quite a simple matter to plot the scattergraph and find out for yourself.

Other coefficients that have been developed include **Kendall's tau** (τ) for monotonically related ranks, the **point biserial** (r_{pb}) for quantitative vs dichotomous variables, the **biserial** (r_b) for quantitative variables where one has been made dichotomous, the **tetrachoric** (r_t) where quantitative variables have both been dichotomized, and the **phi** (ϕ) coefficient where both variables are dichotomous. Interested students are encouraged to consult upper level statistic texts for information on these correlation coefficients.

FOCUS ON RESEARCH

A cross-national survey was conducted by Kalleberg and Rosenfeld (1990)* to examine the interrelationships by gender between domestic work and labor market work in the United States, Canada, Norway, and Sweden. The researchers had several hypotheses they wished to test. For example, they hypothesized that the ways women balance working in and outside the home would differ between countries. Women living in countries where part-time employment is more flexible (e.g. Sweden, Norway) should be better able to balance the two kinds of work than women living in countries where employment outside the home is less flexible (e.g. Canada, US).

The Data
The data were collected by interview and by telephone and mail questionnaire. An attempt to randomly sample was made with certain restrictions.

The Variables
The dependent variables included number of hours worked per week, and a percentage measure of household division of labour. Several variables were controlled in the study. These included spouse employment, children in the home, sex-role attitude, and other demographic factors such as level of education, age, and gender.

The Analyses
Because the researchers were interested in the interrelationships by gender between the various countries, they chose a correlational analysis. The data, number of hours worked and percentage of household tasks, were continuous. The Pearson correlation coefficient was used.

The Results
Here are some of the preliminary results obtained in the study.

---

* Source: Kalleberg, A.L. and Rosenfeld, R.A. (1990). Work in the Family and in the Labor Market: A Cross-National, Reciprocal Analysis, *Journal of Marriage and the Family*, 52, 331–46.

Table 16-1 Results of the study

Variable	US Male	US Female	Canada Male	Canada Female	Norway Male	Norway Female	Sweden Male	Sweden Female
Number of hours employed	47.3	39.7	45.9	35.2	43.0	30.1	42.4	32.2
Percentage of child care claimed by respondent	36.3	64.0	36.7	65.0	29.2	50.8	24.8	53.2
Percentage of household work claimed by respondent	22.5	78.7	21.6	79.8	23.3	77.4	27.1	74.0

Source: Kalleberg and Rosenfeld (1990). Copyright 1990 by the National Council on Family Relations, 3989 Central Avenue, N.E., Suite 550, Minneapolis, MN 55421. Reprinted by permission.

In all cases men worked more hours outside of the home than did women and women did more child care and household work than men.

The dependent variable, number of hours worked, was correlated with percentage of household work and percentage of child care for each country by gender. Here are some of the results of the correlational analysis.

Table 16-2 Analysis of data

Hours worked correlated with	US Male	US Female	Canada Male	Canada Female	Norway Male	Norway Female	Sweden Male	Sweden Female
Percentage of household work	−0.11*	−0.28*	−0.08	−0.15*	−0.18*	−0.26*	−0.28*	−0.45*
Percentage of child care	−0.15*	−0.20	−0.02	−0.10	−0.09	−0.09	−0.23*	−0.17*

* $p < .01$

Source: Kalleberg and Rosenfield (1990), Copyright 1990 by the National Council on Family Relations, 3989 Central Ave., N.E., Suite 550, Minneapolis, MN 55421. Reprinted by permission.

The relationship between hours employed and domestic work was negative in all cases, although not all the relationships were statistically significant at the .01 level. The correlations tend to be larger for women than for men, suggesting that it's more difficult for women to balance work outside and in the home.

SUMMARY OF TERMS AND FORMULAS

Correlation does not imply causation.

Pearson's product-moment correlation coefficient (ρ) is used to determine the extent of relationship between two variables. The numerical size of the coefficient indicates the strength and the sign indicates the direction of the relationship. The square of the coefficient, the **coefficient of determination (ρ^2)**, indicates how much of the total variance in the Y dimension is accounted for by the association of Y with the X variable. Pearson's technique is suitable for describing the relationship between two variables and for making inferences from sample data about the correlation in the population.

Pearson's ρ	Formulas
For raw data	$\rho = \dfrac{\Sigma XY - (\Sigma X)(\Sigma Y)/N}{\sqrt{[\Sigma X^2 - (\Sigma X)^2/N][\Sigma Y^2 - (\Sigma Y)^2/N]}}$
For deviation data	$\rho = \dfrac{\Sigma xy}{\sqrt{(\Sigma x^2)(\Sigma y^2)}}$
For Z-score data	$\rho = \dfrac{\Sigma(Z_x Z_y)}{N}$
t formula for the r statistic	$t = \dfrac{r - \rho}{s_r}$
r for a sample	$r = \dfrac{\Sigma XY - (\Sigma X)(\Sigma Y)/n}{\sqrt{[\Sigma X^2 - (\Sigma X)^2/n][\Sigma Y^2 - (\Sigma Y)^2/n]}}$
Standard error	$s_r = \sqrt{\dfrac{1 - r^2}{n - 2}}$

EXERCISES

1. For the data provided below, plot a scattergraph. What direction is the correlation?

Subject	X	Y
1	12	34
2	12	37
3	14	40
4	17	41
5	18	56
6	20	55
7	21	56
8	25	60

2. For the data provided below, plot a scattergraph. What direction is the correlation?

Subject	X	Y
1	11	102
2	11	100
3	12	98
4	14	90
5	14	92
6	15	84
7	17	79
8	21	65

3. Determine ρ for the data given in Exercise 1. Use the raw score formula. How much of the variance is accounted for by the association?

4. Determine ρ for the data given in Exercise 2. Use the deviation score formula. How much of the variance is accounted for by the association?

5. For the data below, determine ρ using the Z-score formula.

Subject	X	Y
1	1	3
2	2	3
3	4	5
4	6	4
5	7	5
6	10	8

6. An administrator at a small junior college is curious about the relationship between student performance in chemistry (a "hard science") and psychology (a "soft science"). She has the final exam scores for 15 students who took both courses. She finds the correlation (r) between the two exams to be 0.64. At $\alpha = .05$, use a non-directional alternative to test the hypothesis that there is no correlation in the population from which her sample was drawn between performance on the two exams.

7. Determine the correlation between the "intelligence" test scores and the "creativity" test scores given below.

	Intelligence Test	Creativity Test
Peter	122	15
Dan	102	35
Susan	135	20
David	110	22
Larry	140	12
Merrilyn	130	10
Lori	128	15

8. A sociologist was interested in the relationship between the IQ's of fathers and sons. He obtained the IQ scores of twenty fathers and the IQ scores of the oldest son of each. Compute the correlation on his data to see if a relationship exists.

IQ father	IQ son
112	125
123	120
100	89
98	117
109	90
125	123
132	128
120	117
117	100
109	113
110	105
114	112
103	99
115	110
118	117
138	124
128	130
120	100
100	115
101	105

9. The data below reflect mean reaction times of fifteen pilots and their scores on an overall physical fitness test. Compute the correlation.

Fitness Score	R.T.
10	0.4
12	2.5
14	1.2
24	2.4
30	4.5
36	3.0
44	4.2
49	4.6
55	3.8
61	5.9
71	5.3
72	6.0
80	4.9
89	6.2
98	5.6

10. A marriage counsellor tests each of her fifteen couples on a test of marital satisfaction and a test of communication skills. Use Pearson's correlation to determine if these variables are related.

Satisfaction	Communication
2.30	6.0
2.48	7.2
2.64	3.5
3.18	2.4
3.40	5.0
3.58	4.0
3.78	5.8
3.89	6.3
4.01	7.8
4.11	8.0
4.26	6.0
4.28	8.2
4.38	8.9
4.49	7.5
4.58	7.0

# CHAPTER 17

Predictive Techniques

LEARNING OBJECTIVES

After reading this chapter you should be able to:
1. Describe the least squares criterion used to fit the regression line.
2. Calculate the slope for a given set of data.
3. Calculate the Y intercept for a given set of data.
4. Use the regression equation to predict Y for a given set of data.
5. Describe what the standard error of estimate measures.
6. Describe the coefficient of determination in terms of explained variance.
7. Describe and provide an example of regression on the mean.
8. Lay down the regression line for a given set of data.
9. Describe the difference between simple linear regression and multiple regression analyses.
10. Compute MR for a given set of data.
11. Describe when multiple correlation and multiple regression are used.
12. Use the multiple regression equation to predict criterion performance for a given set of data.
13. Define the term "partial correlation."
14. Compute the partial correlations for a given set of data.

When we know that two variables are related, we can use this information to make predictions from one variable to the other. For example, college applicants are accepted on the basis of their high school marks because it has been found that college performance is correlated with high school performance; most students who do well in high school also do well in college. Looking at this another way, we can *predict* how well a person will perform in college if we know his or her high school average. Our prediction is based on how the average student, with that particular high school average, has done in the past in college. Sometimes we will be wrong, of course, but if the correlation is very strong we will usually predict correctly.

The previous chapter discussed the straight line of best fit in a bivariate frequency distribution. Let's look at how that line is determined.

The Regression Line

The straight line of best fit is called the **regression line**. The mathematical equation that defines it is called the **regression equation**. The scattergraph in Figure 17-1 shows the regression line for a set of data.

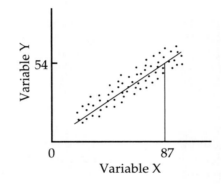

Figure 17-1   The regression line for a bivariate distribution

If we gather data and determine the correlation between two variables, we can use this information in the future to predict from one variable to the other. When we use the correlation between two variables to predict one from the other, we use the regression line as our prediction. We take a particular X value and predict for Y the point on the regression corresponding to that X value. We can take any value of X and predict what Y will be by noting the corresponding Y value on the line. On the scattergraph in Figure 17-1, when X is 87, we would predict that Y is 54.

> **Regression line:** The straight line of best fit.
> **Regression equation:** The mathematical equation that defines the regression line.

Criterion of Best Fit

To fit the straight line to a bivariate frequency distribution, Pearson used the **least squares criterion**. This criterion dictates that the line be laid down in such a way that the sum of the squared distances between the Y values and the line be as small as possible. In other words, *the sum of the squared distances is a minimum*. Consider the scattergraph in Figure 17-2.

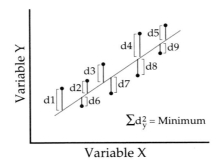

Figure 17-2 The least squares criterion for the regression of Y on X

The points are the actual values of Y found for each value of X. The straight line is called the line of regression of Y on X. Note that the distances are measured in the Y dimension. The line, Y on X, is laid down so that the sum of the distances squared is as small as possible in the Y dimension. This may sound familiar. In Chapter 3, we learned one way to define a mean: the place in a distribution where the sum of the squared deviations about it is a minimum. The regression line is much like a mean.

A different line is fit to the data when we minimize the sum of the squared discrepancies in the X dimension. Consider the scattergraph in Figure 17-3.

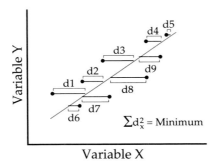

Figure 17-3 The least squares criterion for the regression of X on Y

Here the distances are measured in the X dimension. This regression line of X on Y is different from Y on X. Which line is appropriate is based on how you name your variables and plot your data. We will always assume that X is known and Y is to be predicted; therefore our regression line will always by Y on X. Keep in mind, however, that two lines can always be fit to the same data.

> **Least Squares Criterion:** For the regression line, a mathematical criterion which specifies that the sum of the squared distances of points from the line is a minimum.

The Regression Equation

The regression line is defined by an equation that takes the same general form as the equation for any straight line. You may recall from your high school math that the equation for a straight line is

$$Y = \underbrace{b}_{\text{slope}} X + \underbrace{a}_{\text{Y intercept}}$$

In any equation for a straight line, the slope indicates the amount of increase in Y which accompanies one unit of increase in X. As you can see below, the regression equation can be expressed in raw score, deviation score, and Z-score form. Prime notation (') is used to indicate that Y is a predicted value. The σ_y and σ_x refer to the standard deviation of Y and the standard deviation of X, respectively.

	Regression Equation	
	slope	Y intercept
Raw score:	$Y' = \rho\left(\dfrac{\sigma_y}{\sigma_x}\right)X$	$+ \; \left(-\rho\left(\dfrac{\sigma_y}{\sigma_x}\right)\mu_x + \mu_y\right)$
Deviation score:	$y' = \rho\left(\dfrac{\sigma_y}{\sigma_x}\right)x$	$+ \; 0$
Z-score:	$Z_{y'} = \rho Z_x$	$+ \; 0$

In the deviation score and Z-score formula, the Y intercept is zero. The regression line passes through the ordinate at zero. In general, the regression line always passes through the mean of Y and the mean of X. When data are in deviation or Z-score form, the means are zero and so the regression line must pass through the origin.

In the Z-score regression equation, the value of ρ is the slope. When the data are in Z-score form, ρ indicates what portion of a *standard deviation* Y increases for *one standard deviation* increase in X.

The regression line can be determined by calculating the slope and the Y intercept of a set of data.

Calculating the Slope

When data are in raw score form the formula for the slope is

$$b = \rho\left(\dfrac{\sigma_y}{\sigma_x}\right) \quad \text{slope of the regression line}$$

By substituting the raw score formula for ρ and simplifying the equation, we find that the formula for calculating the slope with raw data is

$$b = \dfrac{\Sigma XY - (\Sigma X)(\Sigma Y)/N}{\Sigma X^2 - (\Sigma X)^2/N} \quad \text{slope for raw data}$$

Let's use this formula to calculate the slope of the regression line for the following data.

	X	Y	XY	X²
	3	5	15	9
	5	7	35	25
	4	4	16	16
	7	8	56	49
	6	9	54	36
	3	5	15	9
	2	3	6	4
	3	4	12	9
	4	3	12	16
	5	7	35	25
Total	42	55	256	198
Mean	4.2	5.5		

Using the formula

$$b = \frac{\Sigma XY - (\Sigma X)(\Sigma Y)/N}{\Sigma X^2 - (\Sigma X)^2/N}$$

$$= \frac{256 - (42)(55)/10}{198 - (42)^2/10}$$

$$= 25/21.6 = 1.16$$

Calculating the Y Intercept
The raw score formula for calculating the Y intercept is

$$a = -\rho\left(\frac{\sigma_y}{\sigma_x}\right)\mu_x + \mu_y \quad \text{Y intercept of the regression line}$$

Since $\rho\left(\frac{\sigma_y}{\sigma_x}\right)$ is the slope, b, we can simplify the formula to

$$a = \mu_y - b\mu_x$$

Let's use the previous example to determine the Y intercept of the regression line:

$$a = 5.5 - (1.16)(4.2) = 0.63$$

The regression line passes through the Y axis at 0.63. You will recall that all regression lines pass through the point of intersection of the mean of Y and the mean of X. We have enough information to lay down the regression line for our example.

Laying Down the Regression Line

Let's lay down the regression line for the example we've been using. We know that the line crosses the Y axis at 0.63 and we know that it passes through the intersection of the mean of X (i.e., 4.2) and the mean of Y (i.e., 5.5). We need only plot these two points and connect them to obtain the regression line. See Figure 17-4.

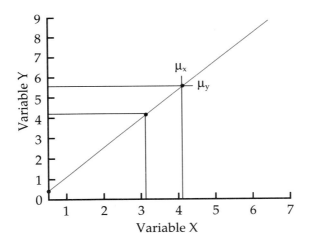

Figure 17-4   Laying down the regression line

Let's verify our work by predicting the value of Y for an X value of 3. The raw score equation is

$$Y' = \rho\left(\frac{\sigma_y}{\sigma_x}\right)X - \rho\left(\frac{\sigma_y}{\sigma_x}\right)\mu_x + \mu_y$$

Since we already know the slope and Y intercept, we can simplify this equation to

$$Y' = bX + a$$
$$= 1.16(3) + 0.63 = 4.11$$

As the illustration above shows, the predicted Y value of 4.11 for an X score of 3 is, indeed, correct.

Using the Regression Equation for Prediction

Let's see how the regression equation can be used to predict Y from X. Suppose a statistics professor kept student test performance scores for many years. She found that performance on the first midterm test correlated reasonably well with the final grade students received in the course. Here are the data:

First test: $\mu_x = 56.45 \quad \sigma_x = 10.25$
Final grade: $\mu_y = 63.12 \quad \sigma_y = 12.14$
The correlation between the two variables: $\rho = 0.60$

A student in her current class scored 76.0 on the first midterm exam.

Let's use the regression equation to predict the final grade this student will receive in the course.

$$Y' = \rho\left(\frac{\sigma_y}{\sigma_x}\right)X - \rho\left(\frac{\sigma_y}{\sigma_x}\right)\mu_x + \mu_y$$

$$= (0.60)\left(\frac{12.14}{10.25}\right)(76.0) - (0.60)\left(\frac{12.14}{10.25}\right)(56.45) + 63.12$$

$$= (0.71)(76.0) - (0.71)(56.45) + 63.12$$

$$= 54.01 - 40.11 + 63.12 = 77.02$$

We would predict a final grade of 77.02 for this student.

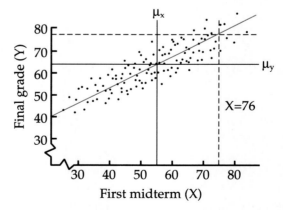

Figure 17-5 Predicting Y' from X

Take a look at Figure 17-5. The regression equation predicts the average final grade received by students who scored 76.0 on the first midterm test. Since the correlation is not perfect there will be some error in prediction.

The predicted value is the point on the line, but the actual points scatter around the regression line to some degree. How far the points vary from the line determines how much error we will make when we use the regression line as our predictor.

Error of Prediction: The Standard Error of Estimate

The regression equation states what value of Y is expected when X has a particular value. Y' is not likely to be the actual value corresponding to X. For example, a regression equation may predict that a man who is 183 cm tall will weigh 79.5 kg. However, we would not expect a particular 183 cm tall man to weigh exactly 79.5 kg. The predicted value is an estimate of weights of men who are 183 cm tall. If the correlation between height and weight is not strong, then we can expect considerable variation in the actual values. Only when there is a perfect correlation, $\rho = \pm 1$, will the actual values precisely equal the predicted values.

The **standard error of estimate** measures the variability of the actual Y values from the predicted Y values. It is denoted as σ_{yx}. Recall that the standard deviation of Y is found by the following formula:

$$\sigma_y = \sqrt{\frac{\Sigma(Y - \mu_y)^2}{N}}$$

To determine the error encountered when we make predictions between two moderately correlated variables, we measure the variability of the actual Y values about the predicted values (Y'). The standard error of estimate indicates the variability of the actual Y values around the regression line. The formula for the standard error of estimate is

$$\sigma_{yx} = \sqrt{\frac{\Sigma(Y - Y')^2}{N}} \qquad \text{standard error of estimate}$$

This measures the magnitude of the error of prediction. When the correlation is perfect, each $Y - Y'$ difference is zero because all the actual Y values fall on the regression line. Therefore, the standard error of estimate is zero and there is no error in prediction. When the correlation is zero, then Y' equals the mean of Y for all X's and

$$\sigma_{yx} = \sqrt{\frac{\Sigma(Y - \mu_y)^2}{N}} = \sigma_y$$

In other words, the standard error of estimate ranges from zero when $\rho = \pm 1$ to the standard deviation of Y when $\rho = 0$.

The standard error of estimate is a standard deviation and has all the properties of one. The sum of the deviations of the Y values about the regression line is zero and the sum of the squared deviations of the Y values about the regression line is minimized.

The standard error of estimate can be calculated more easily with the following formula:

$$\sigma_{yx} = \sigma_y \sqrt{1 - \rho^2} \qquad \text{standard error of estimate}$$

As we saw above, when $\rho = 0$ then $\sigma_{yx} = \sigma_y$; when $\rho = \pm 1$ then $\sigma_{yx} = 0$.

Interpreting the Correlation in Terms of Explained Variance

When X and Y are correlated, Y takes on different values depending on whether X is high or low. If we select a single X value, Y still varies to some extent unless the correlation is perfect. In other words, unless the correlation is ± 1, the actual Y values will vary around the straight line of best fit. With lower correlations, this variability increases.

The total variation in the Y distribution can be partitioned into two components:

1. the variation in Y that is associated with changes in X, and
2. the variation inherent in Y that is independent of changes in X.

Let's take a single Y value and look at how its variation can be partitioned into two parts. See Figure 17-6.

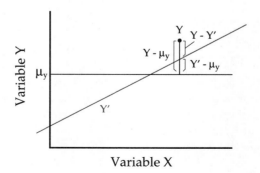

Figure 17-6 Partitioning the Y variance in regression

Remember that the total variation in Y is based on the deviations of the Y values from the mean of the distribution. If all the deviations were squared, summed and divided by N, we would have the Y variance.

Look at the graph above. The Y value differs from the mean of the Y distribution. That discrepancy can be partitioned into (1) the difference between the Y value and the point on the straight line of best fit (i.e., Y'), and (2) the difference between the line (Y') and the mean of the distribution.

If we square all the differences, sum the squares, and then divide each by N, we would have the following:

$$\frac{\Sigma(Y - \mu_y)^2}{N} = \frac{\Sigma(Y - Y')^2}{N} + \frac{\Sigma(Y' - \mu_y)^2}{N}$$

$$\sigma_y^2 = \sigma_{yx}^2 + \sigma_{y'}^2$$

$$\text{Total Y variance} = \begin{pmatrix} \text{Variance in Y} \\ \text{independent of} \\ \text{changes in X} \end{pmatrix} + \begin{pmatrix} \text{Variance in Y} \\ \text{associated with} \\ \text{changes in X} \end{pmatrix}$$

where σ_y^2 is the total variance in the Y distribution; σ_{yx}^2 is the variance of the actual Y values around the straight line (Y'); and $\sigma_{y'}^2$ is the variance of the points on the line of best fit around the mean of the Y distribution.

When the correlation is ±1, all the Y values fall exactly on the straight line of best fit, and there is no variation of the Y values from Y'. The value of σ_{yx}^2 will be zero; all the variation in Y is due to changes in X. When the correlation is 0, none of the variation in Y is due to changes in X. The value of $\sigma_{y'}^2$ will be zero.

The correlation coefficient can be interpreted in terms of the *proportion of the total Y variance which is associated with changes in* X. This proportion is called the **coefficient of determination**. It is determined by

$$\frac{\text{Variance in Y associated with changes in X}}{\text{Total Y variance}} = \frac{\sigma_{y'}^2}{\sigma_y^2} = \rho^2 \quad \text{coefficient of determination}$$

Recall that the coefficient of determination, ρ^2, indicates the strength of the relationship between the two variables. It estimates how much of the total Y variation is due to the correlation Y has with X.

Think of the coefficient of determination in terms of how much of the variance in Y can be *explained* and how much is left unaccounted for. Many people find this a more helpful way to think about correlations. For example, if you have a correlation of 0.50, you know that 25% of the total variability of Y is due to the correlation and the rest is unexplained.

Regression on the Mean

When a value of Y is predicted from a given value of X, Y' can never be further from its mean than X is from its mean. Unless the correlation is perfect, Y' will be closer to its mean than X is to its mean. This is called **regression on the mean**. It can lead us into some peculiar situations.

Consider the correlation between IQ of parents and their offspring. It's about 0.5. Let's predict the IQ of children whose parents' IQ are 2 standard deviations below the mean. We will use our Z-score formula.

$$Z_{y'} = \rho Z_x + 0$$
$$= 0.5(-2) + 0 = -1$$

For parents whose IQ scores are 2 standard deviations below the mean, we will predict their offspring to be only 1 standard deviation below the mean. Similarly, for parents whose scores are 2 standard deviations above the mean, we will predict their offspring to be 1 standard deviation above the mean. As you can see, the predicted values regress toward the mean.

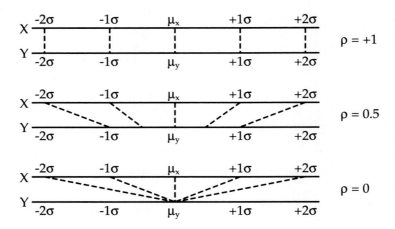

Figure 17-7 Regression on the mean

Figure 17-7 shows the Z-scores of Y we would predict for various Z-scores of X, when ρ is 0, 0.5, and 1. When $\rho = 0$, we predict that the Z-score of Y will be the mean (which in any Z distribution is 0). When $\rho = 1$, the Z-score of Y will be the same as the Z-score of X. But when ρ is 0.5, the predicted value of Y will tend toward the mean.

Regression on the mean occurs because the predicted Y score cannot be further away from the mean of its distribution than its X counterpart. We must always predict that Y will be no further away from its mean than X is from its mean.

Multiple Regression Analysis

In simple linear regression, Y is predicted from knowledge of X. The strength of the correlation between X (often called the **predictor variable**) and Y (often called the **criterion variable**) determines the accuracy of the prediction. A technique that allows prediction of Y from more than one X variable is presented in the following section.

Multiple Regression Analysis (MRA) is a technique used to predict Y (the criterion variable) from a set of predictor variables (X1, X2, etc.). MRA provides an index of the relationship between the criterion variable and each of the predictor variables, in the form of a regression coefficient. Imagine that the Canadian Air Force is interested in screening applicants for military flying school. They might use various measures to predict an applicant's future performance as a pilot trainee. Perhaps they have a standard aptitude test that has been proven to be correlated with success. Perhaps in addition they assess the applicant's general physical fitness. They could use each of these predictor variables to predict the applicant's likelihood of benefiting from training. A multiple regression analysis will provide a measure of the kinds of predictor information most useful in predicting success in training school.

The Multiple Correlation Coefficient

We will use **MR** to stand for the **multiple correlation** between all predictors and the criterion.

The equation for multiple correlation from two predictor variables is as follows:

$$\text{MR} = \sqrt{\frac{\rho^2_{y1} + \rho^2_{y2} - 2\rho_{y1}\rho_{y}\rho_{12}}{1 - \rho^2_{12}}} \qquad \text{multiple correlation coefficient}$$

Here y is the criterion variable; 1 is the first predictor variable; and 2 is the second predictor variable. Therefore,

ρ^2_{y1} is the square of the correlation coefficient between the criterion variable and the first predictor variable.

ρ^2_{y2} is the square of the correlation coefficient between the criterion variable and the second predictor variable.

ρ_{12} is the correlation coefficient between the first and second predictor variables.

Let's use our Air Force example to see how this equation would be used.

Suppose the Air Force had determined that the correlation between the standard aptitude test and success in flying school is 0.58. The correlation between their physical fitness measure and success is 0.52 and the correlation between physical fitness and aptitude is 0.32. You can see that the aptitude measure is a better predictor of flying school success than is the fitness measure. What we will find out with multiple regression is whether combining both predictor measures is a better predictor of success than either alone. We can write:

$\rho_{y1} = 0.58$, the correlation between aptitude and success
$\rho_{y2} = 0.52$, the correlation between physical fitness and success
$\rho_{12} = 0.32$, the correlation between physical fitness and aptitude

Using these values in the multiple correlation equation:

$$MR = \sqrt{\frac{\rho^2_{y1} + \rho^2_{y2} - 2\rho_{y1}\rho_{y2}\rho_{12}}{1 - \rho^2_{12}}}$$

$$= \sqrt{\frac{0.58^2 + 0.52^2 - 2(0.58)(0.52)(0.32)}{1 - 0.32^2}}$$

$$= 0.68$$

You can see that using both predictor measures produces a correlation coefficient that is higher than each separate coefficient, allowing us to better predict success.

Using Multiple Correlation for Prediction

In simple linear regression we used the correlation coefficient to predict from X to Y. We can do the same here. We use a multiple regression equation to predict the criterion variable from predictor variables. As with linear regression we need to determine the Y intercept. Unlike simple linear regression, we need in addition to calculate slopes for each predictor variable. Each slope tells us how much change occurs in Y for a unit change in one X variable when all other predictor variables are held constant. With two predictor variables the multiple regression equation is as follows:

$$Y' = b_1 X_1 + b_2 X_2 + a \quad \text{multiple regression equation with two predictor variables}$$

Here, a is the Y intercept, b_1 is the slope for predictor variable X_1, and b_2 is the slope for predictor variable X_2.

You can see that the predicted value of Y is equal to a linear combination of X's each weighted by a value of b.

The equations for the slopes are as follows:

$$b_1 = \left(\frac{\sigma_y}{\sigma_1}\right)\left(\frac{\rho_{y1} - \rho_{y2}\rho_{12}}{1 - \rho^2_{12}}\right)$$

$$b_2 = \left(\frac{\sigma_y}{\sigma_2}\right)\left(\frac{\rho_{y2} - \rho_{y1}\rho_{12}}{1 - \rho^2_{12}}\right)$$

where σ_y is the standard deviation of the criterion variable, σ_1 is the standard deviation of the first predictor variable, and σ_2 is the standard deviation of the second predictor variable.

The b's, or slopes, indicate the relationship between the criterion variable (Y) and each predictor variable.

The equation for the Y intercept is

$$a = \mu_y - b_1\mu_1 - b_2\mu_2$$

where μ_y is the mean of the criterion variable, μ_1 is the mean of the first predictor variable, and μ_2 is the mean of the second predictor variable.

Let's use our Air Force example to predict performance for two applicants. Suppose the following data have been collected for the aptitude test, the physical fitness test and flying school performance.

Flying school performance (Y)

$\mu_y = 64.8$
$\sigma_y = 12.6$

Aptitude test norms (1)

$\mu_1 = 432$
$\sigma_1 = 65$

Physical fitness norms (2)

$\mu_2 = 7.2$
$\sigma_2 = 1.4$

The correlations were

$\rho_{y1} = 0.58$, the correlation between aptitude and success
$\rho_{y2} = 0.52$, the correlation between physical fitness and success
$\rho_{12} = 0.32$, the correlation between physical fitness and aptitude

Suppose our first candidate for flying school obtained an aptitude score of 390 and a physical fitness score of 8.2. Our second candidate obtained an aptitude score of 512 and a physical fitness score of 7.0. Let's use our equations to predict the flying school performance of each applicant.

Step 1. Determine the slopes.

$$b_1 = \left(\frac{\sigma_y}{\sigma_1}\right)\left(\frac{\rho_{y1} - \rho_{y2}\rho_{12}}{1 - \rho_{12}^2}\right)$$

$$= \left(\frac{12.6}{65}\right)\left(\frac{0.58 - (0.52)(0.32)}{1 - 0.32^2}\right) = 0.09$$

$$b_2 = \left(\frac{\sigma_y}{\sigma_2}\right)\left(\frac{\rho_{y2} - \rho_{y1}\rho_{12}}{1 - \rho_{12}^2}\right)$$

$$= \left(\frac{12.6}{1.4}\right)\left(\frac{0.52 - (0.58)(0.32)}{1 - 0.32^2}\right) = 3.35$$

Step 2. Determine the Y intercept.

$$a = \mu_y - b_1\mu_1 - b_2\mu_2$$

$$= 64.8 - 0.09(432) - 3.35(7.2) = 1.8$$

Step 3. Determine the predicted values of Y for each applicant. For the first applicant:

$$Y' = b_1X_1 + b_2X_2 + a$$

$$= 0.09(390) + 3.35(8.2) + 1.8 = 64.37$$

For the second applicant:

$$Y' = b_1X_1 + b_2X_2 + a$$

$$= 0.09(512) + 3.35(7.0) + 1.8 = 71.33$$

If we had to choose between the two, we might be wise to select the second applicant.

With simple linear regression, the strength of the correlation coefficient determines the amount of predictive error. With multiple regression the strength of the multiple correlation determines predictive error. With simple linear regression predictive error was measured by the standard error of estimate. One formula for the standard error of estimate was

$$\sigma_{yx} = \sigma_y\sqrt{1 - \rho^2}$$

The formula for the standard error of multiple estimate is similar:

$$\sigma_{ME} = \sigma_y\sqrt{1 - MR^2} \quad \text{standard error of multiple estimate}$$

For our above example the standard error of multiple estimate is

$$\sigma_{ME} = 12.6\sqrt{1 - 0.68^2} = 9.24$$

You can see that with a very strong multiple correlation, the standard error of multiple estimate tends toward zero; and with a very weak multiple correlation, the standard error tends toward the standard deviation of the criterion variable, Y.

Partial Correlation

The multiple correlation equation estimates the combined influence of predictor variables on a criterion measure. This may allow the researcher to make a more accurate prediction of the criterion variable.

Partial correlation techniques, on the other hand, are used to measure the relationship between two variables when a third variable has an influence on them both. In other words, it assesses the correlation between the two variables of interest by ruling out the influence of the third variable known to be involved. The formula for partial correlation is as follows:

$$R_p = \frac{\rho_{y1} - \rho_{y2}\rho_{12}}{\sqrt{(1 - \rho^2_{y2})(1 - \rho^2_{12})}} \quad \text{partial correlation}$$

Suppose there is a positive correlation between age and income level. Older people make more money than younger people. This would seem to make sense since the longer a person is in the work force, the more promotions and therefore higher income he or she can obtain. Can you think of another variable that might be correlated with both age and income? How about years of education? We might imagine that older people have more education than younger people and that better educated people earn higher salaries. The question then is what is the true relationship between age and income level if the years of education factor is held constant. This is a problem that could be solved with partial correlation. Suppose that the correlation between age and income is 0.60, the correlation between age and years of education is 0.63, and the correlation between between years of education and income is 0.77. Let's determine the partial correlation between age and income.

$\rho_{y1} = 0.60$, correlation between age and income
$\rho_{y2} = 0.63$, correlation between age and years of education
$\rho_{12} = 0.77$, correlation between years of education and income

$$R_p = \frac{0.60 - (0.63)(0.77)}{\sqrt{(1 - 0.63^2)(1 - 0.77^2)}}$$

$$= 0.35$$

Although the correlation between age and income was quite high (i.e. 0.60), once the influence of years of education is removed, the correlation is not nearly as impressive.

Correlational and regression analyses are gaining popularity in the social sciences, particularly for researchers working in areas where experimental designs are not possible or are ethically unacceptable. Multiple correlation and multiple regression analyses are powerful and complicated techniques that cannot be presented with any degree of detail here. Interested students should consult upper level statistics books for more comprehensive coverage of these useful techniques.

FOCUS ON RESEARCH

Lee, Mancini, and Maxwell (1990)* examined the influence of a variety of variables, such as relationship quality, individual characteristics and family characteristics, on sibling relationships in adulthood.

The Data
The data were collected by telephone and mail-out survey. The sampling procedure attempted to ensure a representative group.

The Variables
The three major dependent (criterion) variables were (i) general patterns of interaction between adult siblings, (ii) obligatory contact motivation, and (iii) discretionary contact motivation. The independent (predictor) variables included emotional closeness, sibling responsibility expectations, sibling conflict, age differences, number of siblings, geographic proximity, gender, and number of children in the home.

The researchers expected on the basis of previous research in the field that sibling contact would be positively related to emotional closeness and sibling responsibility expectations and negatively related to conflict. They further hypothesized that sibling contact would be greater for larger sibling groups who were closer in age and of the same gender. Sibling contact was expected to be greater for women and for those without children in the home and for siblings in closer proximity.

The Analyses
A multiple regression analysis was performed and partial correlations were computed for each of the predictor to criterion variables.

---

* Lee, T.R., Mancini, J.A., and Maxwell, J.W. (1990). Sibling Relationships in Adulthood: Contact Patterns and Motivations, *Journal of Marriage and the Family*, 52, 431–40.

The multiple correlation coefficients for all predictors were as follows:

MR general contact = 0.83
MR obligatory contact motivation = 0.61
MR discretionary contact motivation = 0.81

The partial correlations are shown in Table 17-1.

Table 17-1 Partial Correlations

	General contact	Obligatory contact motivation	Discretionary contact motivation
Emotional closeness	0.39	0.33	0.65
Sibling responsibility expectations	0.10	0.32	0.24
Sibling conflict	0.11	0.02	−0.03
Age difference	−0.07	0.03	0.02
Total number of siblings	−0.18	0.01	−0.07
Geographic proximity	0.61	0.10	−0.13
Gender of sibling pair			
Male/male vs. mixed	0.003	0.013	−0.05
Male/female vs. mixed	0.14	0.016	0.00
Number children at home	−0.02	−0.10	0.03
Gender of respondent	0.01	−0.06	0.10

Source: Lee, Mancini, and Maxwell (1990). Copyright 1990 by the National Council on Family Relations, 3989 Central Ave. N.E., Suite 550, Minneapolis, MN 55421. Reprinted by permission.

As you can see, in terms of the general contact variable, geographic proximity and emotional closeness were the best predictors. With respect to the respondent's perception of contact being due to obligation, the important variables were emotional closeness and a sense of responsibility for the sibling. Those same two variables were the most important with respect to discretionary contact as well. The researchers concluded that the results in general supported most of their hypotheses.

This example illustrates the application of multiple regression analysis. In fields where numerous variables may be involved, such as in the understanding of complex interpersonal relationships, this sort of analysis can be very useful.

SUMMARY OF TERMS AND FORMULAS

When the **correlation** between two variables is known, we may use knowledge of performance on the first variable, to predict performance on the second variable. A **regression line** is fitted to the correlational data and the point that lies on the line is the predicted value of Y for a given X value.

When the correlation between variables is not perfect, some predictive error will occur. The measure of predictive error is called the **standard error of estimate**.

The **coefficient of determination**, ρ^2, can be interpreted in terms of the proportion of the total variance in Y that can be explained or accounted for by the relationship of Y to X.

Regression on the mean occurs in prediction whenever the correlation between X and Y is less than 1. The predicted value will tend to be closer to its mean than was the value used in the prediction.

Multiple correlation is used to predict from several predictor variables to a criterion variable. It often allows a more accurate prediction than simple linear correlation. **Partial correlation** is used to estimate the individual influence of a variable on another by holding constant other variables known to have an effect.

Regression Equation for Predicting Y from X

Raw score: $\qquad Y' = \rho\left(\dfrac{\sigma_y}{\sigma_x}\right)X - \rho\left(\dfrac{\sigma_y}{\sigma_x}\right)\mu_x + \mu_y$

Deviation score: $\qquad y' = \rho\left(\dfrac{\sigma_y}{\sigma_x}\right)x$

Z-score: $\qquad Z_{y'} = \rho Z_x$

Slope of the Regression Line

$$b = \rho\left(\dfrac{\sigma_y}{\sigma_x}\right)$$

Raw Data: $\qquad b = \dfrac{\Sigma XY - (\Sigma X)(\Sigma Y)/N}{\Sigma X^2 - (\Sigma X)^2/N}$

Y Intercept of the Regression Line

$$a = -\rho\left(\frac{\sigma_y}{\sigma_x}\right)\mu_x + \mu_y$$

Standard Error of Estimate

$$\sigma_{yx} = \sqrt{\frac{\Sigma(Y - Y')^2}{N}}$$

$$\sigma_{yx} = \sigma_y\sqrt{1 - \rho^2}$$

Multiple Correlation Coefficient

$$MR = \sqrt{\frac{\rho^2_{y1} + \rho^2_{y2} - 2\rho_{y1}\rho_{y2}\rho_{12}}{1 - \rho^2_{12}}}$$

Multiple Regression Equation

$$Y' = b_1X_1 + b_2X_2 + a$$

Slopes for Multiple Regression

For first predictor variable

$$b_1 = \left(\frac{\sigma_y}{\sigma_1}\right)\left(\frac{\rho_{y1} - \rho_{y2}\rho_{12}}{1 - \rho^2_{12}}\right)$$

For second predictor variable

$$b_2 = \left(\frac{\sigma_y}{\sigma_2}\right)\left(\frac{\rho_{y2} - \rho_{y1}\rho_{12}}{1 - \rho^2_{12}}\right)$$

Standard Error of Multiple Estimate

$$\sigma_{ME} = \sigma_y\sqrt{1 - MR^2}$$

Partial Correlation

$$R_p = \frac{\rho_{y1} - \rho_{y2}\rho_{12}}{\sqrt{(1 - \rho^2_{y2})(1 - \rho^2_{12})}}$$

EXERCISES

1. A professor collected the following data on number of hours per week students spend studying and their scores on tests.

Hours/Week	Test Scores
8	75
8	50
2	50
4	45
4	65
9	60
10	80
10	95
2	35
5	50
7	65
4	60
2	50
1	50
7	70

   a. Calculate the slope for the above data (use the raw score equation).
   b. Calculate the Y intercept for the above data.
   c. Plot the regression line. Be precise.

2. If Russell tells you he studies 7.5 hours/week, circle the test score on the graph from Exercise 1(c) that you would predict for him. Verify the predicted value with your equation.

3. Suppose $\rho = 0.60$, $\sigma_y = 4.2$, $\sigma_x = 3.0$, $\mu_x = 8.6$, and $\mu_y = 12.0$. Determine Y' for an X value of:
   a. 2
   b. 8
   c. 5

4. If $\rho = -0.60$, find the Z-score in Y that should be predicted for:
   a. a score 1/2 a standard deviation below the mean in X
   b. $Z_x = 1.5$
   c. a score equal to the mean of X

5. Consider the following data.

X	Y
22	12
16	16
16	11
15	13
13	10
11	9
11	12
9	7
7	3
4	2

   a. Calculate Pearson's ρ using the raw score formula and the deviation score formula.
   b. How much of the variance is accounted for by the correlation between the two variables?

6. Using the data in Exercise 5, calculate the slope (b) and the Y intercept (a) in order to determine the predicted Y values for each of the following given X values.
   a. X = 9
   b. X = 13
   c. X = 17

7. Consider the following data.

X	Y
43	19
49	18
52	23
61	27
64	34
65	21
70	45
72	46
73	40
77	53
77	52
78	40
80	69
83	67

a. Calculate Pearson's ρ using the deviation score formula.
b. Determine the slope (b) and the Y intercept (a) for the above data.
c. Plot the regression line.

8. A researcher finds that the correlation between psychological disorder in mothers and psychological disorder in their children is 0.45. The correlation between psychological disorder in fathers and their children is 0.25. The correlation between parents in terms of disorder is 0.15. Determine the multiple correlation where the child's psychological health is the criterion and the psychological health of the parents are the predictor variables.

9. If the correlation between the IQ's of mothers and their children is 0.50, the correlation between the IQ's of fathers and their children is 0.45, and the correlation between the IQ's of parents is 0.35, determine the multiple correlation using the child's IQ as the criterion variable.

10. Using the data from Exercise 9, predict the IQ of a child whose mother's IQ is 132 and whose father's IQ is 125. Assume the mean and standard deviation of each distribution of IQ's is 100 and 15 respectively.

11. The correlation between graduating average and IQ is 0.72. The correlation between graduating average and time spent studying is 0.87. The correlation between IQ and time spent studying is 0.65. What is the correlation between graduating average and IQ if the time spent studying variable is removed?

12. The correlation between marital satisfaction and number of years married is 0.50. The correlation between marital satisfaction and frequency of sexual contact is 0.80. The correlation between frequency of sexual contact and number of years married is 0.45. What is the correlation between marital satisfaction and number of years married if the frequency of sexual contact variable is removed?

CHAPTER 18

Choosing the Appropriate Test of Significance

> **LEARNING OBJECTIVES**
>
> After reading this chapter you should be able to:
> 1. Choose the appropriate parametric test of significance for a given research problem.
> 2. Choose the appropriate non-parametric test of significance for a given research problem.

Non-Parametric versus Parametric Analysis

Throughout this book you have been learning how to decide which test of significance is appropriate for a given set of data or research question. As more tests have been introduced this decision-making process has become more complicated. In this chapter, we will go through the steps involved in deciding which, of all the tests of significance we have studied, we should use. This is meant to be a guide in decision-making only. Parametric analyses, for example, although robust may not be appropriate when their assumptions are badly violated. It isn't possible here to cover all the intricacies involved in selecting the appropriate statistical analysis but this chapter should help you with many common research problems and data types.

The following provides a progression of questions and answers that have to be dealt with when deciding on the most appropriate test of significance. The first step is to determine what kinds of data have been collected by the investigator. We need to decide between three possibilities.

First, if the data are measures of performance where means will be computed to compare groups we will choose a parametric test. Parametric tests of significance test hypotheses about specific population parameters, such as the population mean or the difference between population means. These tests assume that measurement is at least on an interval scale and that the population distributions are normal with equal variability.

When the research design or the type of data do not permit us to make the assumptions necessary for a parametric approach, we should use a non-parametric technique to analyze the data. Non-parametric techniques have weaker assumptions. It should be pointed out, however, that parametric analyses can tolerate some violations of their assumptions and may be more powerful than their non-parametric counterparts. Much of the time, though, non-parametric tests will be more powerful than the parametric approach if violations of parametric analysis are serious, such as unequal sample sizes and heterogeneity of variances. In such situations we may choose to convert our measurement data to ranks. Deciding whether parametric assumptions have been violated is a difficult process and we will not include such examples here.

Second, if the data are not measures but are rank order data, we will choose a non-parametric test.

Third, if the data are neither rank orders nor measures, we need to determine if they are frequency counts. When the observations are frequency counts, percentages, or proportions, we will likely be interested in a chi-square analysis. Remember that categorical data are data where subjects have been classified on some variable. In other words the performance measures of subjects will not not analyzed per se, but rather are used to classify subjects into categories.

Once the kind of data has been determined we continue with the steps in choosing the appropriate test.

Choosing the Appropriate Parametric Test of Significance

To determine the appropriate procedure to test a parametric hypothesis, several questions must be answered about the nature of the data and research design.

The following flow diagram shows the progression of steps we follow when deciding on the appropriate parametric test.

Performance measure data

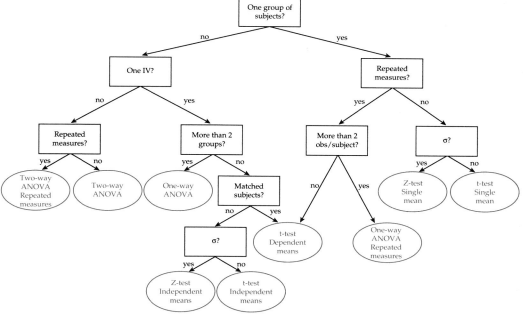

Figure 18-1 Choosing the appropriate parametric test of significance

---

Let's go through each step involved in deciding which test is most appropriate.

One group in the experiment	If there is only one group of subjects, then you must determine whether each subject provides one observation or more than one observation. In other words, you have to determine if repeated measures have been taken.
One group— repeated measures	If each subject contributes more than one data point, then simply determine how many measures each subject contributes. If

each subject contributes two observations, you run a t-test for dependent samples. If each subject contributes more than two observations, you run a one-way ANOVA with repeated measures.

One group—
no repeated measures

If you have determined that each subject in the group provides only one data point or observation, then you should run a Z-test or a t-test for the population mean. A Z-test is appropriate when the population standard deviation is known and a t-test is appropriate if it must be estimated.

More than one group in the experiment

If you have a situation where there are two or more groups in the study, you must determine how many independent variables are involved. Do you have several groups of subjects under different levels of one independent variable, or do you have groups being treated with more than one independent variable?

One independent variable

With more than two groups of subjects, each group under a different level of a single independent variable, you have only one test of significance to choose: one-way ANOVA. With only two groups of subjects, you need to determine whether subjects have been matched, i.e. a matched-groups design. If they have, you run a t-test for dependent means. If subjects have not been matched but, rather, have been independently assigned to the two groups, you have one more question to answer. If you know the population standard deviations, you run a Z-test for independent means. If you do not know the population standard deviations, you run a t-test for independent means.

Two independent variables

If you determine that the experimental design involves two independent variables, then you know you will run an analysis of variance. If subjects have been randomly and independently assigned to all levels of both IV's, you choose a two-way ANOVA.

If one of the independent variables involves measures on the same subjects, i.e. a repeated measures design, then you will run a two-way ANOVA with repeated measures.

Some Examples

Example A
A sociologist wishes to compare the annual salaries of Canadian men and women in similar occupations. She randomly selects 35 women from a variety of occupational groups. She assigns a male in the same occupation as each female to a second group. She wishes to determine if women and men get "equal pay for equal work."

Step 1. How many groups? The sociologist wishes to compare the salaries of men and women in similar occupations. She has two groups in her study.

Step 2. How many independent variables? The issue is whether salary depends on gender. Although gender, as you may recall from Chapter 1, is not truly an independent variable but rather an organismic variable, you may treat it as an IV as far as our statistical analysis is concerned.

Step 3. Are subjects matched or independently assigned? Since the sociologist did not independently assign subjects to groups but rather matched her subjects according to occupation, you will run a t-test for dependent means on the salary data.

Example B
A research team, composed of a nutritionist, a physician, a physical education expert, and a sports psychologist, developed an exercise and diet program designed to improve physical fitness. They randomly select 30 people to participate in the program and 30 others to serve as a control group. The physical fitness of all subjects is measured first. Physical fitness of the experimental subjects is measured again halfway through the program, at the end of the program, and 6 months later. The subjects in the control group are evaluated at the same times as the subjects in the experimental group. The researchers are interested in improvement of experimental subjects and in whether any gains in physical fitness are maintained once the program is finished.

Step 1. You have more than one group of subjects since you have an experimental and a control group.

Step 2. This example has two independent variables. One IV is participation in the fitness program. The other is time of testing. This study is a pre-test post-test kind of study. Recall that the dependent variable, fitness, is measured at different times throughout and after the program for both groups of subjects.

Step 3. You are testing the same subjects for fitness at different times, so you have a repeated measures design. Measures are repeated on the time of testing variable. You will run a two-way repeated measures ANOVA with participation between subjects and time of measurement within subjects.

Example C
The mayor of a small town in Newfoundland is concerned about the standard of living of his townspeople. From Statistics Canada he discovers that the mean income of people living in similar small towns across the country is $22 000 with a standard deviation of $6500. He randomly selects 100 people from the census files for his town and records the annual income of each. He finds the mean income of his sample is only $18 000. How would he determine the significance of his findings?

Step 1. This study is a good exercise in differentiating between a sample and a population. Many students think that there are two groups, one from Newfoundland and the other from towns across Canada. However, the mayor randomly selected one group of subjects from his town and that is the sample. The information obtained from Statistics Canada is population information. The mayor did not randomly select subjects from towns across Canada. Rather, he is asking whether the people in his town are a random sample from the population of all townspeople.

Step 2. There are no repeated measures in this study. The mayor recorded income for each member of his sample.

Step 3. You do know the population standard deviation and so you will run a Z-test for a single mean. The mayor wants to know if his townspeople differ in annual income from the national norms available.

Choosing the Appropriate Non-Parametric Test of Significance

Let's now go through the decision-making steps to choose the appropriate non-parametric test of significance. We will first consider situations in which the data do not satisfy the requirements of a parametric approach.

Testing for Identical Rank-Order Populations
The following flow diagram illustrates the steps involved in choosing the appropriate test of significance when data are rank orders.

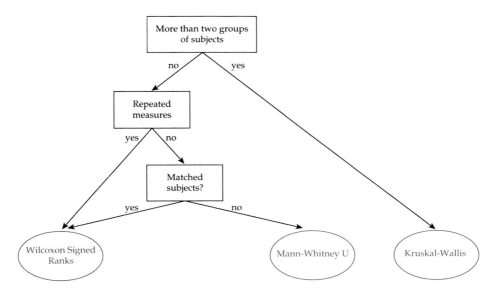

Figure 18-2 Choosing the appropriate test for rank-order data

Let's go through each step involved in deciding which test is most appropriate.

More than two groups in the experiment	The appropriate analysis for experiments with more than two groups of rank-order data is the Kruskal-Wallis procedure. This is analogous to a one-way ANOVA.
Two groups or less in the experiment	You must determine if repeated measures have been taken, or if subjects have been matched in some way.
Repeated measures	If subjects have contributed more than one observation, then you will use the Wilcoxon signed-ranks procedure for repeated measures. This is analogous to a t-test for dependent groups.
Matched subjects	When subjects have been matched on some variable, then the Wilcoxon signed-ranks procedure is appropriate. This is analogous to a t-test for dependent groups.

Subjects not matched — When subjects have not been matched, you will run the non-parametric equivalent of a t-test for independent groups, the Mann-Whitney U test.

Some Examples

Example A
A rating scale was used to evaluate the morale of fifteen employees at a meat-packing plant before and after several new policies regarding working conditions were put into effect. The psychologist in charge of this study wanted to know if the new policies improved morale.

Step 1. How many groups? There is one group of fifteen people in the study.

Step 2. Have repeated measures been taken? Since each subject is tested before and after the new policies were implemented, this is a repeated measures design. The appropriate analysis is a Wilcoxon signed-ranks test.

Example B
Five groups of eight rats each were used to investigate the effects of exercise on caloric intake. The exercise level of each group was controlled by access time to a running wheel. The lowest exercise group was allowed two minutes access to the wheel, the next group five minutes, the next group eight minutes, etc. Caloric intake was recorded for each animal in terms of the number of pellets of rat chow consumed per day.

Step 1. How many groups? Since we have five groups of subjects in this study we need go no further. The appropriate non-parametric analysis is the Krukal-Wallis test.

Example C
A graduate student in special education was interested in the effects of French immersion education on the reading of Grade I children. She compared 18 children from a French immersion program with 18 children in a regular Grade I program by recording the number of books each child borrowed from the library in a week.

Step 1. How many groups? There are 2 groups of children in this study.

Step 2. Were repeated measures taken? The children were measured once only.

Step 3. Were subjects matched? The children were not matched on a variable, and so the Mann-Whitney U test is the appropriate analysis for this study.

Example D
An experimental reading program was being introduced in an inner-city school in response to complaints from parents that their children were below average in reading skills. In order to evaluate the effectiveness of the new program, 15 children were selected to participate in the experimental program. Each child was evaluated for reading level and paired with a child of equal ability from a class that would not be using the new program. After the program was completed, all the children were again evaluated for reading skills and the results of this final evaluation were used to evaluate program effectiveness.

Step 1. How many groups? There are two groups of subjects in this study: an experimental group and a control group.

Step 2. Were repeated measures taken? Although two measures were taken from each child, the first measure was used only to match children of equal ability. The analysis only looked at the final measure of reading ability.

Step 3. Were subjects matched? The initial measure of reading ability was used to match each experimental child with a control child. This is a dependent groups design and the appropriate analysis is the Wilcoxon signed-ranks test.

Testing for Differences between Obtained and Expected Frequencies

When a research design uses percentage, proportion, or frequency as its dependent measure, then a chi-square analysis is likely to be the most appropriate procedure. In these designs, subjects are classified into categories based on some measure. Chi-square analyses compare obtained frequencies with those expected, given a particular hypothesis. Deciding which chi-square test is appropriate involves answering a series of questions about the nature of the data.

The following flow diagram illustrates this process.

Testing for differences between obtained and expected frequencies

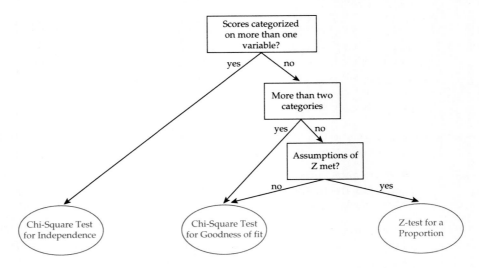

Figure 18-3 Choosing the appropriate test for comparing obtained and expected frequencies

Let's go through the steps to decide on a chi-square analysis.

One variable classification	If the scores have been classified into categories of one variable only, you must determine how many categories were used.
Two categories	With one variable and only 2 categories, you may run a chi-square test for goodness of fit with 1 df. If the assumptions required for a Z-test have been met, then a Z-test for a proportion is also an appropriate analysis.
More than two categories	With one variable and more than 2 categories, a chi-square test for goodness of fit is appropriate, with the number of degrees of freedom = number of categories − 1.
Two variable classification	If the scores have been classified on 2 variables simultaneously and all categories are mutually exclusive, the appropriate analysis is a chi-square test for independence. The degrees of freedom = (number of rows − 1)(number of columns − 1).

Some Examples

Example A
A city planner, whose job involves making decisions about traffic over city bridges, decides to gather some data on bridge use. He wants to know if there is a difference in bridge use depending on the day of the week. He monitors flow over each of the five bridges in the city by counting the number of cars passing over each bridge from 5 p.m. to 8 p.m. each day of the week.

Step 1. How many variables? In this case the city planner has 2 variables of interest, day of the week and bridge. He will run a chi-square test for independence to determine if bridge use depends on day of the week. He has 24 df (6x4).

Example B
A sociologist interviews 150 randomly selected citizens to determine their opinion about the Free-Trade agreement between Canada and the U.S. He places each individual into one of 5 categories: strongly in favor of, moderately in favor of, no opinion about, moderately against, and strongly against the Free-Trade agreement. He also places each individual into one of 3 socio-economic groups: upper class, middle class, and lower class. He is interested in knowing whether socioeconomic status and opinion are related.

Step 1. The researcher classified his subjects simultaneously on 2 variables, opinion and S.E.S. He will run a chi-square test for independence with 8 df.

Example C
A blue-jeans manufacturer randomly selects 100 young women and asks them if they prefer stone-washed or acid-treated blue jeans.

Step 1. How many variables? The women are classified on one variable: preference.

Step 2. How many categories? There are 2 categories of the preference variable and so a chi-square test for goodness of fit is appropriate. A Z-test for a proportion is also appropriate.

Example D
A botanist plants 100 seeds in each of three planters. Each planter is exposed to different amounts of light for a 3-week period. She then counts the number of seeds that germinate under high light, moderate light and low light conditions.

Step 1. There is one variable: light condition.

Step 2. There are 3 categories of the light variable and so a chi-square test for goodness of fit with 2 df will be used.

EXERCISES

Part A: For each of the following research studies, determine the most appropriate parametric test of significance.

A-1. A research group of behavior analysts is interested in the effects of diet and exercise on the development of anorexia nervosa in laboratory animals. An initial study is designed to determine the relationship between caloric intake and amount of exercise on weight loss. They randomly assign 12 laboratory rats to each of 6 treatment groups. Animals in three of the six groups receive a low-calorie diet, while the rest receive a moderate-calorie diet. In addition , one group from each diet type is put on a low-exercise program, one group is put on a moderate exercise program, and the last group is put on a high-exercise program. The researchers measure the weight of each animal before and after the program. They will use amount of weight loss as their measure.

A-2. A speech pathologist is concerned about the influence of sign-language training on speech development in hearing-impaired children. Specifically, he wonders if training children by means of signs may reduce their speech learning, since they may come to rely on the signing technique for communication. He randomly selects and independently assigns 15 children to each of two groups. All children learn lists of common nouns paired with numbers. The experimenter presents the word by pronouncing it out loud and the child is expected to respond with the number that goes with the word. For the signing group, the experimenter accompanies each pronounced word with its sign. For the control group, the sign is not given. The experimenter measures the number of trials it takes each child to learn the responses correctly.

A-3. A social psychologist is investigating group-helping behavior. She randomly assigns 20 subjects to each of three groups. Each subject is left in a waiting room and told that the experimenter will arrive shortly. In the Alone group subjects are alone in the waiting room. In the One-Other group the subject waits with another person who, unbeknownst to the subject, is a confederate of the experimenter. In the Five-Others group the real subject is in the waiting room with five other people, all confederates. Three minutes after the subject has been waiting, a loud crash and a moan are heard outside the waiting room. The confederates of the experiment ignore them. The experimenter records how long it takes for the real subjects to respond to the sounds of distress. She suspects that as the number of bystanders increases, so will the time taken to help.

A-4. A forward-thinking farmer decides to experiment on crop yield by comparing his usual fertilizer with a new type just on the market. He selects two fields each of corn, wheat, and barley, and uses his old fertilizer on one field of each type and the new fertilizer on the other field of each type. He compares the yield, i.e. average number of bushels per acre, of each of the six fields.

A-5. A physician is interested in the relationship between maternal weight-gain and birth weight. Although the fashion has been for pregnant women to gain less weight than they used to, the physician is worried about the effects of this trend on the weight of newborns. She randomly selects 50 women from her practice. At the time of birth she compares the weight of the newborns of the 35 women who gained 10 kg or more with the weight of the children born to the 15 women who gained less than 10 kg.

A-6. An educator in bilingual immersion programs randomly selects 45 children in French immersion kindergarten and 45 children in regular kindergarten. At the end of the year he gives each child a standard achievement test for which he has national norms.

A-7. A bilingual school has decided to respond to the recent criticism that the children in French immersion are behind in certain areas of English, such as reading and writing. A researcher randomly selects 20 French immersion children starting kindergarten and gives them a standard English language knowledge test. She gives the same English test to several children starting English kindergarten. Using these scores she matches an English child with each French immersion child. At the end of Grade 1 she re-tests all the children with a standard English language knowledge test. She will compare the performance of the French immersion and English children on this last test.

A-8. Bell Canada has decided to do a study on the effects of different kinds of incentives on staff performance. The research team randomly assigns 20 staffers to each of four groups. One group serves as a control group. The other three groups are given an incentive to increase their productivity, as measured by number of jobs completed per unit time. The Pay-Incentive group receives a bonus at the end of each month in which they have increased their productivity. The Share-Incentive group receives shares in the company for increasing productivity. The Praise-Incentive group receives public praise for their increase in productivity. Productivity is measured before the incentive program begins, and again at the end of 3, 6, 9 and 12 months.

Part B: For each of the following research studies, determine the most appropriate non-parametric test of significance.

B-1. A junior college was concerned about class attendance. The head of student services decided to do a study to see if attendance differed between faculties. She monitored classes in the sciences, the arts, and commerce and recorded student absences over a period of several weeks. Her data suggested that attendance was poorest in science classes. What non-parametric technique could she use to see if there was a significant difference in attendance?

B-2. An obedience school instructor was gathering data about which kinds of dogs respond best to training. He used a rating scale to evaluate the performance of six breeds of dogs that had completed an 8-week course. He suspected that certain breeds were less intelligent and therefore would benefit more from a longer course. He compared Golden Retrievers, Irish Setters, Poodles, Old English Sheepdogs, Spaniels and Beagles.

B-3. A sports psychologist randomly selected 25 people from the city of Edmonton phone book. She interviewed each person about the Gretzky trade to Los Angeles, immediately after the trade was announced, to determine whether they believed that it was Gretzky or the team owner, Peter Pocklington, who had initiated the trade. Two weeks later, the psychologist re-interviewed the 25 people to determine if the enormous amount of media speculation had influenced their beliefs about the trade.

B-4. Eighteen musicians and 18 engineers participated in an experiment to study the hypothesis that dream recall differed between the two groups. All participants slept in a sleep-lab where they could be monitored with physiological devices. Whenever a subject entered REM (rapid eye movement indicating dreaming) the subject was awakened and asked to report the dream. The ability of the subject to describe the dream content was evaluated by the researcher on a rating scale devised for that purpose.

B-5. Eight sets of identical twins suffering from a mild form of dyslexia participated in a study to investigate the effects of a new bio-feedback program developed to increase attention span. All of the children learned a series of tasks involving motor, perceptual and cognitive skills. One twin from each set was given bio-feedback during the learning sessions; the other twin was not. Several measures of the rate and quality of learning were taken. What non-parametric procedure should be used to evaluate the effectiveness of the bio-feedback training?

Part C: For each of the following research studies, determine the frequency test you would use and specify the number of degrees of freedom.

- **C-1.** A day care worker offers two kinds of toys to her class of 35 children. Action toys are toys requiring active participation on the part of the children. Examples of action toys are building blocks, puzzles, etc. Cuddly toys are toys that fill a nurturing need such as dolls, stuffed animals, etc. The day care worker wonders if gender (girls vs boys) makes a difference in choice (action vs cuddly).

- **C-2.** A mathematics instructor keeps track of who attends class and who doesn't the day before his weekly quiz. He wants to know if passing or failing the quiz depends on attendance.

- **C-3.** A professor of women's studies polls a random sample of 300 women and asks them how they feel about the abortion issue. She categorizes them into one of six groups based on whether they have any children (yes or no) and how they feel about abortion on demand (pro, con or undecided). She wishes to know if having children makes a difference on how women feel about abortion on demand.

- **C-4.** A ski manufacturer keeps track of the number of people who purchase "shorty" skis vs regular length skis and their level of ability (expert, intermediate or novice).

- **C-5.** A researcher has found that twice as many middle-aged students prefer studying at home through correspondence courses to attending night school. She randomly selects 150 young marrieds and asks them which they would prefer. She wants to know if the younger group resembles the older group in preference.

- **C-6.** The matching law in operant conditioning says that an animal will match the number of responses it makes to the rate of reinforcement it receives in a choice situation. For example, a pigeon faced with two keys to peck, one of which delivers twice as many reinforcements as the other, will make twice as many responses on that key. How would you use a chi-square analysis to test this law?

APPENDIX A

Toolbox

This appendix consists of two parts. The first section presents most of the computational formulas used in the text. This provides you with a handy reference. The second section contains all the test summaries found in the text. Both sections are arranged in alphabetical order. You are encouraged to refer to the appropriate chapter before beginning any analysis.

Toolbox of Computational Formulas

Analysis of Variance

One-Way ANOVA
Sums of Squares

Total
$$SS_{TOT} = \Sigma X_{tot}^2 - \frac{(\Sigma X_{tot})^2}{n_{tot}}$$

Between Groups
$$SS_{BG} = \frac{(\Sigma X_1)^2}{n_1} + \frac{(\Sigma X_2)^2}{n_2} + \ldots + \frac{(\Sigma X_k)^2}{n_k} - \frac{(\Sigma X_{tot})^2}{n_{tot}}$$

Within Groups
$$SS_{WG} = SS_{TOT} - SS_{BG}$$

Mean Squares

Between Groups
$$MS_{BG} = \frac{SS_{BG}}{k-1}$$

Within Groups
$$MS_{WG} = \frac{SS_{WG}}{n_{tot} - k}$$

F Ratio
$$F = MS_{BG}/MS_{WG}$$

Two-Way ANOVA

Sums of Squares

Total
$$SS_{TOT} = \Sigma X_{tot}^2 - \frac{(\Sigma X_{tot})^2}{n_{tot}}$$

Between Groups
$$SS_{BG} = \frac{(\Sigma A_1 B_1)^2 + (\Sigma A_1 B_2)^2 + \ldots + (\Sigma A_a B_b)^2}{n} - \frac{(\Sigma X_{tot})^2}{n_{tot}}$$

A
$$SS_A = \frac{(\Sigma A_1)^2 + (\Sigma A_2)^2 + \ldots + (\Sigma A_a)^2}{bn} - \frac{(\Sigma X_{tot})^2}{n_{tot}}$$

B
$$SS_B = \frac{(\Sigma B_1)^2 + (\Sigma B_2)^2 + \ldots + (\Sigma B_b)^2}{an} - \frac{(\Sigma X_{tot})^2}{n_{tot}}$$

AXB
$$SS_{AXB} = SS_{BG} - SS_A - SS_B$$

Within Groups
$$SS_{WG} = SS_{TOT} - SS_{BG}$$

Mean Squares

A
$$MS_A = \frac{SS_A}{a - 1}$$

B
$$MS_B = \frac{SS_B}{b - 1}$$

AXB
$$MS_{AXB} = \frac{SS_{AXB}}{(a - 1)(b - 1)}$$

WG
$$MS_{WG} = \frac{SS_{WG}}{n_{tot} - k}$$

F Ratios

$$F_A = MS_A / MS_{WG}$$

$$F_B = MS_B / MS_{WG}$$

$$F_{AXB} = MS_{AXB} / MS_{WG}$$

One-Way ANOVA with Repeated Measures

Sums of Squares

Total
$$SS_{TOT} = \Sigma X_{tot}^2 - \frac{(\Sigma X_{tot})^2}{kn}$$

Between Subject
$$SS_S = \frac{(\Sigma S_1)^2 + (\Sigma S_2)^2 + ... + (\Sigma S_n)^2}{k} - \frac{(\Sigma X_{tot})^2}{kn}$$

Within Subject
$$SS_{WS} = SS_{TOT} - SS_S$$

Treatment
$$SS_S = \frac{(\Sigma S_1)^2 + (\Sigma S_2)^2 + ... + (\Sigma S_n)^2}{k} - \frac{(\Sigma X_{tot})^2}{kn}$$

Subject by Treatment
$$SS_{SXT} = SS_{WS} - SS_T$$

Mean Squares

Treatment
$$MS_T = \frac{SS_T}{k-1}$$

Subject by Treatment
$$MS_{SXT} = \frac{SS_{SXT}}{(n-1)(k-1)}$$

F-Ratio

$$F = \frac{MS_T}{MS_{SXT}}$$

Two-Way ANOVA with Repeated Measures

Sums of Squares

Total
$$SS_{TOT} = \Sigma X_{tot}^2 - \frac{(\Sigma X_{tot})^2}{abn}$$

Between Subjects
$$SS_S = \frac{(\Sigma S_1)^2 + (\Sigma S_2)^2 + ... + (\Sigma S_{an})^2}{b} - \frac{(\Sigma X_{tot})^2}{abn}$$

A
$$SS_A = \frac{(\Sigma A_1)^2 + (\Sigma A_2)^2 + ... + (\Sigma A_a)^2}{bn} - \frac{(\Sigma X_{tot})^2}{abn}$$

Subjects within Groups
$$SS_{S(gps)} = SS_S - SS_A$$

B
$$SS_B = \frac{(\Sigma B_1)^2 + (\Sigma B_2)^2 + ... + (\Sigma B_b)^2}{an} - \frac{(\Sigma X_{tot})^2}{abn}$$

AXB
$$SS_{AXB} = \frac{(\Sigma A_1 B_1)^2 + (\Sigma A_1 B_2)^2 + ... + (\Sigma A_a B_b)^2}{n} - \frac{(\Sigma X_{tot})^2}{abn} - SS_A - SS_B$$

Subjects within GroupsXB $SS_{S(gps)XB} = SS_{WS} - SS_B - SS_{AXB}$

Mean Squares

A $MS_A = \dfrac{SS_A}{a-1}$

Subjects within Groups $MS_{S(gps)} = \dfrac{SS_{S(gps)}}{a(n-1)}$

B $MS_B = \dfrac{SS_B}{b-1}$

AXB $MS_{AXB} = \dfrac{SS_{AXB}}{(a-1)(b-1)}$

Subjects within GroupsXB $MS_{S(gps)XB} = \dfrac{SS_{S(gps)XB}}{a(n-1)(b-1)}$

F-Ratios

$$F_A = \dfrac{MS_A}{MS_{S(gps)}}$$

$$F_B = \dfrac{MS_B}{MS_{S(gps)XB}}$$

$$F_{AXB} = \dfrac{MS_{AXB}}{MS_{S(gps)XB}}$$

Chi-Square Formula

$$\chi^2 = \Sigma \dfrac{(O-E)^2}{E}$$

Combinations

$$_nC_r = \dfrac{n!}{(n-r)!r!}$$

Confidence Intervals

Difference: $\mu_1 - \mu_2 = (\overline{X}_1 - \overline{X}_2) \pm Z(\sigma_{\overline{x}_1 - \overline{x}_2})$

Mean: $\mu = \overline{X} \pm Z(\sigma_{\overline{x}})$

Proportion: $P = p \pm Z(\sigma_p)$

When σ is estimated with s

Difference-Independent: $\mu_1 - \mu_2 = (\overline{X}_1 - \overline{X}_2) \pm t_{crit}(s_{\overline{x}_1 - \overline{x}_2})$

Difference-Dependent: $\mu_{\overline{D}} = \overline{D} \pm t_{crit}(s_{\overline{D}})$

Mean: $\mu = \overline{X} \pm t_{crit}(s_{\overline{x}})$

Deviation Score $\quad x = X - \mu$

Kruskal-Wallis H

$$H = \frac{12}{n_{tot}(n_{tot}+1)}\left[\frac{(\Sigma R_1)^2}{n_1} + \frac{(\Sigma R_2)^2}{n_2} + \ldots + \frac{(\Sigma R_k)^2}{n_k}\right] - 3(n_{tot}+1)$$

Mann-Whitney U

$$U_1 = n_1 n_2 + \frac{n_1(n_1+1)}{2} - \Sigma R_1$$

$$U_2 = n_1 n_2 + \frac{n_2(n_2+1)}{2} - \Sigma R_2$$

Mean

Population

Raw Score: $\quad \mu = \frac{\Sigma X}{N}$

Data in a Frequency Distribution: $\quad \mu = \frac{\Sigma fX}{N}$

Mean for Combined Subgroups:

when sums are known: $\quad \mu_c = \frac{\Sigma X + \Sigma Y}{N_x + N_y}$

when means are known: $\quad \mu_c = \frac{N_x \mu_x + N_y \mu_y}{N_x + N_y}$

when $N_x = N_y$: $\quad \mu_c = \frac{\mu_x + \mu_y}{2}$

Sample

Raw Score: $\quad \overline{X} = \frac{\Sigma X}{n}$

Data in a Frequency Distribution: $\quad \overline{X} = \frac{\Sigma fX}{n}$

Median

$$Mdn = L + \frac{\left[N\left(\frac{50}{100}\right) - f_b\right]i}{f_w}$$

Pearson's Coefficient of Correlation

Raw Score: $$\rho = \frac{\Sigma XY - (\Sigma X)(\Sigma Y)/N}{\sqrt{[\Sigma X^2 - (\Sigma X)^2/N][\Sigma Y^2 - (\Sigma Y)^2/N]}}$$

Deviation Score: $$\rho = \frac{\Sigma xy}{\sqrt{(\Sigma x^2)(\Sigma y^2)}}$$

Z-Score Data: $$\rho = \frac{\Sigma(Z_x Z_y)}{N}$$

When estimating ρ with r:

$$r = \frac{\Sigma XY - (\Sigma X)(\Sigma Y)/n}{\sqrt{[\Sigma X^2 - (\Sigma X)^2/n][\Sigma Y^2 - (\Sigma Y)^2/n]}}$$

Percentile

$$P_{PR} = L + \frac{\left[N\left(\frac{PR}{100}\right) - f_b\right]i}{f_w}$$

Percentile Rank

$$PR_X = \frac{\left[f_w \frac{(X - L)}{i} + f_b\right]100}{N}$$

Permutations

$$_nP_r = \frac{n!}{(n - r)!}$$

Probability

Binomial Probability

$$_nC_r\, p^r q^{n-r} = \frac{n!}{(n - r)!r!} p^r q^{n-r}$$

Compound
  p (A and B)
    Dependent events: $p(A) \cdot p(B/A)$

    Independent events: $p(A) \cdot p(B)$

  p (A or B)
    Not mutually
      exclusive: $p(A) + p(B) - p(A \text{ and } B)$

    Mutually exclusive: $p(A) + p(B)$

Conditional $p(B/A) = \dfrac{\#B/A \text{ has occurred}}{\#O/A \text{ has occurred}}$

Simple $\quad p(A) = \dfrac{\#A}{\#O}$

Range $\quad H - L + 1$

Regression Formulas

Simple linear regression

Raw Score: $\quad Y' = \rho\left(\dfrac{\sigma_y}{\sigma_x}\right)X - \rho\left(\dfrac{\sigma_y}{\sigma_x}\right)\mu_x + \mu_y$

Deviation Score: $\quad y' = \rho\left(\dfrac{\sigma_y}{\sigma_x}\right)x$

Z-Score: $\quad Z_{y'} = \rho Z_x$

Slope of the Regression Line: $\quad b = \rho\left(\dfrac{\sigma_y}{\sigma_x}\right)$

Slope for Raw Data: $\quad b = \dfrac{\Sigma XY - (\Sigma X)(\Sigma Y)/N}{\Sigma X^2 - (\Sigma X)^2/N}$

Y Intercept of the Regression Line: $\quad a = -\rho\left(\dfrac{\sigma_y}{\sigma_x}\right)\mu_x + \mu_y$

Multiple Regression

Multiple Correlation Coefficient: $\quad MR = \sqrt{\dfrac{\rho^2_{y1} + \rho^2_{y2} - 2\rho_{y1}\rho_{y2}\rho_{12}}{1 - \rho^2_{12}}}$

Multiple Regression Equation: $\quad Y' = b_1 X_1 + b_2 X_2 + a$

Partial Correlation: $\quad R_p = \dfrac{\rho_{y1} - \rho_{y2}\rho_{12}}{\sqrt{(1 - \rho^2_{y2})(1 - \rho^2_{12})}}$

Slope

First Predictor Variable: $\quad b_1 = \left(\dfrac{\sigma_y}{\sigma_1}\right)\left(\dfrac{\rho_{y1} - \rho_{y2}\rho_{12}}{1 - \rho^2_{12}}\right)$

Second Predictor Variable: $\quad b_2 = \left(\dfrac{\sigma_y}{\sigma_2}\right)\left(\dfrac{\rho_{y2} - \rho_{y1}\rho_{12}}{1 - \rho^2_{12}}\right)$

Scheffé

F' Statistic: $\quad F' = C/s_c$

Scheffé's Critical F: $\quad F_s = \sqrt{(k-1)F_{crit}}$

Comparison: $\quad C = c_1\overline{X}_1 + c_2\overline{X}_2 + ... + c_k\overline{X}_k$

Standard Error: $\quad s_c = \sqrt{MS_{error}\left(\dfrac{c_1^2}{n_1} + \dfrac{c_2^2}{n_2} + ... + \dfrac{c_k^2}{n_k}\right)}$

Spearman Rank-Order Correlation Coefficient

$$\text{rho} = 1 - \dfrac{6\Sigma d^2}{n(n^2 - 1)}$$

Standard Deviation

Population

Raw Data: $\quad \sigma = \sqrt{\dfrac{\Sigma X^2 - (\Sigma X)^2/N}{N}}$

Data in Frequency Distribution: $\quad \sigma = \sqrt{\dfrac{\Sigma fX^2 - (\Sigma fX)^2/N}{N}}$

Estimate of σ:

$$s = \sqrt{\dfrac{\Sigma X^2 - (\Sigma X)^2/n}{n - 1}}$$

Standard Errors for Z-tests

Difference $\quad \sigma_{\bar{x}_1 - \bar{x}_2} = \sqrt{\dfrac{\Sigma x_1^2 + \Sigma x_2^2}{n_1 + n_2}\left(\dfrac{1}{n_1} + \dfrac{1}{n_2}\right)}$

$\quad \sigma_{\bar{x}_1 - \bar{x}_2} = \sqrt{\dfrac{\Sigma x_1^2 + \Sigma x_2^2}{n(n)}} \quad \text{if } n_1 = n_2$

where $\Sigma x^2 = \Sigma X^2 - (\Sigma X)^2/n$

Mean $\quad \sigma_{\bar{x}} = \sigma/\sqrt{n}$

Proportion $\quad \sigma_p = \sqrt{PQ/n}$

Standard Errors: Estimates for t-tests

Difference

Independent Samples

$$s_{\bar{x}_1 - \bar{x}_1} = \sqrt{s_{\bar{x}_1}^2 + s_{\bar{x}_2}^2}$$

$$s_{\bar{x}_1 - \bar{x}_2} = \sqrt{\frac{\Sigma x_1^2 + \Sigma x_2^2}{n_1 + n_2 - 2}\left(\frac{1}{n_1} + \frac{1}{n_2}\right)}$$

$$s_{\bar{x}_1 - \bar{x}_2} = \sqrt{\frac{\Sigma x_1^2 + \Sigma x_2^2}{n(n-1)}} \quad \text{if } n_1 = n_2$$

where $\Sigma x^2 = \Sigma X^2 - (\Sigma X)^2/n$

Dependent Samples

$$s_{\bar{D}} = \sqrt{\frac{\Sigma D^2 - (\Sigma D)^2/n}{n(n-1)}}$$

Mean

$$s_{\bar{x}} = s/\sqrt{n}$$

$$s_{\bar{x}} = \sqrt{\frac{\Sigma X^2 - (\Sigma X)^2/n}{n(n-1)}}$$

Standard Error of Estimate

$$\sigma_{yx} = \sqrt{\frac{\Sigma(Y - Y')^2}{N}}$$

$$\sigma_{yx} = \sigma_y\sqrt{1 - \rho^2}$$

Standard Error of Multiple Estimate

$$\sigma_{ME} = \sigma_y\sqrt{1 - MR^2}$$

Standard Error for Pearson's r

$$s_r = \sqrt{\frac{1 - r^2}{n - 2}}$$

t-Ratios

Mean

$$t = \frac{\bar{X} - \mu_{\bar{x}}}{s_{\bar{x}}}$$

Difference: Independent Means

$$t = \frac{\bar{X}_1 - \bar{X}_2}{s_{\bar{x}_1 - \bar{x}_2}}$$

Difference: Dependent Means		$t = \dfrac{\overline{D} - \mu_{\overline{D}}}{s_{\overline{D}}}$
r		$t = \dfrac{r - \rho}{s_r}$
Planned Comparison		$t = \dfrac{\overline{X}_1 - \overline{X}_2}{\sqrt{2MS_{error}/n}}$

Treatment Effect Estimate

$$\hat{\omega}^2 = \dfrac{t^2 - 1}{t^2 + df + 1}$$

Tukey $\quad HSD = q(\alpha, df_{error}, k)\sqrt{MS_{error}/n}$

Variance

Population

Raw Score $\quad \sigma^2 = \dfrac{\Sigma X^2 - (\Sigma X)^2/N}{N}$

Data in Frequency Distribution $\quad \sigma^2 = \dfrac{\Sigma fX^2 - (\Sigma fX)^2/N}{N}$

Pooled Variance for Three Combined Subgroups

$$\sigma_c^2 = \dfrac{N_w\sigma_w^2 + N_x\sigma_x^2 + N_y\sigma_y^2 + N_w(\mu_w - \mu_c)^2 + N_x(\mu_x - \mu_c)^2 + N_y(\mu_y - \mu_c)^2}{N_w + N_x + N_y}$$

Estimate of σ^2 $\quad s^2 = \dfrac{\Sigma X^2 - (\Sigma X)^2/n}{n - 1}$

Wilcoxon $\quad Z = \dfrac{T - \mu_T}{\sigma_T}$

Z-Ratios

Difference $\quad Z = \dfrac{\overline{X}_1 - \overline{X}_2}{\sigma_{\overline{x}_1 - \overline{x}_2}}$

Mean $\quad Z = \dfrac{\overline{X} - \mu_{\overline{x}}}{\sigma_{\overline{x}}}$

Proportion $\quad Z = \dfrac{p - P}{\sigma_p}$

Score $\quad Z = \dfrac{X - \mu}{\sigma}$

Mann-Whitney U $\quad Z = \dfrac{U - n_1 n_2/2}{\sqrt{\dfrac{n_1 n_2 (n_1 + n_2 + 1)}{12}}}$

Wilcoxon T $\quad Z = \dfrac{T - n(n + 1)/4}{\sqrt{\dfrac{n(n + 1)(2n + 1)}{24}}}$

Toolbox of Test Summaries

Summary of One-Way ANOVA

Hypotheses
H_o: $\mu_1 = \mu_2 = \ldots = \mu_k$
H_a: H_o is false

Assumptions
1. Subjects are randomly selected and independently assigned to groups.
2. Population distributions are normal.
3. Population variances are homogeneous.

Decision Rules
$df_{bg} = k - 1 \quad df_{wg} = n_{tot} - k$
If $F_{obt} \geq F_{crit}$, reject the H_o
If $F_{obt} < F_{crit}$, do not reject H_o

Formula
$$F = \dfrac{MS_{BG}}{MS_{WG}}$$

Summary of Two-Way ANOVA

Hypotheses
   H_o: No main effects and no interaction
   H_a: H_o is false

Assumptions
  1. Subjects are randomly selected and independently assigned to groups.
  2. Population distributions are normal.
  3. Population variances are homogeneous.

Decision Rules
   $df_a = a - 1 \quad df_b = b - 1 \quad df_{axb} = (a - 1)(b - 1)$
   If $F_{obt} \geq F_{crit}$, reject the H_o
   If $F_{obt} < F_{crit}$, do not reject H_o

Formulas
$$F_A = \frac{MS_A}{MS_{WG}}$$
$$F_B = \frac{MS_B}{MS_{WG}}$$
$$F_{AXB} = \frac{MS_{AXB}}{MS_{WG}}$$

Summary of One-Way ANOVA with Repeated Measures

Hypotheses
   H_o: $\mu_1 = \mu_2 = \ldots = \mu_k$
   H_a: H_o is false

Assumptions
  1. Subjects are randomly selected.
  2. Population distributions are normal.
  3. Population variances are homogeneous.
  4. Population covariances are equal.

Decision Rules
   $df_t = k - 1 \quad df_{sxt} = (n - 1)(k - 1)$
   If $F_{obt} \geq F_{crit}$, reject the H_o
   If $F_{obt} < F_{crit}$, do not reject H_o

Formula
$$F = \frac{MS_T}{MS_{SXT}}$$

Summary of Two-Way ANOVA with Repeated Measures

Hypotheses
H_o: No main effects and no interaction
H_a: H_o is false

Assumptions
1. Subjects are randomly selected with repeated measures on factor B.
2. Population distributions are normal.
3. Population variances are homogeneous.
4. Population covariances are equal.

Decision Rules
$df_a = a - 1 \quad df_b = b - 1 \quad df_{axb} = (a-1)(b-1)$
$df_{s(gps)} = a(n-1) \quad df_{s(gps)xb} = a(n-1)(b-1)$
If $F_{obt} \geq F_{crit}$, reject the H_o
If $F_{obt} < F_{crit}$, do not reject H_o

Formulas
$$F_A = \frac{MS_A}{MS_{S(gps)}}$$
$$F_B = \frac{MS_B}{MS_{S(gps)XB}}$$
$$F_{AXB} = \frac{MS_{AXB}}{MS_{S(gps)XB}}$$

Summary of the Chi-Square Test for Goodness of Fit

Hypotheses
H_o: O's = E's
H_a: O's ≠ E's

Assumptions
1. Subjects are randomly selected.
2. Categories are mutually exclusive.

Decision Rules
df = number of categories − 1
If $\chi^2_{obt} \geq \chi^2_{crit}$, reject H_o
If $\chi^2_{obt} < \chi^2_{crit}$, do not reject H_o

Formula
$$\chi^2 = \sum \frac{(O - E)^2}{E}$$

Summary of the Chi-Square Test for Independence

Hypotheses
 H_o: The variables are independent
 H_a: The variables are dependent

Assumptions
1. Subjects are randomly selected.
2. Observations have been classified simultaneously on two independent categories.

Decision Rules
 df = (number of rows − 1)(number of columns − 1)
 If $\chi^2_{obt} \geq \chi^2_{crit}$, reject H_o
 If $\chi^2_{obt} < \chi^2_{crit}$, do not reject H_o

Formula
$$\chi^2 = \Sigma \frac{(O - E)^2}{E}$$

Summary of the Mann-Whitney U Test

Hypotheses
 H_o: Populations are identical
 H_a: Populations are not identical

Assumptions
1. Subjects are randomly selected and independently assigned to groups.
2. Measurement scale is at least ordinal.

Decision Rules
 If $U_{obt} \leq U_{crit}$, reject the H_o
 If $U_{obt} > U_{crit}$, do not reject the H_o

Formulas
$$U_1 = n_1 n_2 + \frac{n_1(n_1 + 1)}{2} - \Sigma R_1$$

$$U_2 = n_1 n_2 + \frac{n_2(n_2 + 1)}{2} - \Sigma R_2$$

U_{obt} is smaller of U_1 and U_2

Summary of the Pearson Correlation Test

Hypotheses
H_o: $\rho = 0$
H_a: $\rho \neq 0$, $\rho < 0$, $\rho > 0$

Assumptions
1. Subjects are randomly selected.
2. Both populations are normally distributed.

Decision Rules
If $t_{obt} \geq t_{crit}$, reject H_o
If $t_{obt} < t_{crit}$, do not reject H_o

Formula
$$t = \frac{r - \rho}{\sqrt{\dfrac{1 - r^2}{n - 2}}}$$

Summary of Planned Comparisons

Hypotheses
H_o: No difference between population means
H_a: H_o is false

Assumptions
The outcome of the ANOVA need not be significant.

Decision Rules
If $t_{obt} > t_{crit}$, reject H_o
If $t_{obt} < t_{crit}$, do not reject H_o

Summary of the Scheffé Test

Hypotheses
 H_o: No difference between population means
 H_a: H_o is false

Assumptions
 The outcome of the ANOVA was significant.

Decision Rules
 If $F' \geq F_s$, reject the H_o
 If $F' < F_s$, do not reject H_o

Formulas
 $F' = C/s_c$
 $F_s = \sqrt{(k-1)(F_{crit})}$

Summary of the Spearman Rank-Order Correlation Test

Hypotheses
 H_o: Rho $= 0$
 H_a: Rho $\neq 0$, Rho < 0, Rho > 0

Assumptions
 1. Subjects are randomly selected.
 2. Observations are rank-ordered.

Decision Rules
 n = number of pairs of ranks
 If $rho_{obt} \geq rho_{crit}$, reject H_o
 If $rho_{obt} < rho_{crit}$, do not reject H_o

Formula
 $$rho = 1 - \frac{6\Sigma d^2}{n(n^2 - 1)}$$

Summary of t-Test for a Single Mean

Hypotheses
 H_o: μ = specified value
 H_a: $\mu \neq$ or $>$ or $<$ specified value

Assumptions
 1. Subjects are randomly selected.
 2. Population distribution is normal.

Decision Rules
 df = n − 1
 If $t_{obt} \geq t_{crit}$, reject the H_o
 If $t_{obt} < t_{crit}$, do not reject H_o

Formula
$$t = \frac{\overline{X} - \mu}{\sqrt{\dfrac{\Sigma X^2 - (\Sigma X)^2/n}{n(n-1)}}}$$

Summary of t-Test for Dependent Means

Hypotheses
 H_o: $\mu_1 = \mu_2$
 H_a: $\mu_1 \neq \mu_2$, $\mu_1 < \mu_2$, $\mu_1 > \mu_2$

Assumptions
 1. Subjects are randomly selected.
 2. Population distributions are normal.
 3. Population variances are homogeneous.
 4. Repeated measures or matched subjects are used.

Decision Rules
 df = n_{pairs} − 1
 If $t_{obt} \geq t_{crit}$, reject H_o
 If $t_{obt} < t_{crit}$, do not reject H_o

Formula
$$t = \frac{\overline{D}}{\sqrt{\dfrac{\Sigma D^2 - (\Sigma D)^2/n}{n(n-1)}}}$$

Summary of t-Test for Independent Means

Hypotheses
H_o: $\mu_1 = \mu_2$
H_a: $\mu_1 \neq \mu_2$, $\mu_1 < \mu_2$, $\mu_1 > \mu_2$

Assumptions
1. Subjects are randomly selected and independently assigned to groups.
2. Population variances are homogeneous.
3. Population distributions are normal.

Decision Rules
df = $n_1 + n_2 - 2$
If $t_{obt} \geq t_{crit}$, reject H_o
If $t_{obt} < t_{crit}$, do not reject H_o

Formula
$$t = \frac{\overline{X}_1 - \overline{X}_2}{\sqrt{\left(\frac{\Sigma x_1^2 + \Sigma x_2^2}{n_1 + n_2 - 2}\right)\left(\frac{1}{n_1} + \frac{1}{n_2}\right)}}$$
where $\Sigma x^2 = \Sigma X^2 - (\Sigma X)^2/n$

Summary of the Tukey Test

Hypotheses
H_o: No difference between population means
H_a: H_o is false

Assumptions
The outcome of the ANOVA was significant.

Decision Rules
Any mean difference $\geq$ HSD, reject the H_o

Formula
$HSD = q(\alpha, df_{error}, k) \sqrt{MS_{error}/n}$

Summary of the Wilcoxon Test

Hypotheses
H_o: Populations are identical
H_a: Populations are not identical

Assumptions
1. Subjects are randomly selected.
2. Same or matched subjects.
3. Measurement scale is at least ordinal.

Decision Rules
If $T_{obt} \leq T_{crit}$, reject the H_o
If $T_{obt} > T_{crit}$, do not reject the H_o

Formula
N = number of pairs with non-zero differences
T is the sum of the absolute ranks with the less frequently appearing sign

Summary of Z-Test for Independent Means

Hypotheses
H_o: $\mu_1 = \mu_2$
H_a: $\mu_1 \neq \mu_2$, $\mu_1 < \mu_2$, $\mu_1 > \mu_2$

Assumptions
1. Subjects are randomly selected and independently assigned to groups.
2. Population distributions are normal.
3. Population standard deviations are known.

Decision Rules
If $Z_{obt} \geq Z_{crit}$, reject H_o
If $Z_{obt} < Z_{crit}$, do not reject H_o

Formula
$$Z = \frac{\overline{X}_1 - \overline{X}_2}{\sqrt{\left(\frac{\Sigma x_1^2 + \Sigma x_2^2}{n_1 + n_2}\right)\left(\frac{1}{n_1} + \frac{1}{n_2}\right)}}$$
where $\Sigma x^2 = \Sigma X^2 - (\Sigma X)^2/n$

Summary of Z-Test for a Proportion

Hypotheses
 H_o: P = specified value
 H_a: P ≠ or < or > specified value

Assumptions
 1. Subjects are randomly selected.
 2. Sampling distribution of the statistic is normal.
 3. Observations are dichotomous.

Decision Rules
 If $Z_{obt} \geq Z_{crit}$, reject the H_o
 If $Z_{obt} < Z_{crit}$, do not reject H_o

Formula
$$Z = \frac{p - P}{\sqrt{PQ/n}}$$

Summary of Z-Test for a Single Mean

Hypotheses
 H_o: μ = specified value
 H_a: μ ≠ or < or > specified value

Assumptions
 1. Subjects are randomly selected.
 2. Population distribution is normal.
 3. Population standard deviation is known.

Decision Rules
 If $Z_{obt} \geq Z_{crit}$, reject the H_o
 If $Z_{obt} < Z_{crit}$, do not reject H_o

Formula
$$Z = \frac{\overline{X} - \mu}{\sigma/\sqrt{n}}$$

APPENDIX B

Statistical Tables

Table B-1 Areas under the normal curve

z	0 to z	beyond z	z	0 to z	beyond z	z	0 to z	beyond z
0.00	.0000	.5000	0.55	.2088	.2912	1.10	.3643	.1357
0.01	.0040	.4960	0.56	.2123	.2877	1.11	.3665	.1335
0.02	.0080	.4920	0.57	.2157	.2843	1.12	.3686	.1314
0.03	.0120	.4880	0.58	.2190	.2810	1.13	.3708	.1292
0.04	.0160	.4840	0.59	.2224	.2776	1.14	.3729	.1271
0.05	.0199	.4801	0.60	.2257	.2743	1.15	.3749	.1251
0.06	.0239	.4761	0.61	.2291	.2709	1.16	.3770	.1230
0.07	.0279	.4721	0.62	.2324	.2676	1.17	.3790	.1210
0.08	.0319	.4681	0.63	.2357	.2643	1.18	.3810	.1190
0.09	.0359	.4641	0.64	.2389	.2611	1.19	.3830	.1170
0.10	.0398	.4602	0.65	.2422	.2578	1.20	.3849	.1151
0.11	.0438	.4562	0.66	.2454	.2546	1.21	.3869	.1131
0.12	.0478	.4522	0.67	.2486	.2514	1.22	.3888	.1112
0.13	.0517	.4483	0.68	.2517	.2483	1.23	.3907	.1093
0.14	.0557	.4443	0.69	.2549	.2451	1.24	.3925	.1075
0.15	.0596	.4404	0.70	.2580	.2420	1.25	.3944	.1056
0.16	.0636	.4364	0.71	.2611	.2389	1.26	.3962	.1038
0.17	.0675	.4325	0.72	.2642	.2358	1.27	.3980	.1020
0.18	.0714	.4286	0.73	.2673	.2327	1.28	.3997	.1003
0.19	.0753	.4247	0.74	.2704	.2296	1.29	.4015	.0985
0.20	.0793	.4207	0.75	.2734	.2266	1.30	.4032	.0968
0.21	.0832	.4168	0.76	.2764	.2236	1.31	.4049	.0951
0.22	.0871	.4129	0.77	.2794	.2206	1.32	.4066	.0934
0.23	.0910	.4090	0.78	.2823	.2177	1.33	.4082	.0918
0.24	.0948	.4052	0.79	.2852	.2148	1.34	.4099	.0901
0.25	.0987	.4013	0.80	.2881	.2119	1.35	.4115	.0885
0.26	.1026	.3974	0.81	.2910	.2090	1.36	.4131	.0869
0.27	.1064	.3936	0.82	.2939	.2061	1.37	.4147	.0853
0.28	.1103	.3897	0.83	.2967	.2033	1.38	.4162	.0838
0.29	.1141	.3859	0.84	.2995	.2005	1.39	.4177	.0823
0.30	.1179	.3821	0.85	.3023	.1977	1.40	.4192	.0808
0.31	.1217	.3783	0.86	.3051	.1949	1.41	.4207	.0793
0.32	.1255	.3745	0.87	.3078	.1922	1.42	.4222	.0778
0.33	.1293	.3707	0.88	.3106	.1894	1.43	.4236	.0764
0.34	.1331	.3669	0.89	.3133	.1867	1.44	.4251	.0749
0.35	.1368	.3632	0.90	.3159	.1841	1.45	.4265	.0735
0.36	.1406	.3594	0.91	.3186	.1814	1.46	.4279	.0721
0.37	.1443	.3557	0.92	.3212	.1788	1.47	.4292	.0708
0.38	.1480	.3520	0.93	.3238	.1762	1.48	.4306	.0694
0.39	.1517	.3483	0.94	.3264	.1736	1.49	.4319	.0681
0.40	.1554	.3446	0.95	.3289	.1711	1.50	.4332	.0668
0.41	.1591	.3409	0.96	.3315	.1685	1.51	.4345	.0655
0.42	.1628	.3372	0.97	.3340	.1660	1.52	.4357	.0643
0.43	.1664	.3336	0.98	.3365	.1635	1.53	.4370	.0630
0.44	.1700	.3300	0.99	.3389	.1611	1.54	.4382	.0618
0.45	.1736	.3264	1.00	.3413	.1587	1.55	.4394	.0606
0.46	.1772	.3228	1.01	.3438	.1562	1.56	.4406	.0594
0.47	.1808	.3192	1.02	.3461	.1539	1.57	.4418	.0582
0.48	.1844	.3156	1.03	.3485	.1515	1.58	.4429	.0571
0.49	.1879	.3121	1.04	.3508	.1492	1.59	.4441	.0559
0.50	.1915	.3085	1.05	.3531	.1469	1.60	.4452	.0548
0.51	.1950	.3050	1.06	.3554	.1446	1.61	.4463	.0537
0.52	.1985	.3015	1.07	.3577	.1423	1.62	.4474	.0526
0.53	.2019	.2981	1.08	.3599	.1401	1.63	.4484	.0516
0.54	.2054	.2946	1.09	.3621	.1379	1.64	.4495	.0505

Table B-1 (cont'd)

z	0 to z	beyond z	z	0 to z	beyond z	z	0 to z	beyond z
1.65	.4505	.0495	2.22	.4868	.0132	2.79	.4974	.0026
1.66	.4515	.0485	2.23	.4871	.0129	2.80	.4974	.0026
1.67	.4525	.0475	2.24	.4875	.0125	2.81	.4975	.0025
1.68	.4535	.0465	2.25	.4878	.0122	2.82	.4976	.0024
1.69	.4545	.0455	2.26	.4881	.0119	2.83	.4977	.0023
1.70	.4554	.0446	2.27	.4884	.0116	2.84	.4977	.0023
1.71	.4564	.0436	2.28	.4887	.0113	2.85	.4978	.0022
1.72	.4573	.0427	2.29	.4890	.0110	2.86	.4979	.0021
1.73	.4582	.0418	2.30	.4893	.0107	2.87	.4979	.0021
1.74	.4591	.0409	2.31	.4896	.0104	2.88	.4980	.0020
1.75	.4599	.0401	2.32	.4898	.0102	2.89	.4981	.0019
1.76	.4608	.0392	2.33	.4901	.0099	2.90	.4981	.0019
1.77	.4616	.0384	2.34	.4904	.0096	2.91	.4982	.0018
1.78	.4625	.0375	2.35	.4906	.0094	2.92	.4982	.0018
1.79	.4633	.0367	2.36	.4909	.0091	2.93	.4983	.0017
1.80	.4641	.0359	2.37	.4911	.0089	2.94	.4984	.0016
1.81	.4649	.0351	2.38	.4913	.0087	2.95	.4984	.0016
1.82	.4656	.0344	2.39	.4916	.0084	2.96	.4985	.0015
1.83	.4664	.0336	2.40	.4918	.0082	2.97	.4985	.0015
1.84	.4671	.0329	2.41	.4920	.0080	2.98	.4986	.0014
1.85	.4678	.0322	2.42	.4922	.0078	2.99	.4986	.0014
1.86	.4686	.0314	2.43	.4925	.0075	3.00	.4987	.0013
1.87	.4693	.0307	2.44	.4927	.0073	3.01	.4987	.0013
1.88	.4699	.0301	2.45	.4929	.0071	3.02	.4987	.0013
1.89	.4706	.0294	2.46	.4931	.0069	3.03	.4988	.0012
1.90	.4713	.0287	2.47	.4932	.0068	3.04	.4988	.0012
1.91	.4719	.0281	2.48	.4934	.0066	3.05	.4989	.0011
1.92	.4726	.0274	2.49	.4936	.0064	3.06	.4989	.0011
1.93	.4732	.0268	2.50	.4938	.0062	3.07	.4989	.0011
1.94	.4738	.0262	2.51	.4940	.0060	3.08	.4990	.0010
1.95	.4744	.0256	2.52	.4941	.0059	3.09	.4990	.0010
1.96	.4750	.0250	2.53	.4943	.0057	3.10	.4990	.0010
1.97	.4756	.0244	2.54	.4945	.0055	3.11	.4991	.0009
1.98	.4761	.0239	2.55	.4946	.0054	3.12	.4991	.0009
1.99	.4767	.0233	2.56	.4948	.0052	3.13	.4991	.0009
2.00	.4772	.0228	2.57	.4949	.0051	3.14	.4992	.0008
2.01	.4778	.0222	2.58	.4951	.0049	3.15	.4992	.0008
2.02	.4783	.0217	2.59	.4952	.0048	3.16	.4992	.0008
2.03	.4788	.0212	2.60	.4953	.0047	3.17	.4992	.0008
2.04	.4793	.0207	2.61	.4955	.0045	3.18	.4993	.0007
2.05	.4798	.0202	2.62	.4956	.0044	3.19	.4993	.0007
2.06	.4803	.0197	2.63	.4957	.0043	3.20	.4993	.0007
2.07	.4808	.0192	2.64	.4959	.0041	3.21	.4993	.0007
2.08	.4812	.0188	2.65	.4960	.0040	3.22	.4994	.0006
2.09	.4817	.0183	2.66	.4961	.0039	3.23	.4994	.0006
2.10	.4821	.0179	2.67	.4962	.0038	3.24	.4994	.0006
2.11	.4826	.0174	2.68	.4963	.0037	3.25	.4994	.0006
2.12	.4830	.0170	2.69	.4964	.0036	3.30	.4995	.0005
2.13	.4834	.0166	2.70	.4965	.0035	3.35	.4996	.0004
2.14	.4838	.0162	2.71	.4966	.0034	3.40	.4997	.0003
2.15	.4842	.0158	2.72	.4967	.0033	3.45	.4997	.0003
2.16	.4846	.0154	2.73	.4968	.0032	3.50	.4998	.0002
2.17	.4850	.0150	2.74	.4969	.0031	3.60	.4998	.0002
2.18	.4854	.0146	2.75	.4970	.0030	3.70	.4999	.0001
2.19	.4857	.0143	2.76	.4971	.0029	3.80	.4999	.0001
2.20	.4861	.0139	2.77	.4972	.0028	3.90	.49995	.00005
2.21	.4864	.0136	2.78	.4973	.0027	4.00	.49997	.00003

Source: Richard Runyon and Audrey Haber, *Fundamentals of Behavioral Statistics*, 2nd edition (Reading, Mass.: Addison-Wesley Inc., 1971). Copyright by Random House, Inc. Reprinted by permission.

Table B-2 Critical values of t

df	Level of significance for a directional (one-tailed) test					
	.10	.05	.025	.01	.005	.0005
	Level of significance for a non-directional (two-tailed) test					
	.20	.10	.05	.02	.01	.001
1	3.078	6.314	12.706	31.821	63.657	636.619
2	1.886	2.920	4.303	6.965	9.925	31.598
3	1.638	2.353	3.182	4.541	5.841	12.941
4	1.533	2.132	2.776	3.747	4.604	8.610
5	1.476	2.015	2.571	3.365	4.032	6.859
6	1.440	1.943	2.447	3.143	3.707	5.959
7	1.415	1.895	2.365	2.998	3.499	5.405
8	1.397	1.860	2.306	2.896	3.355	5.041
9	1.383	1.833	2.262	2.821	3.250	4.781
10	1.372	1.812	2.228	2.764	3.169	4.587
11	1.363	1.796	2.201	2.718	3.106	4.437
12	1.356	1.782	2.179	2.681	3.055	4.318
13	1.350	1.771	2.160	2.650	3.012	4.221
14	1.345	1.761	2.145	2.624	2.977	4.140
15	1.341	1.753	2.131	2.602	2.947	4.073
16	1.337	1.746	2.120	2.583	2.921	4.015
17	1.333	1.740	2.110	2.567	2.898	3.965
18	1.330	1.734	2.101	2.552	2.878	3.922
19	1.328	1.729	2.093	2.539	2.861	3.883
20	1.325	1.725	2.086	2.528	2.845	3.850
21	1.323	1.721	2.080	2.518	2.831	3.819
22	1.321	1.717	2.074	2.508	2.819	3.792
23	1.319	1.714	2.069	2.500	2.807	3.767
24	1.318	1.711	2.064	2.492	2.797	3.745
25	1.316	1.708	2.060	2.485	2.787	3.725
26	1.315	1.706	2.056	2.479	2.779	3.707
27	1.314	1.703	2.052	2.473	2.771	3.690
28	1.313	1.701	2.048	2.467	2.763	3.674
29	1.311	1.699	2.045	2.462	2.756	3.659
30	1.310	1.697	2.042	2.457	2.750	3.646
40	1.303	1.684	2.021	2.423	2.704	3.551
60	1.296	1.671	2.000	2.390	2.660	3.460
120	1.289	1.658	1.980	2.358	2.617	3.373
∞	1.282	1.645	1.960	2.326	2.576	3.291

Source: From Table III of Fisher and Yates, *Statistical Tables for Biological, Agricultural and Medical Research*, published by Longman Group UK Ltd., London (previously published by Oliver and Boyd Ltd., Edinburgh), with permission of the authors and publishers.

Table B-3 Critical values of F

(.05 level in roman type, .01 level in **bold face**)

Degrees of freedom for the denominator (rows) × Degrees of freedom for the numerator (columns)

	1	2	3	4	5	6	7	8	9	10	11	12	14	16	20	24	30	40	50	75	100	200	500	∞
1	161 **4,052**	200 **4,999**	216 **5,403**	225 **5,625**	230 **5,764**	234 **5,859**	237 **5,928**	239 **5,981**	241 **6,022**	242 **6,056**	243 **6,082**	244 **6,106**	245 **6,142**	246 **6,169**	248 **6,208**	249 **6,234**	250 **6,261**	251 **6,286**	252 **6,302**	253 **6,323**	253 **6,334**	254 **6,352**	254 **6,361**	254 **6,366**
2	18.51 **98.49**	19.00 **99.00**	19.16 **99.17**	19.25 **99.25**	19.30 **99.30**	19.33 **99.33**	19.36 **99.36**	19.37 **99.37**	19.38 **99.39**	19.39 **99.40**	19.40 **99.41**	19.41 **99.42**	19.42 **99.43**	19.43 **99.44**	19.44 **99.45**	19.45 **99.46**	19.46 **99.47**	19.47 **99.48**	19.47 **99.48**	19.48 **99.49**	19.49 **99.49**	19.49 **99.49**	19.50 **99.50**	19.50 **99.50**
3	10.13 **34.12**	9.55 **30.82**	9.28 **29.46**	9.12 **28.71**	9.01 **28.24**	8.94 **27.91**	8.88 **27.67**	8.84 **27.49**	8.81 **27.34**	8.78 **27.23**	8.76 **27.13**	8.74 **27.05**	8.71 **26.92**	8.69 **26.83**	8.66 **26.69**	8.64 **26.60**	8.62 **26.50**	8.60 **26.41**	8.58 **26.35**	8.57 **26.27**	8.56 **26.23**	8.54 **26.18**	8.54 **26.14**	8.53 **26.12**
4	7.71 **21.20**	6.94 **18.00**	6.59 **16.69**	6.39 **15.98**	6.26 **15.52**	6.16 **15.21**	6.09 **14.98**	6.04 **14.80**	6.00 **14.66**	5.96 **14.54**	5.93 **14.45**	5.91 **14.37**	5.87 **14.24**	5.84 **14.15**	5.80 **14.02**	5.77 **13.93**	5.74 **13.83**	5.71 **13.74**	5.70 **13.69**	5.68 **13.61**	5.66 **13.57**	5.65 **13.52**	5.64 **13.48**	5.63 **13.46**
5	6.61 **16.26**	5.79 **13.27**	5.41 **12.06**	5.19 **11.39**	5.05 **10.97**	4.95 **10.67**	4.88 **10.45**	4.82 **10.29**	4.78 **10.15**	4.74 **10.05**	4.70 **9.96**	4.68 **9.89**	4.64 **9.77**	4.60 **9.68**	4.56 **9.55**	4.53 **9.47**	4.50 **9.38**	4.46 **9.29**	4.44 **9.24**	4.42 **9.17**	4.40 **9.13**	4.38 **9.07**	4.37 **9.04**	4.36 **9.02**
6	5.99 **13.74**	5.14 **10.92**	4.76 **9.78**	4.53 **9.15**	4.39 **8.75**	4.28 **8.47**	4.21 **8.26**	4.15 **8.10**	4.10 **7.98**	4.06 **7.87**	4.03 **7.79**	4.00 **7.72**	3.96 **7.60**	3.92 **7.52**	3.87 **7.39**	3.84 **7.31**	3.81 **7.23**	3.77 **7.14**	3.75 **7.09**	3.72 **7.02**	3.71 **6.99**	3.69 **6.94**	3.68 **6.90**	3.67 **6.88**
7	5.59 **12.25**	4.74 **9.55**	4.35 **8.45**	4.12 **7.85**	3.97 **7.46**	3.87 **7.19**	3.79 **7.00**	3.73 **6.84**	3.68 **6.71**	3.63 **6.62**	3.60 **6.54**	3.57 **6.47**	3.52 **6.35**	3.49 **6.27**	3.44 **6.15**	3.41 **6.07**	3.38 **5.98**	3.34 **5.90**	3.32 **5.85**	3.29 **5.78**	3.28 **5.75**	3.25 **5.70**	3.24 **5.67**	3.23 **5.65**
8	5.32 **11.26**	4.46 **8.65**	4.07 **7.59**	3.84 **7.01**	3.69 **6.63**	3.58 **6.37**	3.50 **6.19**	3.44 **6.03**	3.39 **5.91**	3.34 **5.82**	3.31 **5.74**	3.28 **5.67**	3.23 **5.56**	3.20 **5.48**	3.15 **5.36**	3.12 **5.28**	3.08 **5.20**	3.05 **5.11**	3.03 **5.06**	3.00 **5.00**	2.98 **4.96**	2.96 **4.91**	2.94 **4.88**	2.93 **4.86**
9	5.12 **10.56**	4.26 **8.02**	3.86 **6.99**	3.63 **6.42**	3.48 **6.06**	3.37 **5.80**	3.29 **5.62**	3.23 **5.47**	3.18 **5.35**	3.13 **5.26**	3.10 **5.18**	3.07 **5.11**	3.02 **5.00**	2.98 **4.92**	2.93 **4.80**	2.90 **4.73**	2.86 **4.64**	2.82 **4.56**	2.80 **4.51**	2.77 **4.45**	2.76 **4.41**	2.73 **4.36**	2.72 **4.33**	2.71 **4.31**
10	4.96 **10.04**	4.10 **7.56**	3.71 **6.55**	3.48 **5.99**	3.33 **5.64**	3.22 **5.39**	3.14 **5.21**	3.07 **5.06**	3.02 **4.95**	2.97 **4.85**	2.94 **4.78**	2.91 **4.71**	2.86 **4.60**	2.82 **4.52**	2.77 **4.41**	2.74 **4.33**	2.70 **4.25**	2.67 **4.17**	2.64 **4.12**	2.61 **4.05**	2.59 **4.01**	2.56 **3.96**	2.55 **3.93**	2.54 **3.91**
11	4.84 **9.65**	3.98 **7.20**	3.59 **6.22**	3.36 **5.67**	3.20 **5.32**	3.09 **5.07**	3.01 **4.88**	2.95 **4.74**	2.90 **4.63**	2.86 **4.54**	2.82 **4.46**	2.79 **4.40**	2.74 **4.29**	2.70 **4.21**	2.65 **4.10**	2.61 **4.02**	2.57 **3.94**	2.53 **3.86**	2.50 **3.80**	2.47 **3.74**	2.45 **3.70**	2.42 **3.66**	2.41 **3.62**	2.40 **3.60**
12	4.75 **9.33**	3.88 **6.93**	3.49 **5.95**	3.26 **5.41**	3.11 **5.06**	3.00 **4.82**	2.92 **4.65**	2.85 **4.50**	2.80 **4.39**	2.76 **4.30**	2.72 **4.22**	2.69 **4.16**	2.64 **4.05**	2.60 **3.98**	2.54 **3.86**	2.50 **3.78**	2.46 **3.70**	2.42 **3.61**	2.40 **3.56**	2.36 **3.49**	2.35 **3.46**	2.32 **3.41**	2.31 **3.38**	2.30 **3.36**
13	4.67 **9.07**	3.80 **6.70**	3.41 **5.74**	3.18 **5.20**	3.02 **4.86**	2.92 **4.62**	2.84 **4.44**	2.77 **4.30**	2.72 **4.19**	2.67 **4.10**	2.63 **4.02**	2.60 **3.96**	2.55 **3.85**	2.51 **3.78**	2.46 **3.67**	2.42 **3.59**	2.38 **3.51**	2.34 **3.42**	2.32 **3.37**	2.28 **3.30**	2.26 **3.27**	2.24 **3.21**	2.22 **3.18**	2.21 **3.16**

Table B-3 (cont'd)

											Degrees of freedom for the numerator											
	1	2	3	4	5	6	7	8	9	10	11	12	14	16	20	24	30	40	50	75	100	200	500	∞
14	4.60 8.86	3.74 6.51	3.34 5.56	3.11 5.03	2.96 4.69	2.85 4.46	2.77 4.28	2.70 4.14	2.65 4.03	2.60 3.94	2.56 3.86	2.53 3.80	2.48 3.70	2.44 3.62	2.39 3.51	2.35 3.43	2.31 3.34	2.27 3.26	2.24 3.21	2.21 3.14	2.19 3.11	2.16 3.06	2.14 3.02	2.13 3.00
15	4.54 8.68	3.68 6.36	3.29 5.42	3.06 4.89	2.90 4.56	2.79 4.32	2.70 4.14	2.64 4.00	2.59 3.89	2.55 3.80	2.51 3.73	2.48 3.67	2.43 3.56	2.39 3.48	2.33 3.36	2.29 3.29	2.25 3.20	2.21 3.12	2.18 3.07	2.15 3.00	2.12 2.97	2.10 2.92	2.08 2.89	2.07 2.87
16	4.49 8.53	3.63 6.23	3.24 5.29	3.01 4.77	2.85 4.44	2.74 4.20	2.66 4.03	2.59 3.89	2.54 3.78	2.49 3.69	2.45 3.61	2.42 3.55	2.37 3.45	2.33 3.37	2.28 3.25	2.24 3.18	2.20 3.10	2.16 3.01	2.13 2.96	2.09 2.98	2.07 2.86	2.04 2.80	2.02 2.77	2.01 2.75
17	4.45 8.40	3.59 6.11	3.20 5.18	2.96 4.67	2.81 4.34	2.70 4.10	2.62 3.93	2.55 3.79	2.50 3.68	2.45 3.59	2.41 3.52	2.38 3.45	2.33 3.35	2.29 3.27	2.23 3.16	2.19 3.08	2.15 3.00	2.11 2.92	2.08 2.86	2.04 2.79	2.02 2.76	1.99 2.70	1.97 2.67	1.96 2.65
18	4.41 8.28	3.55 6.01	3.16 5.09	2.93 4.58	2.77 4.25	2.66 4.01	2.58 3.85	2.51 3.71	2.46 3.60	2.41 3.51	2.37 3.44	2.34 3.37	2.29 3.27	2.25 3.19	2.19 3.07	2.15 3.00	2.11 2.91	2.07 2.83	2.04 2.78	2.00 2.71	1.98 2.68	1.95 2.62	1.93 2.59	1.92 2.57
19	4.38 8.18	3.52 5.93	3.13 5.01	2.90 4.50	2.74 4.17	2.63 3.94	2.55 3.77	2.48 3.63	2.43 3.52	2.38 3.43	2.34 3.36	2.31 3.30	2.26 3.19	2.21 3.12	2.15 3.00	2.11 2.92	2.07 2.84	2.02 2.76	2.00 2.70	1.96 2.63	1.94 2.60	1.91 2.54	1.90 2.51	1.88 2.49
20	4.35 8.10	3.49 5.85	3.10 4.94	2.87 4.43	2.71 4.10	2.60 3.87	2.52 3.71	2.45 3.56	2.40 3.45	2.35 3.37	2.31 3.30	2.28 3.23	2.23 3.13	2.18 3.05	2.12 2.94	2.08 2.86	2.04 2.77	1.99 2.69	1.96 2.63	1.92 2.56	1.90 2.53	1.87 2.47	1.85 2.44	1.84 2.42
21	4.32 8.02	3.47 5.78	3.07 4.87	2.84 4.37	2.68 4.04	2.57 3.81	2.49 3.65	2.42 3.51	2.37 3.40	2.32 3.31	2.28 3.24	2.25 3.17	2.20 3.07	2.15 2.99	2.09 2.88	2.05 2.80	2.00 2.72	1.96 2.63	1.93 2.58	1.89 2.51	1.87 2.47	1.84 2.42	1.82 2.38	1.81 2.36
22	4.30 7.94	3.44 5.72	3.05 4.82	2.82 4.31	2.66 3.99	2.55 3.76	2.47 3.59	2.40 3.45	2.35 3.35	2.30 3.26	2.26 3.18	2.23 3.12	2.18 3.02	2.13 2.94	2.07 2.83	2.03 2.75	1.98 2.67	1.93 2.58	1.91 2.53	1.87 2.46	1.84 2.42	1.81 2.37	1.80 2.33	1.78 2.31
23	4.28 7.88	3.42 5.66	3.03 4.76	2.80 4.26	2.64 3.94	2.53 3.71	2.45 3.54	2.38 3.41	2.32 3.30	2.28 3.21	2.24 3.14	2.20 3.07	2.14 2.97	2.10 2.89	2.04 2.78	2.00 2.70	1.96 2.62	1.91 2.53	1.88 2.48	1.84 2.41	1.82 2.37	1.79 2.32	1.77 2.28	1.76 2.26
24	4.26 7.82	3.40 5.61	3.01 4.72	2.78 4.22	2.62 3.90	2.51 3.67	2.43 3.50	2.36 3.36	2.30 3.25	2.26 3.17	2.22 3.09	2.18 3.03	2.13 2.93	2.09 2.85	2.02 2.74	1.98 2.66	1.94 2.58	1.89 2.49	1.86 2.44	1.82 2.36	1.80 2.33	1.76 2.27	1.74 2.23	1.73 2.21
25	4.24 7.77	3.38 5.57	2.99 4.68	2.76 4.18	2.60 3.86	2.49 3.63	2.41 3.46	2.34 3.32	2.28 3.21	2.24 3.13	2.20 3.05	2.16 2.99	2.11 2.89	2.06 2.81	2.00 2.70	1.96 2.62	1.92 2.54	1.87 2.45	1.84 2.40	1.80 2.32	1.77 2.29	1.74 2.23	1.72 2.19	1.71 2.17
26	4.22 7.72	3.37 5.53	2.98 4.64	2.74 4.14	2.59 3.82	2.47 3.59	2.39 3.42	2.32 3.29	2.27 3.17	2.22 3.09	2.18 3.02	2.15 2.96	2.10 2.86	2.05 2.77	1.99 2.66	1.95 2.58	1.90 2.50	1.85 2.41	1.82 2.36	1.78 2.28	1.76 2.25	1.72 2.19	1.70 2.15	1.69 2.13

Degrees of freedom for the denominator

Table B-3 (cont'd)

									Degrees of freedom for the numerator												
	1	2	3	4	5	6	7	8	9	10	11	12	14	16	20	24	30	40	50	75	100	200	500	∞
27	4.21 / 7.68	3.35 / 5.49	2.96 / 4.60	2.73 / 4.11	2.57 / 3.79	2.46 / 3.56	2.37 / 3.39	2.30 / 3.26	2.25 / 3.14	2.20 / 3.06	2.16 / 2.98	2.13 / 2.93	2.08 / 2.83	2.03 / 2.74	1.97 / 2.63	1.93 / 2.55	1.88 / 2.47	1.84 / 2.38	1.80 / 2.33	1.76 / 2.25	1.74 / 2.21	1.71 / 2.16	1.68 / 2.12	1.67 / 2.10
28	4.20 / 7.64	3.34 / 5.45	2.95 / 4.57	2.71 / 4.07	2.56 / 3.76	2.44 / 3.53	2.36 / 3.36	2.29 / 3.23	2.24 / 3.11	2.19 / 3.03	2.15 / 2.95	2.12 / 2.90	2.06 / 2.80	2.02 / 2.71	1.96 / 2.60	1.91 / 2.52	1.87 / 2.44	1.81 / 2.35	1.78 / 2.30	1.75 / 2.22	1.72 / 2.18	1.69 / 2.13	1.67 / 2.09	1.65 / 2.06
29	4.18 / 7.60	3.33 / 5.42	2.93 / 4.54	2.70 / 4.04	2.54 / 3.73	2.43 / 3.50	2.35 / 3.33	2.28 / 3.20	2.22 / 3.08	2.18 / 3.00	2.14 / 2.92	2.10 / 2.87	2.05 / 2.77	2.00 / 2.68	1.94 / 2.57	1.90 / 2.49	1.85 / 2.41	1.80 / 2.32	1.77 / 2.27	1.73 / 2.19	1.71 / 2.15	1.68 / 2.10	1.65 / 2.06	1.64 / 2.03
30	4.17 / 7.56	3.32 / 5.39	2.92 / 4.51	2.69 / 4.02	2.53 / 3.70	2.42 / 3.47	2.34 / 3.30	2.27 / 3.17	2.21 / 3.06	2.16 / 2.98	2.12 / 2.90	2.09 / 2.84	2.04 / 2.74	1.99 / 2.66	1.93 / 2.55	1.89 / 2.47	1.84 / 2.38	1.79 / 2.29	1.76 / 2.24	1.72 / 2.16	1.69 / 2.13	1.66 / 2.07	1.64 / 2.03	1.62 / 2.01
32	4.15 / 7.50	3.30 / 5.34	2.90 / 4.46	2.67 / 3.97	2.51 / 3.66	2.40 / 3.42	2.32 / 3.25	2.25 / 3.12	2.19 / 3.01	2.14 / 2.94	2.10 / 2.86	2.07 / 2.80	2.02 / 2.70	1.97 / 2.62	1.91 / 2.51	1.86 / 2.42	1.82 / 2.34	1.76 / 2.25	1.74 / 2.20	1.69 / 2.12	1.67 / 2.08	1.64 / 2.02	1.61 / 1.98	1.59 / 1.96
34	4.13 / 7.44	3.28 / 5.29	2.88 / 4.42	2.65 / 3.93	2.49 / 3.61	2.38 / 3.38	2.30 / 3.21	2.23 / 3.08	2.17 / 2.97	2.12 / 2.89	2.08 / 2.82	2.05 / 2.76	2.00 / 2.66	1.95 / 2.58	1.89 / 2.47	1.84 / 2.38	1.80 / 2.30	1.74 / 2.21	1.71 / 2.15	1.67 / 2.08	1.64 / 2.04	1.61 / 1.98	1.59 / 1.94	1.57 / 1.91
36	4.11 / 7.39	3.26 / 5.25	2.86 / 4.38	2.63 / 3.89	2.48 / 3.58	2.36 / 3.35	2.28 / 3.18	2.21 / 3.04	2.15 / 2.94	2.10 / 2.86	2.06 / 2.78	2.03 / 2.72	1.98 / 2.62	1.93 / 2.54	1.87 / 2.43	1.82 / 2.35	1.78 / 2.26	1.72 / 2.17	1.69 / 2.12	1.65 / 2.04	1.62 / 2.00	1.59 / 1.94	1.56 / 1.90	1.55 / 1.87
38	4.10 / 7.35	3.25 / 5.21	2.85 / 4.34	2.62 / 3.86	2.46 / 3.54	2.35 / 3.32	2.26 / 3.15	2.19 / 3.02	2.14 / 2.91	2.09 / 2.82	2.05 / 2.75	2.02 / 2.69	1.96 / 2.59	1.92 / 2.51	1.85 / 2.40	1.80 / 2.32	1.76 / 2.22	1.71 / 2.14	1.67 / 2.08	1.63 / 2.00	1.60 / 1.97	1.57 / 1.90	1.54 / 1.86	1.53 / 1.84
40	4.08 / 7.31	3.23 / 5.18	2.84 / 4.31	2.61 / 3.83	2.45 / 3.51	2.34 / 3.29	2.25 / 3.12	2.18 / 2.99	2.12 / 2.88	2.07 / 2.80	2.04 / 2.73	2.00 / 2.66	1.95 / 2.56	1.90 / 2.49	1.84 / 2.37	1.79 / 2.29	1.74 / 2.20	1.69 / 2.11	1.66 / 2.05	1.61 / 1.97	1.59 / 1.94	1.55 / 1.88	1.53 / 1.84	1.51 / 1.81
42	4.07 / 7.27	3.22 / 5.15	2.83 / 4.29	2.59 / 3.80	2.44 / 3.49	2.32 / 3.26	2.24 / 3.10	2.17 / 2.96	2.11 / 2.86	2.06 / 2.77	2.02 / 2.70	1.99 / 2.64	1.94 / 2.54	1.89 / 2.46	1.82 / 2.35	1.78 / 2.26	1.73 / 2.17	1.68 / 2.08	1.64 / 2.02	1.60 / 1.94	1.57 / 1.91	1.54 / 1.85	1.51 / 1.80	1.49 / 1.78
44	4.06 / 7.24	3.21 / 5.12	2.82 / 4.26	2.58 / 3.78	2.43 / 3.46	2.31 / 3.24	2.23 / 3.07	2.16 / 2.94	2.10 / 2.84	2.05 / 2.75	2.01 / 2.68	1.98 / 2.62	1.92 / 2.52	1.88 / 2.44	1.81 / 2.32	1.76 / 2.24	1.72 / 2.15	1.66 / 2.06	1.63 / 2.00	1.58 / 1.92	1.56 / 1.88	1.52 / 1.82	1.50 / 1.78	1.48 / 1.75
46	4.05 / 7.21	3.20 / 5.10	2.81 / 4.24	2.57 / 3.76	2.42 / 3.44	2.30 / 3.22	2.22 / 3.05	2.14 / 2.92	2.09 / 2.82	2.04 / 2.73	2.00 / 2.66	1.97 / 2.60	1.91 / 2.50	1.87 / 2.42	1.80 / 2.30	1.75 / 2.22	1.71 / 2.13	1.65 / 2.04	1.62 / 1.98	1.57 / 1.90	1.54 / 1.86	1.51 / 1.80	1.48 / 1.76	1.46 / 1.72
48	4.04 / 7.19	3.19 / 5.08	2.80 / 4.22	2.56 / 3.74	2.41 / 3.42	2.30 / 3.20	2.21 / 3.04	2.14 / 2.90	2.08 / 2.80	2.03 / 2.71	1.99 / 2.64	1.96 / 2.58	1.90 / 2.48	1.86 / 2.40	1.79 / 2.28	1.74 / 2.20	1.70 / 2.11	1.64 / 2.02	1.61 / 1.96	1.56 / 1.88	1.53 / 1.84	1.50 / 1.78	1.47 / 1.73	1.45 / 1.70

Degrees of freedom for the denominator

Table B-3 (cont'd)

Degrees of freedom for the numerator

	1	2	3	4	5	6	7	8	9	10	11	12	14	16	20	24	30	40	50	75	100	200	500	∞	
50	4.03 7.17	3.18 5.06	2.79 4.20	2.56 3.72	2.40 3.41	2.29 3.18	2.20 3.02	2.13 2.88	2.07 2.78	2.02 2.70	1.98 2.62	1.95 2.56	1.90 2.46	1.85 2.39	1.78 2.26	1.74 2.18	1.69 2.10	1.63 2.00	1.60 1.94	1.55 1.86	1.52 1.82	1.48 1.76	1.46 1.71	1.44 1.68	50
55	4.02 7.12	3.17 5.01	2.78 4.16	2.54 3.68	2.38 3.37	2.27 3.15	2.18 2.98	2.11 2.85	2.05 2.75	2.00 2.66	1.97 2.59	1.93 2.53	1.88 2.43	1.83 2.35	1.76 2.23	1.72 2.15	1.67 2.06	1.61 1.96	1.58 1.90	1.52 1.82	1.50 1.78	1.46 1.71	1.43 1.66	1.41 1.64	55
60	4.00 7.08	3.15 4.98	2.76 4.13	2.52 3.65	2.37 3.34	2.25 3.12	2.17 2.95	2.10 2.82	2.04 2.72	1.99 2.63	1.95 2.56	1.92 2.50	1.86 2.40	1.81 2.32	1.75 2.20	1.70 2.12	1.65 2.03	1.59 1.93	1.56 1.87	1.50 1.79	1.48 1.74	1.44 1.68	1.41 1.63	1.39 1.60	60
65	3.99 7.04	3.14 4.95	2.75 4.10	2.51 3.62	2.36 3.31	2.24 3.09	2.15 2.93	2.08 2.79	2.02 2.70	1.98 2.61	1.94 2.54	1.90 2.47	1.85 2.37	1.80 2.30	1.73 2.18	1.68 2.09	1.63 2.00	1.57 1.90	1.54 1.84	1.49 1.76	1.46 1.71	1.42 1.64	1.39 1.60	1.37 1.56	65
70	3.98 7.01	3.13 4.92	2.74 4.08	2.50 3.60	2.35 3.29	2.23 3.07	2.14 2.91	2.07 2.77	2.01 2.67	1.97 2.59	1.93 2.51	1.89 2.45	1.84 2.35	1.79 2.28	1.72 2.15	1.67 2.07	1.62 1.98	1.56 1.88	1.53 1.82	1.47 1.74	1.45 1.69	1.40 1.62	1.37 1.56	1.35 1.53	70
80	3.96 6.96	3.11 4.88	2.72 4.04	2.48 3.56	2.33 3.25	2.21 3.04	2.12 2.87	2.05 2.74	1.99 2.64	1.95 2.55	1.91 2.48	1.88 2.41	1.82 2.32	1.77 2.24	1.70 2.11	1.65 2.03	1.60 1.94	1.54 1.84	1.51 1.78	1.45 1.70	1.42 1.65	1.38 1.57	1.35 1.52	1.32 1.49	80
100	3.94 6.90	3.09 4.82	2.70 3.98	2.46 3.51	2.30 3.20	2.19 2.99	2.10 2.82	2.03 2.69	1.97 2.59	1.92 2.51	1.88 2.43	1.85 2.36	1.79 2.26	1.75 2.19	1.68 2.06	1.63 1.98	1.57 1.89	1.51 1.79	1.48 1.73	1.42 1.64	1.39 1.59	1.34 1.51	1.30 1.46	1.28 1.43	100
125	3.92 6.84	3.07 4.78	2.68 3.94	2.44 3.47	2.29 3.17	2.17 2.95	2.08 2.79	2.01 2.65	1.95 2.56	1.90 2.47	1.86 2.40	1.83 2.33	1.77 2.23	1.72 2.15	1.65 2.03	1.60 1.94	1.55 1.85	1.49 1.75	1.45 1.68	1.39 1.59	1.36 1.54	1.31 1.46	1.27 1.40	1.25 1.37	125
150	3.91 6.81	3.06 4.75	2.67 3.91	2.43 3.44	2.27 3.14	2.16 2.92	2.07 2.76	2.00 2.62	1.94 2.53	1.89 2.44	1.85 2.37	1.82 2.30	1.76 2.20	1.71 2.12	1.64 2.00	1.59 1.91	1.54 1.83	1.47 1.72	1.44 1.66	1.37 1.56	1.34 1.51	1.29 1.43	1.25 1.37	1.22 1.33	150
200	3.89 6.76	3.04 4.71	2.65 3.88	2.41 3.41	2.26 3.11	2.14 2.90	2.05 2.73	1.98 2.60	1.92 2.50	1.87 2.41	1.83 2.34	1.80 2.28	1.74 2.17	1.69 2.09	1.62 1.97	1.57 1.88	1.52 1.79	1.45 1.69	1.42 1.62	1.35 1.53	1.32 1.48	1.26 1.39	1.22 1.33	1.19 1.28	200
400	3.86 6.70	3.02 4.66	2.62 3.83	2.39 3.36	2.23 3.06	2.12 2.85	2.03 2.69	1.96 2.55	1.90 2.46	1.85 2.37	1.81 2.29	1.78 2.23	1.72 2.12	1.67 2.04	1.60 1.92	1.54 1.84	1.49 1.74	1.42 1.64	1.38 1.57	1.32 1.47	1.28 1.42	1.22 1.32	1.16 1.24	1.13 1.19	400
1000	3.85 6.66	3.00 4.62	2.61 3.80	2.38 3.34	2.22 3.04	2.10 2.82	2.02 2.66	1.95 2.53	1.89 2.43	1.84 2.34	1.80 2.26	1.76 2.20	1.70 2.09	1.65 2.01	1.58 1.89	1.53 1.81	1.47 1.71	1.41 1.61	1.36 1.54	1.30 1.44	1.26 1.38	1.19 1.28	1.13 1.19	1.08 1.11	1000
∞	3.84 6.64	2.99 4.60	2.60 3.78	2.37 3.32	2.21 3.02	2.09 2.80	2.01 2.64	1.94 2.51	1.88 2.41	1.83 2.32	1.79 2.24	1.75 2.18	1.69 2.07	1.64 1.99	1.57 1.87	1.52 1.79	1.46 1.69	1.40 1.59	1.35 1.52	1.28 1.41	1.24 1.36	1.17 1.25	1.11 1.15	1.00 1.00	∞

Degrees of freedom for the denominator

Source: Reprinted by permission from G.W. Snedecor and W.G. Cochran, *Statistical Methods* (6th edition), Ames, Iowa: Iowa State University Press, © 1967. Courtesy of the authors and the publisher.

Table B-4 Critical values of chi-square

df	\multicolumn{6}{c}{Level of significance for a non-directional test}
	.20	.10	.05	.02	.01	.001
1	1.64	2.71	3.84	5.41	6.64	10.83
2	3.22	4.60	5.99	7.82	9.21	13.82
3	4.64	6.25	7.82	9.84	11.34	16.27
4	5.99	7.78	9.49	11.67	13.28	18.46
5	7.29	9.24	11.07	13.39	15.09	20.52
6	8.56	10.64	12.59	15.03	16.81	22.46
7	9.80	12.02	14.07	16.62	18.48	24.32
8	11.03	13.36	15.51	18.17	20.09	26.12
9	12.24	14.68	16.92	19.68	21.67	27.88
10	13.44	15.99	18.31	21.16	23.21	29.59
11	14.63	17.28	19.68	22.62	24.72	31.26
12	15.81	18.55	21.03	24.05	26.22	32.91
13	16.98	19.81	22.36	25.47	27.69	34.53
14	18.15	21.06	23.68	26.87	29.14	36.12
15	19.31	22.31	25.00	28.26	30.58	37.70
16	20.46	23.54	26.30	29.63	32.00	39.29
17	21.62	24.77	27.59	31.00	33.41	40.75
18	22.76	25.99	28.87	32.35	34.80	42.31
19	23.90	27.20	30.14	33.69	36.19	43.82
20	25.04	28.41	31.41	35.02	37.57	45.32
21	26.17	29.62	32.67	36.34	38.93	46.80
22	27.30	30.81	33.92	37.66	40.29	48.27
23	28.43	32.01	35.17	38.97	41.64	49.73
24	29.55	33.20	36.42	40.27	42.98	51.18
25	30.68	34.38	37.65	41.57	44.31	52.62
26	31.80	35.56	38.88	42.86	45.64	54.05
27	32.91	36.74	40.11	44.14	46.96	55.48
28	34.03	37.92	41.34	45.42	48.28	56.89
29	35.14	39.09	42.69	46.69	49.59	58.30
30	36.25	40.26	43.77	47.96	50.89	59.70
32	38.47	42.59	46.19	50.49	53.49	62.49
34	40.68	44.90	48.60	53.00	56.06	65.25
36	42.88	47.21	51.00	55.49	58.62	67.99
38	45.08	49.51	53.38	57.97	61.16	70.70
40	47.27	51.81	55.76	60.44	63.69	73.40
44	51.64	56.37	60.48	65.34	68.71	78.75
48	55.99	60.91	65.17	70.20	73.68	84.04
52	60.33	65.42	69.83	75.02	78.62	89.27
56	64.66	69.92	74.47	79.82	83.51	94.46
60	68.97	74.40	79.08	84.58	88.38	99.61

Source: From Fisher and Yates, *Statistical Tables for Biological, Agricultural and Medical Research*, published by Longman Group UK Ltd., London (previously published by Oliver and Boyd Ltd., Edinburgh), with permission of the authors and the publishers.

Table B-5 Studentized range points for Tukey test

Error df	α	\multicolumn{10}{c}{r = number of means or number of steps between ordered means}
		2	3	4	5	6	7	8	9	10	11
5	.05	3.64	4.60	5.22	5.67	6.03	6.33	6.58	6.80	6.99	7.17
	.01	5.70	6.98	7.80	8.42	8.91	9.32	9.67	9.97	10.24	10.48
6	.05	3.46	4.34	4.90	5.30	5.63	5.90	6.12	6.32	6.49	6.65
	.01	5.24	6.33	7.03	7.56	7.97	8.32	8.61	8.87	9.10	9.30
7	.05	3.34	4.16	4.68	5.06	5.36	5.61	5.82	6.00	6.16	6.30
	.01	4.95	5.92	6.54	7.01	7.37	7.68	7.94	8.17	8.37	8.55
8	.05	3.26	4.04	4.53	4.89	5.17	5.40	5.60	5.77	5.92	6.05
	.01	4.75	5.64	6.20	6.62	6.96	7.24	7.47	7.68	7.86	8.03
9	.05	3.20	3.95	4.41	4.76	5.02	5.24	5.43	5.59	5.74	5.87
	.01	4.60	5.43	5.96	6.35	6.66	6.91	7.13	7.33	7.49	7.65
10	.05	3.15	3.88	4.33	4.65	4.91	5.12	5.30	5.46	5.60	5.72
	.01	4.48	5.27	5.77	6.14	6.43	6.67	6.87	7.05	7.21	7.36
11	.05	3.11	3.82	4.26	4.57	4.82	5.03	5.20	5.35	5.49	5.61
	.01	4.39	5.15	5.62	5.97	6.25	6.48	6.67	6.84	6.99	7.13
12	.05	3.08	3.77	4.20	4.51	4.75	4.95	5.12	5.27	5.39	5.51
	.01	4.32	5.05	5.50	5.84	6.10	6.32	6.51	6.67	6.81	6.94
13	.05	3.06	3.73	4.15	4.45	4.69	4.88	5.05	5.19	5.32	5.43
	.01	4.26	4.96	5.40	5.73	5.98	6.19	6.37	6.53	6.67	6.79
14	.05	3.03	3.70	4.11	4.41	4.64	4.83	4.99	5.13	5.25	5.36
	.01	4.21	4.89	5.32	5.63	5.88	6.08	6.26	6.41	6.54	6.66
15	.05	3.01	3.67	4.08	4.37	4.59	4.78	4.94	5.08	5.20	5.31
	.01	4.17	4.84	5.25	5.56	5.80	5.99	6.16	6.31	6.44	6.55
16	.05	3.00	3.65	4.05	4.33	4.56	4.74	4.90	5.03	5.15	5.26
	.01	4.13	4.79	5.19	5.49	5.72	5.92	6.08	6.22	6.35	6.46
17	.05	2.98	3.63	4.02	4.30	4.52	4.70	4.86	4.99	5.11	5.21
	.01	4.10	4.74	5.14	5.43	5.66	5.85	6.01	6.15	6.27	6.38
18	.05	2.97	3.61	4.00	4.28	4.49	4.67	4.82	4.96	5.07	5.17
	.01	4.07	4.70	5.09	5.38	5.60	5.79	5.94	6.08	6.20	6.31
19	.05	2.96	3.59	3.98	4.25	4.47	4.65	4.79	4.92	5.04	5.14
	.01	4.05	4.67	5.05	5.33	5.55	5.73	5.89	6.02	6.14	6.25
20	.05	2.95	3.58	3.96	4.23	4.45	4.62	4.77	4.90	5.01	5.11
	.01	4.02	4.64	5.02	5.29	5.51	5.69	5.84	5.97	6.09	6.19
24	.05	2.92	3.53	3.90	4.17	4.37	4.54	4.68	4.81	4.92	5.01
	.01	3.96	4.55	4.91	5.17	5.37	5.54	5.69	5.81	5.92	6.02
30	.05	2.89	3.49	3.85	4.10	4.30	4.46	4.60	4.72	4.82	4.92
	.01	3.89	4.45	4.80	5.05	5.24	5.40	5.54	5.65	5.76	5.85
40	.05	2.86	3.44	3.79	4.04	4.23	4.39	4.52	4.63	4.73	4.82
	.01	3.82	4.37	4.70	4.93	5.11	5.26	5.39	5.50	5.60	5.69
60	.05	2.83	3.40	3.74	3.98	4.16	4.31	4.44	4.55	4.65	4.73
	.01	3.76	4.28	4.59	4.82	4.99	5.13	5.25	5.36	5.45	5.53
120	.05	2.80	3.36	3.68	3.92	4.10	4.24	4.36	4.47	4.56	4.64
	.01	3.70	4.20	4.50	4.71	4.87	5.01	5.12	5.21	5.30	5.37
∞	.05	2.77	3.31	3.63	3.86	4.03	4.17	4.29	4.39	4.47	4.55
	.01	3.64	4.12	4.40	4.60	4.76	4.88	4.99	5.08	5.16	5.23

Table B-5 (cont'd)

r = number of means or number of steps between ordered means									α	Error df
12	13	14	15	16	17	18	19	20		
7.32	7.47	7.60	7.72	7.83	7.93	8.03	8.12	8.21	.05	5
10.70	10.89	11.08	11.24	11.40	11.55	11.68	11.81	11.93	.01	
6.79	6.92	7.03	7.14	7.24	7.34	7.43	7.51	7.59	.05	6
9.48	9.65	9.81	9.95	10.08	10.21	10.32	10.43	10.54	.01	
6.43	6.55	6.66	6.76	6.85	6.94	7.02	7.10	7.17	.05	7
8.71	8.86	9.00	9.12	9.24	9.35	9.46	9.55	9.65	.01	
6.18	6.29	6.39	6.48	6.57	6.65	6.73	6.80	6.87	.05	8
8.18	8.31	8.44	8.55	8.66	8.76	8.85	8.94	9.03	.01	
5.98	6.09	6.19	6.28	6.36	6.44	6.51	6.58	6.64	.05	9
7.78	7.91	8.03	8.13	8.23	8.33	8.41	8.49	8.57	.01	
5.83	5.93	6.03	6.11	6.19	6.27	6.34	6.40	6.47	.05	10
7.49	7.60	7.71	7.81	7.91	7.99	8.08	8.15	8.23	.01	
5.71	5.81	5.90	5.98	6.06	6.13	6.20	6.27	6.33	.05	11
7.25	7.36	7.46	7.56	7.65	7.73	7.81	7.88	7.95	.01	
5.61	5.71	5.80	5.88	5.95	6.02	6.09	6.15	6.21	.05	12
7.06	7.17	7.26	7.36	7.44	7.52	7.59	7.66	7.73	.01	
5.53	5.63	5.71	5.79	5.86	5.93	5.99	6.05	6.11	.05	13
6.90	7.01	7.10	7.19	7.27	7.35	7.42	7.48	7.55	.01	
5.46	5.55	5.64	5.71	5.79	5.85	5.91	5.97	6.03	.05	14
6.77	6.87	6.96	7.05	7.13	7.20	7.27	7.33	7.39	.01	
5.40	5.49	5.57	5.65	5.72	5.78	5.85	5.90	5.96	.05	15
6.66	6.76	6.84	6.93	7.00	7.07	7.14	7.20	7.26	.01	
5.35	5.44	5.52	5.59	5.66	5.73	5.79	5.84	5.90	.05	16
6.56	6.66	6.74	6.82	6.90	6.97	7.03	7.09	7.15	.01	
5.31	5.39	5.47	5.54	5.61	5.67	5.73	5.79	5.84	.05	17
6.48	6.57	6.66	6.73	6.81	6.87	6.94	7.00	7.05	.01	
5.27	5.35	5.43	5.50	5.57	5.63	5.69	5.74	5.79	.05	18
6.41	6.50	6.58	6.65	6.73	6.79	6.85	6.91	6.97	.01	
5.23	5.31	5.39	5.46	5.53	5.59	5.65	5.70	5.75	.05	19
6.34	6.43	6.51	6.58	6.65	6.72	6.78	6.84	6.89	.01	
5.20	5.28	5.36	5.43	5.49	5.55	5.61	5.66	5.71	.05	20
6.28	6.37	6.45	6.52	6.59	6.65	6.71	6.77	6.82	.01	
5.10	5.18	5.25	5.32	5.38	5.44	5.49	5.55	5.59	.05	24
6.11	6.19	6.26	6.33	6.39	6.45	6.51	6.56	6.61	.01	
5.00	5.08	5.15	5.21	5.27	5.33	5.38	5.43	5.47	.05	30
5.93	6.01	6.08	6.14	6.20	6.26	6.31	6.36	6.41	.01	
4.90	4.98	5.04	5.11	5.16	5.22	5.27	5.31	5.36	.05	40
5.76	5.83	5.90	5.96	6.02	6.07	6.12	6.16	6.21	.01	
4.81	4.88	4.94	5.00	5.06	5.11	5.15	5.20	5.24	.05	60
5.60	5.67	5.73	5.78	5.84	5.89	5.93	5.97	6.01	.01	
4.71	4.78	4.84	4.90	4.95	5.00	5.04	5.09	5.13	.05	120
5.44	5.50	5.56	5.61	5.66	5.71	5.75	5.79	5.83	.01	
4.62	4.68	4.74	4.80	4.85	4.89	4.93	4.97	5.01	.05	∞
5.29	5.35	5.40	5.45	5.49	5.54	5.57	5.61	5.65	.01	

Source: *Biometrika Tables for Statisticians*, 3rd edition (New York: Cambridge University Press, 1966) volume 1. Copyright by the Biometrika Trustees. Reprinted by permission.

Table B-6 Critical values of Mann-Whitney U

Critical Values of the Mann–Whitney U. For a one-tailed test at $\alpha = 0.01$ (roman type) and $\alpha = 0.005$ (boldface type) and for a two-tailed test at $\alpha = 0.02$ (roman type) and $\alpha = 0.01$ (boldface type).

n_2 \ n_1	1	2	3	4	5	6	7	8	9	10	11	12	13	14	15	16	17	18	19	20
1	—[b]	—	—	—	—	—	—	—	—	—	—	—	—	—	—	—	—	—	—	—
2	—	—	—	—	—	—	—	—	—	—	—	—	0	0	0	0	0	0	1	1
	—	—	—	—	—	—	—	—	—	—	—	—	—	—	—	—	—	—	**0**	**0**
3	—	—	—	—	—	—	0	0	1	1	1	2	2	2	3	3	4	4	4	5
	—	—	—	—	—	—	—	—	**0**	**0**	**0**	**1**	**1**	**1**	**2**	**2**	**2**	**2**	**3**	**3**
4	—	—	—	—	0	1	1	2	3	3	4	5	5	6	7	7	8	9	9	10
	—	—	—	—	—	**0**	**0**	**1**	**1**	**2**	**2**	**3**	**3**	**4**	**5**	**5**	**6**	**6**	**7**	**8**
5	—	—	—	0	1	2	3	4	5	6	7	8	9	10	11	12	13	14	15	16
	—	—	—	—	**0**	**1**	**1**	**2**	**3**	**4**	**5**	**6**	**7**	**7**	**8**	**9**	**10**	**11**	**12**	**13**
6	—	—	—	1	2	3	4	6	7	8	9	11	12	13	15	16	18	19	20	22
	—	—	—	**0**	**1**	**2**	**3**	**4**	**5**	**6**	**7**	**9**	**10**	**11**	**12**	**13**	**15**	**16**	**17**	**18**
7	—	—	0	1	3	4	6	7	9	11	12	14	16	17	19	21	23	24	26	28
	—	—	—	**0**	**1**	**3**	**4**	**6**	**7**	**9**	**10**	**12**	**13**	**15**	**16**	**18**	**19**	**21**	**22**	**24**
8	—	—	0	2	4	6	7	9	11	13	15	17	20	22	24	26	28	30	32	34
	—	—	—	**1**	**2**	**4**	**6**	**7**	**9**	**11**	**13**	**15**	**17**	**18**	**20**	**22**	**24**	**26**	**28**	**30**
9	—	—	1	3	5	7	9	11	14	16	18	21	23	26	28	31	33	36	38	40
	—	—	**0**	**1**	**3**	**5**	**7**	**9**	**11**	**13**	**16**	**18**	**20**	**22**	**24**	**27**	**29**	**31**	**33**	**36**
10	—	—	1	3	6	8	11	13	16	19	22	24	27	30	33	36	38	41	44	47
	—	—	**0**	**2**	**4**	**6**	**9**	**11**	**13**	**16**	**18**	**21**	**24**	**26**	**29**	**31**	**34**	**37**	**39**	**42**
11	—	—	1	4	7	9	12	15	18	22	25	28	31	34	37	41	44	47	50	53
	—	—	**0**	**2**	**5**	**7**	**10**	**13**	**16**	**18**	**21**	**24**	**27**	**30**	**33**	**36**	**39**	**42**	**45**	**48**
12	—	—	2	5	8	11	14	17	21	24	28	31	35	38	42	46	49	53	56	60
	—	—	**1**	**3**	**6**	**9**	**12**	**15**	**18**	**21**	**24**	**27**	**31**	**34**	**37**	**41**	**44**	**47**	**51**	**54**
13	—	0	2	5	9	12	16	20	23	27	31	35	39	43	47	51	55	59	63	67
	—	—	**1**	**3**	**7**	**10**	**13**	**17**	**20**	**24**	**27**	**31**	**34**	**38**	**42**	**45**	**49**	**53**	**56**	**60**
14	—	0	2	6	10	13	17	22	26	30	34	38	43	47	51	56	60	65	69	73
	—	—	**1**	**4**	**7**	**11**	**15**	**18**	**22**	**26**	**30**	**34**	**38**	**42**	**46**	**50**	**54**	**58**	**63**	**67**
15	—	0	3	7	11	15	19	24	28	33	37	42	47	51	56	61	66	70	75	80
	—	—	**2**	**5**	**8**	**12**	**16**	**20**	**24**	**29**	**33**	**37**	**42**	**46**	**51**	**55**	**60**	**64**	**69**	**73**
16	—	0	3	7	12	16	21	26	31	36	41	46	51	56	61	66	71	76	82	87
	—	—	**2**	**5**	**9**	**13**	**18**	**22**	**27**	**31**	**36**	**41**	**45**	**50**	**55**	**60**	**65**	**70**	**74**	**79**
17	—	0	4	8	13	18	23	28	33	38	44	49	55	60	66	71	77	82	88	93
	—	—	**2**	**6**	**10**	**15**	**19**	**24**	**29**	**34**	**39**	**44**	**49**	**54**	**60**	**65**	**70**	**75**	**81**	**86**
18	—	0	4	9	14	19	24	30	36	41	47	53	59	65	70	76	82	88	94	100
	—	—	**2**	**6**	**11**	**16**	**21**	**26**	**31**	**37**	**42**	**47**	**53**	**58**	**64**	**70**	**75**	**81**	**87**	**92**
19	—	1	4	9	15	20	26	32	38	44	50	56	63	69	75	82	88	94	101	107
	—	**0**	**3**	**7**	**12**	**17**	**22**	**28**	**33**	**39**	**45**	**51**	**56**	**63**	**69**	**74**	**81**	**87**	**93**	**99**
20	—	1	5	10	16	22	28	34	40	47	53	60	67	73	80	87	93	100	107	114
	—	**0**	**3**	**8**	**13**	**18**	**24**	**30**	**36**	**42**	**48**	**54**	**60**	**67**	**73**	**79**	**86**	**92**	**99**	**105**

Table B-6 (cont'd)

Critical values for a one-tailed test at $\alpha = 0.05$ (roman type) and $\alpha = 0.025$ (boldface type) and for a two-tailed test at $\alpha = 0.10$ (roman type) and $\alpha = 0.05$ (boldface type).

n_2 \ n_1	1	2	3	4	5	6	7	8	9	10	11	12	13	14	15	16	17	18	19	20
1	—	—	—	—	—	—	—	—	—	—	—	—	—	—	—	—	—	—	0	0
	—	—	—	—	—	—	—	—	—	—	—	—	—	—	—	—	—	—	—	—
2	—	—	—	—	0	0	0	1	1	1	1	2	2	2	3	3	3	4	4	4
	—	—	—	—	—	—	**0**	**0**	**0**	**0**	**1**	**1**	**1**	**1**	**1**	**2**	**2**	**2**	**2**
3	—	—	0	0	1	2	2	3	3	4	5	5	6	7	7	8	9	9	10	11
	—	—	—	—	**0**	**1**	**1**	**2**	**2**	**3**	**3**	**4**	**4**	**5**	**5**	**6**	**6**	**7**	**7**	**8**
4	—	—	0	1	2	3	4	5	6	7	8	9	10	11	12	14	15	16	17	18
	—	—	—	**0**	**1**	**2**	**3**	**4**	**4**	**5**	**6**	**7**	**8**	**9**	**10**	**11**	**11**	**12**	**13**	**13**
5	—	0	1	2	4	5	6	8	9	11	12	13	15	16	18	19	20	22	23	25
	—	—	**0**	**1**	**2**	**3**	**5**	**6**	**7**	**8**	**9**	**11**	**12**	**13**	**14**	**15**	**17**	**18**	**19**	**20**
6	—	0	2	3	5	7	8	10	12	14	16	17	19	21	23	25	26	28	30	32
	—	—	**1**	**2**	**3**	**5**	**6**	**8**	**10**	**11**	**13**	**14**	**16**	**17**	**19**	**21**	**22**	**24**	**25**	**27**
7	—	0	2	4	6	8	11	13	15	17	19	21	24	26	28	30	33	35	37	39
	—	—	**1**	**3**	**5**	**6**	**8**	**10**	**12**	**14**	**16**	**18**	**20**	**22**	**24**	**26**	**28**	**30**	**32**	**34**
8	—	1	3	5	8	10	13	15	18	20	23	26	28	31	33	36	39	41	44	47
	—	**0**	**2**	**4**	**6**	**8**	**10**	**13**	**15**	**17**	**19**	**22**	**24**	**26**	**29**	**31**	**34**	**36**	**38**	**41**
9	—	1	3	6	9	12	15	18	21	24	27	30	33	36	39	42	45	48	51	54
	—	**0**	**2**	**4**	**7**	**10**	**12**	**15**	**17**	**20**	**23**	**26**	**28**	**31**	**34**	**37**	**39**	**42**	**45**	**48**
10	—	1	4	7	11	14	17	20	24	27	31	34	37	41	44	48	51	55	58	62
	—	**0**	**3**	**5**	**8**	**11**	**14**	**17**	**20**	**23**	**26**	**29**	**33**	**36**	**39**	**42**	**45**	**48**	**52**	**55**
11	—	1	5	8	12	16	19	23	27	31	34	38	42	46	50	54	57	61	65	69
	—	**0**	**3**	**6**	**9**	**13**	**16**	**19**	**23**	**26**	**30**	**33**	**37**	**40**	**44**	**47**	**51**	**55**	**58**	**62**
12	—	2	5	9	13	17	21	26	30	34	38	42	47	51	55	60	64	68	72	77
	—	**1**	**4**	**7**	**11**	**14**	**18**	**22**	**26**	**29**	**33**	**37**	**41**	**45**	**49**	**53**	**57**	**61**	**65**	**69**
13	—	2	6	10	15	19	24	28	33	37	42	47	51	56	61	65	70	75	80	84
	—	**1**	**4**	**8**	**12**	**16**	**20**	**24**	**28**	**33**	**37**	**41**	**45**	**50**	**54**	**59**	**63**	**67**	**72**	**76**
14	—	2	7	11	16	21	26	31	36	41	46	51	56	61	66	71	77	82	87	92
	—	**1**	**5**	**9**	**13**	**17**	**22**	**26**	**31**	**36**	**40**	**45**	**50**	**55**	**59**	**64**	**67**	**74**	**78**	**83**
15	—	3	7	12	18	23	28	33	39	44	50	55	61	66	72	77	83	88	94	100
	—	**1**	**5**	**10**	**14**	**19**	**24**	**29**	**34**	**39**	**44**	**49**	**54**	**59**	**64**	**70**	**75**	**80**	**85**	**90**
16	—	3	8	14	19	25	30	36	42	48	54	60	65	71	77	83	89	95	101	107
	—	**1**	**6**	**11**	**15**	**21**	**26**	**31**	**37**	**42**	**47**	**53**	**59**	**64**	**70**	**75**	**81**	**86**	**92**	**98**
17	—	3	9	15	20	26	33	39	45	51	57	64	70	77	83	89	96	102	109	115
	—	**2**	**6**	**11**	**17**	**22**	**28**	**34**	**39**	**45**	**51**	**57**	**63**	**67**	**75**	**81**	**87**	**93**	**99**	**105**
18	—	4	9	16	22	28	35	41	48	55	61	68	75	82	88	95	102	109	116	123
	—	**2**	**7**	**12**	**18**	**24**	**30**	**36**	**42**	**48**	**55**	**61**	**67**	**74**	**80**	**86**	**93**	**99**	**106**	**112**
19	0	4	10	17	23	30	37	44	51	58	65	72	80	87	94	101	109	116	123	130
	—	**2**	**7**	**13**	**19**	**25**	**32**	**38**	**45**	**52**	**58**	**65**	**72**	**78**	**85**	**92**	**99**	**106**	**113**	**119**
20	0	4	11	18	25	32	39	47	54	62	69	77	84	92	100	107	115	123	130	138
	—	**2**	**8**	**13**	**20**	**27**	**34**	**41**	**48**	**55**	**62**	**69**	**76**	**83**	**90**	**98**	**105**	**112**	**119**	**127**

Source: From *Introductory Statistics*, by R. E. Kirk. Copyright © 1978 by Wadsworth, Inc. Reprinted by permission of Brooks/Cole Publishing Company, Pacific Grove, CA 93950.

Table B-7 Critical values of Wilcoxon T

	Level of Significance for a One-Tailed Test			
	0.05	0.025	0.01	0.005
	Level of Significance for a Two-Tailed Test			
n	0.10	0.05	0.02	0.01
5	0	—	—	—
6	2	0	—	—
7	3	2	0	—
8	5	3	1	0
9	8	5	3	1
10	10	8	5	3
11	13	10	7	5
12	17	13	9	7
13	21	17	12	9
14	25	21	15	12
15	30	25	19	15
16	35	29	23	19
17	41	34	27	23
18	47	40	32	27
19	53	46	37	32
20	60	52	43	37

Source: From *Introductory Statistics*, by R. E. Kirk. Copyright © 1978 by Wadsworth, Inc. Reprinted by permission of Brooks/Cole Publishing Company, Pacific Grove, CA 93950.

Table B-8 Critical values of Spearman rho

N	Significance level for a directional test at			
	.05	.025	.005	.001
	Significance level for a non-directional test at			
	.10	.05	.01	.002
5	.900	1.000		
6	.829	.886	1.000	
7	.715	.786	.929	1.000
8	.620	.715	.881	.953
9	.600	.700	.834	.917
10	.564	.649	.794	.879
11	.537	.619	.764	.855
12	.504	.588	.735	.826
13	.484	.561	.704	.797
14	.464	.539	.680	.772
15	.447	.522	.658	.750
16	.430	.503	.636	.730
17	.415	.488	.618	.711
18	.402	.474	.600	.693
19	.392	.460	.585	.676
20	.381	.447	.570	.661
21	.371	.437	.556	.647
22	.361	.426	.544	.633
23	.353	.417	.532	.620
24	.345	.407	.521	.608
25	.337	.399	.511	.597
26	.331	.391	.501	.587
27	.325	.383	.493	.577
28	.319	.376	.484	.567
29	.312	.369	.475	.558
30	.307	.363	.467	.549

Source: Reprinted with permission from *CRC Handbook of Tables for Probability and Statistics* (2nd edition). Copyright 1968, CRC Press, Inc., Boca Raton, Florida.

Table B-9 Values of r at the 5% and 1% levels of significance (two-tailed test)

Degrees of Freedom (df)	5%	1%	Degrees of Freedom (df)	5%	1%
1	.997	1.000	24	.388	.496
2	.950	.990	25	.381	.487
3	.878	.959	26	.374	.478
4	.811	.917	27	.367	.470
5	.754	.874	28	.361	.463
6	.707	.834	29	.355	.456
7	.666	.798	30	.349	.449
8	.632	.765	35	.325	.418
9	.602	.735	40	.304	.393
10	.576	.708	45	.288	.372
11	.553	.684	50	.273	.354
12	.532	.661	60	.250	.325
13	.514	.641	70	.232	.302
14	.497	.623	80	.217	.283
15	.482	.606	90	.205	.267
16	.468	.590	100	.195	.254
17	.456	.575	125	.174	.228
18	.444	.561	150	.159	.208
19	.433	.549	200	.138	.181
20	.423	.537	300	.113	.148
21	.413	.526	400	.098	.128
22	.404	.515	500	.088	.115
23	.396	.505	1000	.062	.081

Source: R. A. Fisher and F. Yates, *Statistical Tables for Biological, Agricultural and Medical Research* (London: Longman Group Ltd., 1978; earlier edition, Edinburgh: Oliver & Boyd Ltd.). Reprinted by permission of the authors and publishers. Part of this table is reprinted by permission from *Statistical Methods* by George W. Snedecor and William G. Cochran, 6th edition © 1967 by Iowa State University Press, Ames, Iowa.

APPENDIX C

Exercises for MYSTAT software

EXERCISES

1. Sort Data Set A below in ascending order.

    Data Set A
    80
    75
    65
    75
    70
    85
    80
    90
    95
    80
    70
    60
    70
    75
    50
    55
    85
    80
    90
    95

2. Compute all statistics for Data Set A above.
3. Use the list format to create a frequency table for Data Set A above.
4. Create a stem and leaf diagram for Data Set A above.

5. For the data below run a t-test with a null hypothesis of $\mu = 60$.

X
65
70
60
60
78
90
58
85
86
59
62
61
75
65
54

6. For the data below run a dependent t-test.

X	Y
80	75
75	75
65	60
75	75
70	60
85	85
80	70
90	85
95	90
80	60
70	75
60	55
70	75
75	80
50	45
55	50
85	80
80	80
90	80
95	90

7. For the data below run an independent t-test.

X	Y
12	8
10	6
9	9
9	8
9	4
8	5
10	5
7	6
11	6
5	7
5	4
9	4
4	3
2	
1	

8. For the data below compute Pearson's correlation and create a scattergraph.

X	Y
80	75
75	75
65	60
75	75
70	60
85	85
80	70
90	85
95	90
80	60
70	75
60	55
70	75
75	80
50	45
55	50
85	80
80	80
90	80
95	90

9. For the data below run an ANOVA.

Group One	Group Two	Group Three
12.0	5.0	8.0
10.0	5.0	4.0
9.0	9.0	5.0
9.0	4.0	5.0
9.0	2.0	6.0
8.0	1.0	6.0
10.0	8.0	7.0
7.0	6.0	4.0
11.0	9.0	4.0

10. For the data below run independent t-tests between the two groups for each of the three variables.

IQ	Average (AVE)	Grade-point average (GPA)	Group
108	66	6.5	1
122	74	6.6	1
111	65	7.0	1
123	82	7.2	1
114	75	6.9	1
100	68	6.5	1
105	66	5.9	1
117	60	6.2	1
128	73	7.8	1
126	85	7.5	1
100	56	6.0	2
101	61	5.6	2
110	60	5.8	2
98	57	7.5	2
103	64	6.8	2
102	60	5.7	2
111	59	7.0	2
109	57	5.9	2
107	58	6.4	2

11. Run a chi-square analysis for the data below concerning the performance of students with different majors.

	Science	Arts	Business	Total
Pass	56	75	42	173
Fail	35	24	35	94
Total	91	99	77	267

12. Construct a stem and leaf diagram for each data set below.

Set A	Set B
34	40
23	30
56	55
46	50
33	40
38	39
13	25
26	30
22	25
37	43
19	36
27	34
45	50
33	47
29	38
30	25
20	15
25	38
15	31
50	42

13. Run a chi-square analysis on the data below.

	1	2	3	Total
1	40	30	55	125
2	50	40	39	129
3	25	30	25	80
Total	115	100	119	334

14. Run a one-way ANOVA on the data below.

Group 1	Group 2	Group 3
65.0	55.0	45.0
77.0	80.0	60.0
69.0	55.0	56.0
50.0	50.0	72.0
70.0	80.0	56.0
75.0	75.0	54.0
63.0	50.0	61.0
69.0	60.0	60.0
89.0	70.0	50.0
92.0	60.0	70.0
70.0	50.0	65.0
60.0	50.0	71.0
70.0	80.0	61.0
80.0	90.0	51.0
60.0	85.0	60.0

15. Run an independent t-test on the data below.

Group 1	Group 2
90	85
95	70
95	80
85	80
95	90
85	70
85	85
80	65
85	65
95	30
90	60
85	75
70	70
90	80
75	75

16. Run a t-test for a single mean on the data below. Your null hypothesis will state that $\mu = 85$.

Score
85
70
80
80
90
70
85
65
65
30
60
75
70
80
75

17. The following data are the rental cost per hour and the rental cost per mile for 10 cars. Five of the cars are compact (size 1), and the other five are luxury (size 2). Compute descriptive statistics for the cars by size.

Cost per hour (dollars)	Cost per mile (cents)	Size
10	5	1
10	5	1
12	0	2
15	0	2
10	5	2
9	10	1
8	10	1
15	0	2
12	2	2
10	5	1

18. Create a frequency distribution for the following data.

Score	f
10	3
11	4
15	8
13	7
18	10
20	6
25	4
8	2
5	2
30	2

19. Sort and rank the following data.

Data
22
56
41
89
34
52
11
69
81
75
75
75
46
23
25
62
35
30
58
56

454   Appendix C

20. Create a scattergraph for the following data.

X	Y
3	75
5	75
8	60
5	75
4	60
2	85
6	70
6	85
6	90
9	60
10	75
4	55
7	75
8	80
8	45
8	50
2	80
2	80
2	80
2	90

SOLUTIONS

1. 50
55
60
65
70
70
70
75
75
75
80
80
80
80
85
85
90
90
95
95

2. Number of cases: 20
Minimum: 50.00
Maximum: 95.00
Range: 45.00
Mean: 76.25
Variance: 154.93
Standard deviation: 12.45
Standard error: 2.78
Skewness: −0.40
Kurtosis: −0.46
Sum: 1525.00

3.

Count	CUM Count	Percentage	CUM Percentage	X
1	1	5.0	5.0	50
1	2	5.0	10.0	55
1	3	5.0	15.0	60
1	4	5.0	20.0	65
3	7	15.0	35.0	70
3	10	15.0	50.0	75
4	14	20.0	70.0	80
2	16	10.0	80.0	85
2	18	10.0	90.0	90
2	20	10.0	100.0	95

4. Stem and leaf plot of variable: X, N = 20

Minimum: 50
Lower hinge is: 70
Median is: 77.5
Upper hinge is: 85
Maximum is: 95

```
5    0
5    5
6    0
6    5
7H   000
7M   555
8    0000
8H   55
9    00
9    55
```

5. Paired samples t-test on X vs. M60 with 15 cases.

Mean difference = 14.667
SD difference = 11.412
DF = 14
T = 4.977
Prob = 0.000

6. Pair samples t-test on X vs. Y with 20 cases.

   Mean difference =   4
   SD difference =   5.982
   DF =   19
   T =   2.99
   Prob =   0.008

7. Independent samples t-test on SCORE grouped by GROUP.

Group	N	Mean	SD
1.000	15	7.400	3.291
2.000	13	5.769	1.833

   Separate variances: t =   1.647
                      df = 22.5
                  prob = .114

   Pooled variances: t =   1.584
                   df = 25
                 prob = .125

8. Pearson correlation matrix

	X	Y
X	1.000	
Y	0.891	1.000

   Number of observations: 20

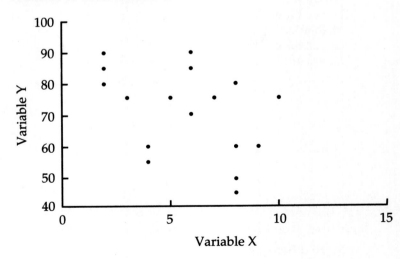

9. Dep var: SCORE
   N: 27
   Multiple R: .699
   Squared multiple R: .488

   Analysis of Variance

Source	Sum-of-squares	DF	Mean-square	F-ratio	P
GROUP	96.000	2	48.000	11.444	0.000
Error	100.667	24	4.194		

10. Independent samples t-test on IQ grouped by GROUP:

Group	N	Mean	SD
1	10	115	9
2	9	105	5

    Separate variances: t = 3.215
                        df = 13.6
                        prob = .007

    Pooled variances: t = 3.111
                      df = 17
                      prob = .006

    Independent samples t-test on AVE grouped by GROUP:

Group	N	Mean	SD
1	10	71	8
2	9	59	2

    Separate variances: t = 4.676
                        df = 10.9
                        prob = .001

    Pooled variances: t = 4.468
                      df = 17
                    prob = 0.000

    Independent samples t-test on GPA grouped by GROUP:

Group	N	Mean	SD
1	10	7	1
2	9	6	1

    Separate variances: t = 1.765
                        df = 16.1
                        prob = .097

    Pooled variances: t = 1.778
                      df = 17
                    prob = .093

11. Table of PERF (row) by MAJOR (columns)

	Frequencies			
	1	2	3	Total
1	56	75	42	173
2	35	24	35	94
Total	91	99	77	267

Test statistic	Value	DF	Prob
Pearson chi-square	9.185	2	.010
Likelihood ratio chi-square	9.378	2	.009

Coefficient	Value	Asymptotic standard error
Phi	.1855	
Cramer V	.1855	
Contingency	.1824	
Goodman-Kruskal gamma	.0749	.10750
Kendall tau-B	.0421	.06064
Stuart tau-C	.0463	.06675
Spearman rho	.0447	.06366
Somers D (column dependent)	.0508	.07313
Lambda (column dependent)	.0655	.04420
Uncertainty (column dependent)	.0161	.01030

12. Stem and leaf plot of variable: VAR1, N = 20

Minimum is: 13.000
Lower hinge is: 22.500
Median is: 29.500
Upper hinge is: 37.500
Maximum is: 56.000

```
1     3
1     59
2H    023
2M    5679
3     0334
3H    78
4
4     56
5     0
5     6
```

Stem and leaf plot of variable: VAR2, N = 20
Minimum is: 15.000
Lower hinge is: 30.000
Median is: 38.000
Upper hinge is: 42.500
Maximum is: 55.000

```
1     5
2
2     555
3H    0014
3M    6889
4H    0023
4     7
5     00
5     5
```

13. Table of VAR1 (row) by VAR2 (columns)

	Frequencies			
	1	2	3	Total
1	40	30	55	125
2	50	40	39	129
3	25	30	25	80
Total	115	100	119	334

Test statistic	Value	DF	Prob
Pearson chi-square	8.144	4	.086
Likelihood ratio chi-square	8.027	4	.091
McNemar symmetry chi-square	17.424	4	.001

Coefficient	Value	Asymptotic standard error
Phi	.1562	
Cramer V	.1104	
Contingency	.1543	
Goodman-Kruskal gamma	−.0959	.07302
Kendall tau-B	−.0636	.04860
Stuart tau-C	−.0629	.04802
Cohen kappa	−.0231	.03739
Spearman rho	−.0725	.05425
Somers D (column dependent)	−.0642	.04904
Lambda (column dependent)	.0744	.05370
Uncertainty (column dependent)	.0110	.00776

14. Dep var: SCORE
    N: 45
    Multiple R: .382
    Squared multiple R: .146

    ### Analysis of Variance

Source	Sum-of-squares	DF	Mean-square	F-ratio	P
GROUP	938.98	2	469.49	3.58	0.04
Error	5511.33	42	131.22		

15. Independent samples t-test on SCORE grouped by GROUP:

Group	N	Mean	SD
1.000	15	86.667	7.480
2.000	15	72.000	14.368

    Pooled variances: t = 3.507
    df = 28
    prob = .002

16. Paired samples t-test on SC vs. M85 with 15 cases.

    Mean difference = −13.000
    SD difference = 14.368
    DF = 14
    T = 3.504
    Prob = .004

17. The following results are for SIZE = 1

    Total observations: 5

	Cost per hour	Cost per mile
N of cases	5	5
Minimum	8.000	5.000
Maximum	10.000	10.000
Mean	9.400	7.000
Standard dev	0.894	2.739

    The following results are for SIZE = 2

    Total observations: 5

	Cost per hour	Cost per mile
N of cases	5	5
Minimum	10.000	0.000
Maximum	15.000	5.000
Mean	12.800	1.400
Standard dev	2.168	2.191

18.

Count	CUM Count	Percentage	CUM Percentage	
2	2	4.2	4.2	
2	4	4.2	8.3	8
3	7	6.3	14.6	10
4	11	8.3	22.9	11
7	18	14.6	37.5	13
8	26	16.7	54.2	15
10	36	20.8	75.0	18
6	42	12.5	87.5	20
4	46	8.3	95.8	25
2	48	4.2	100.0	30

19.

Sorted Data	Ranked Data
11	1
22	2
23	3
25	4
30	5
34	6
35	7
41	8
46	9
52	10
56	11.5
56	11.5
58	13
62	14
69	15
75	17
75	17
75	17
81	19
89	20

20.

Answers to Selected Exercises

Chapter 1

1. a. Each value differs from the others in some qualitative way.
   b. The values differ in quantity. X_2 is larger than X_1.
   c. The difference between X_2 and X_1 is the same amount as the difference between X_3 and X_2.
   d. X_4 is twice as large as X_3.

2. a. Ordinal b. Interval c. Ratio d. Nominal

4. a. constant   d. constant
   b. constant   e. variable
   c. variable

6. a. continuous   d. continuous   g. continuous
   b. discrete   e. discrete   h. discrete
   c. continuous   f. discrete   i. discrete

7. Brand of pain reliever-IV; rating-DV.

9. a. 11   b. 4   c. 6   d. 2

10. a. observation   d. verbal report
    b. observation   e. standardized test
    c. verbal report   f. observation

12. This is an example of a study with no hope for internal validity. The teacher has no control group. She didn't test her subjects before she introduced her new technique. If she finds they do well, she has no way of knowing what the responsible variables are.

14. This investigator has taken some trouble to control for factors affecting internal validity by using random selection, by using a placebo control group, and by using a double-blind technique. He could not randomly assign subjects to groups, but his placebo control will help to mitigate changes in memory due to maturation etc. The major problem here will be with attrition. The experiment spans a two-year period. Thus, we would expect that the group of 80 to 90 year-olds may lose more subjects than the younger groups.

Chapter 2

1. a.

Table 1. Simple frequency distribution of weights

X	f	X	f	X	f	X	f
164	1	144	0	124	1	104	2
163	0	143	0	123	2	103	3
162	0	142	1	122	1	102	2
161	0	141	1	121	2	101	2
160	0	140	0	120	0	100	3
159	2	139	0	119	3	99	0
158	0	138	1	118	1	98	3
157	1	137	1	117	3	97	2
156	0	136	3	116	4	96	1
155	2	135	1	115	2	95	0
154	1	134	2	114	2	94	1
153	1	133	3	113	1	93	1
152	0	132	1	112	0	92	0
151	1	131	2	111	2	91	2
150	1	130	2	110	2	90	2
149	0	129	3	109	3	89	0
148	0	128	2	108	3	88	1
147	0	127	1	107	0	87	0
146	0	126	0	106	3	86	1
145	0	125	1	105	3	85	1

b.

Table 2. Grouped frequency distribution of weights

Apparent limits	Exact limits	M.P.	f	rel. f	cum. f	rel. cf
160–164	159.5–164.5	162	1	0.01	100	1.00
155–159	154.5–159.5	157	5	0.05	99	0.99
150–154	149.5–154.5	152	4	0.04	94	0.94
145–149	144.5–149.5	147	0	0.00	90	0.90
140–144	139.5–144.5	142	2	0.02	90	0.90
135–139	134.5–139.5	137	6	0.06	88	0.88
130–134	129.5–134.5	132	10	0.10	82	0.82
125–129	124.5–129.5	127	7	0.07	72	0.72
120–124	119.5–124.5	122	6	0.06	65	0.65
115–119	114.5–119.5	117	13	0.13	59	0.59
110–114	109.5–114.5	112	7	0.07	46	0.46
105–109	104.5–109.5	107	12	0.12	39	0.39
100–104	99.5–104.5	102	12	0.12	27	0.27
95–99	94.5–99.5	97	6	0.06	15	0.15
90–94	89.5–94.5	92	6	0.06	9	0.09
85–89	84.5–89.5	87	3	0.03	3	0.03

Answers to Selected Exercises

2. a.

Class interval	Before	After
64–66	1	0
61–63	0	0
58–60	0	0
55–57	2	0
52–54	0	0
49–51	0	1
46–48	3	1
43–45	0	0
40–42	4	4
37–39	1	2
34–36	2	0
31–33	4	2
28–30	3	3
25–27	1	3
22–24	2	5
19–21	2	2
16–18	0	2

3.

X	f
25	1
24	0
23	0
22	0
21	0
20	0
19	0
18	1
17	0
16	0
15	3
14	1
13	1
12	1
11	1
10	1
9	1
8	2
7	1
6	1

5.

X	cf
21	25
20	24
19	23
18	21
17	20
16	18
15	14
14	11
13	8
12	4
11	4
10	3

8.

Empathy towards students	Knowledge of subject matter			
	Excellent (1)	Good (2)	Fair (3)	Poor (4)
Very empathetic (1)	4	2	0	3
Moderately empathetic (2)	2	3	3	1
Somewhat empathetic (3)	3	1	4	0
Not empathetic (4)	1	0	1	2

9.

Interval	f
46–50	1
41–45	2
36–40	2
31–35	0
26–30	0
21–25	1
16–20	0
11–15	2
6–10	5
1– 5	1

13.

Interval	Rel. f
84–90	0.04
77–83	0.03
70–76	0.00
63–69	0.09
56–62	0.15
49–55	0.19
42–48	0.13
35–41	0.10
28–34	0.06
21–27	0.10
14–20	0.04
7–13	0.04
0– 6	0.05

15.
- **a.** 1.95 to 2.05
- **b.** 2.55 to 2.65
- **c.** 1.5 to 4.5
- **d.** 24.5 to 29.5
- **e.** 24.45 to 29.55
- **f.** 24.495 to 29.505

16. Bar graph. Relative frequency.

19.

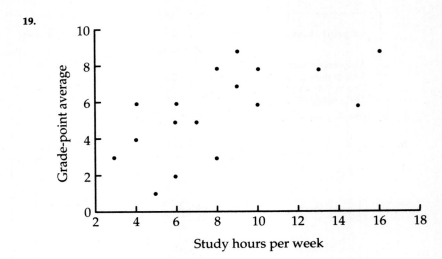

21.

```
1 | 0 1 1 5 6
2 | 1 3 3 5 6 7 8
3 | 1 2 3 7 7 8 9 9
4 | 2 2 3 6 6 8 9 9
5 | 0 1 2 8 9 9 9 9
6 | 1 4 4 5 6 7 7 8
7 | 2 3 3 4 5 7
8 | 4 5 5 6 7 8
9 | 0 0 3 4 5 6
```

Chapter 3

1.

DATA SET A
a. $\Sigma X = 114$
b. $N = 15$
c. $\mu = 7.60$
d. $Mo = 11, 9, 8, 7, 5, 3$
e. $Mdn = 7.75$
f. Negative skew

DATA SET B
a. $\Sigma X = 22$
b. $N = 10$
c. $\mu = 2.20$
d. $Mo = 2$
e. $Mdn = 1.83$
f. Positive skew

3.

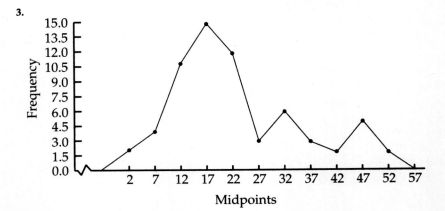

4. $\mu = 7$ Mo = 8   Mdn = 7.67   negative skew

6. $\mu_c = 5.44$

7. $\mu = 19.73$ Mdn = 18.5   Mo = 12   positive skew

8. $\mu = 6.79$ Mo = 5   Mdn = 6.2   positive skew

10. Mo = 8   Mdn = 9.5   Mean = 10.1   positive skew

12. **a.** It is limited at zero.   **b.** Mean

13. Mean = 12.7   Mdn = 12.46   Mo = 11.8

Chapter 4

1.
   DATA SET A
   a. $\Sigma X = 200$
   b. $\Sigma(X - \mu) = 0$
   c. $\Sigma(X - \mu)^2 = 1198$
   d. $N = 10$
   e. $\mu = 20$
   f. $\sigma^2 = 119.80$
   g. $\sigma = 10.94$

   DATA SET B
   a. $\Sigma X = 49$
   b. $\Sigma(X - \mu) = 0$
   c. $\Sigma(X - \mu)^2 = 104$
   d. $N = 7$
   e. $\mu = 7$
   f. $\sigma^2 = 14.86$
   g. $\sigma = 3.85$

3.

X	x
2	−2
4	0
6	2
7	3
4	0
3	−1
2	−2
$\mu = 4$	

Y	y
12	−16
23	−5
50	22
35	7
20	−8
$\mu = 28$	

5. $\mu = 3$ $\sigma^2 = 7.25$ $\sigma = 2.69$ Range = 9

7. $\sigma^2 = 3.22$ $\sigma = 1.79$ Range = 6

9. $\sigma_c^2 = 9.16$

468 Answers to Selected Exercises

11.

	Group 1	Group 2
μ	23.42	21.53
σ	1.95	3.31
Median	23.92	21.92
Skew	slight negative	slight negative

13. $\mu = 6.40$ $\sigma = 1.43$ Skew: slight postive

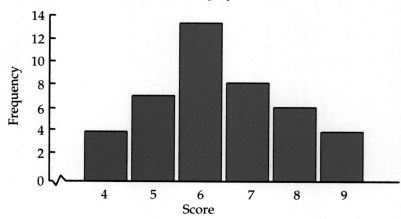

Chapter 5

1. $P_{50} = 121.5$ $P_{75} = 129.5$ $P_{90} = 133.25$ $PR_{117} = 30.83$

2. $Z = -2$

4. Mary did better on her math test.
Z grammar = 1.
Z math = 1.5.

6. 62% of the scores were at or below a score value of 89%.

8. X = 63

10. **a.** $P_{30} = 59.25$ $P_{45} = 71.93$ $P_{85} = 84.50$
   b. $PR_{83} = 81.25$ $PR_{54} = 16.25$ $PR_{78} = 66.25$

c. and **d.**

X	f	fX	X²	fX²	X − μ	Z
98	1	98	9604	9604	27.5	1.93
93	3	279	8649	25947	22.5	1.58
88	1	88	7744	7744	17.5	1.23
83	5	415	6889	34445	12.5	0.88
78	7	546	6084	42588	7.5	0.53
73	7	511	5329	37303	2.5	0.18
68	1	68	4624	4624	−2.5	−0.18
63	2	126	3969	7938	−7.5	−0.53
58	4	232	3364	13456	−12.5	−0.88
53	5	265	2809	14045	−17.5	−1.23
48	4	192	2304	9216	−22.5	−1.58
Sum		2820		206910		

$$\mu = 70.50$$
$$\sigma = 14.23$$

12.

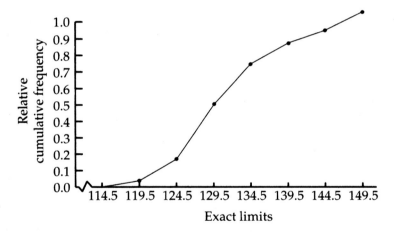

$PR_{130} = 52.6$

$Mdn = 129.5$

14. **a.** Z-score Test One = 0.33   Z-Score Test Two = 0.4
   b. Ben's Z = 2.83   Tom's Z = 3.13

Chapter 6

1. 0.9876

3. 0.0250

5. +1.28

7. a. Z = 0.66   Area = 25.14%   e. 250
   b. Z = −0.5   Area = 31%   f. 0.0008   X ≅ 109
   c. X = 61.92 and 82.08   g. X = 63.96
   d. X = 52.35

9. Z = −0.84 P_{20} = 41.6

11. Z = ±1.28

13. 0.005   Z = −2.58   X = 395.20

Chapter 7

1. a, c, d

3. a. p = 0.56   b. p = 0.94

5. a. p = 0.025   b. p = 0.325

7. p = 0.32

9. 56

11. a. 1/48   b. 1/48   c. 2/48   d. 46/48   e. 4/48

13. a. 36   b. 4

15. 1/4, 2/4

17. a. Row totals: 4, 13, 33, 25, 45, 6, 0, 2, 1
    Column totals: 58, 37, 34
    Total = 129
    b. p = 0.45   c. p = 0.09   d. p = 0.01   e. p = 0.98

Chapter 8

1. **a.** $\Sigma X = 130$ **d.** $\Sigma X^2 = 2708$
    b. $(\Sigma X)^2/N = 2414.29$ **e.** $\mu = 18.57$
    c. $N = 7$ **f.** $\sigma = 6.48$

3.

Samples

1, 1	1, 2	1, 4	1, 7	1, 11
2, 1	2, 2	2, 4	2, 7	2, 11
4, 1	4, 2	4, 4	4, 7	4, 11
7, 1	7, 2	7, 4	7, 7	7, 11
11, 1	11, 2	11, 4	11, 7	11, 11

Sample means

1.00	1.50	2.50	4.00	6.00
1.50	2.00	3.00	4.50	6.50
2.50	3.00	4.00	5.50	7.50
4.00	4.50	5.50	7.00	9.00
6.00	6.50	7.50	9.00	11.00

4. $\mu_{\bar{x}} = 5.0$ $\sigma_{\bar{x}} = 2.57$

6. **a.** $\mu_{\bar{x}} = 75$ and $\sigma_{\bar{x}} = 1$
    b. $\mu_{\bar{x}} = 75$ and $\sigma_{\bar{x}} = 1.5$
    c. $\mu_{\bar{x}} = 75$ and $\sigma_{\bar{x}} = 3$

8. Standard error of the mean $= 3.20$
    a. $Z = 3.75$ **b.** $Z = -1.56$ **c.** $Z = -3.125$
    $p \cong 0.0001$ $p = 0.8812$ $p \cong 0.0009$

10. Standard error of the difference $= 18.28$
    a. $Z = 1.20$ **b.** $Z = 1.64$ **c.** $Z = 2.58$
    $p = 0.1151$ $p = 0.0505$ $p = 0.0049$

11. Standard error of the difference $= 0.97$
    a. $Z = -0.30$ **b.** $Z = -2.06$ **c.** $Z = -0.51$
    $p = 0.3821$ $p = 0.0197$ $p = 0.3050$

12. Standard error of the proportion $= 0.06$
    a. $Z = 1.41$ **b.** $Z = -0.28$ **c.** $Z = -1.97$
    $p = 0.0793$ $p = 0.3897$ $p \cong 0.0244$

Chapter 9

1. $H_o: \mu = 79$ $H_a: \mu \neq 79$ $Z = 2.14$ Fail to reject.

3. $H_o: P = 0.50$ $H_a: P > 0.50$ $p = 0.56$ $Z = 0.86$ Fail to reject.

5. $H_o: P = 0.75$ $H_a: P > 0.75$ $p = 0.81$ $Z = 1.39$ Fail to reject.

7. $H_o: P = 0.70$ $H_a: P \neq 0.70$ $p = 0.60$ $Z = -1.54$ Fail to reject.

9. **a.** $H_o: \mu = 70$
   $H_a: \mu < 70$
   b. Critical Z value $= -1.64$
   c. Obtained Z value $= -2.00$
   d. Reject

11. **a.** $H_o: \mu = 1.1$
    $H_a: \mu \neq 1.1$
    b. Critical Z value $= \pm 2.58$
    c. Obtained Z value $= -2.53$
    d. Fail to reject

Chapter 10

1. t-test for dependent means (this is a within subjects design).

3. t-test for independent means (subjects have not been matched; the population of interest is male children with IQ's over 120).

5. $H_o: \mu_A = \mu_B$ $H_a: \mu_A \neq \mu_B$ $t_{.01} = \pm 2.98$ $t = -1.03$

7. $H_o: \mu_1 = \mu_2$ $H_a: \mu_1 \neq \mu_2$ $df = 14$ $t_{.05} = \pm 2.145$
   $t = 3.813$ Fail to reject.

9. **a.** Rejecting a true null hypothesis.
   b. Failing to reject a false null hypothesis.
   c. The probability of rejecting a false null hypothesis.

11. **a.** $H_o: \mu = 28$
    $H_a: \mu \neq 28$
    b. $df = 15$
    c. Critical t value $= \pm 2.131$
    d. $s = 6.74$
    e. Obtained t value $= -1.33$
    f. Fail to reject

13. **a.** $H_o: \mu_1 = \mu_2$
    $H_a: \mu_1 > \mu_2$
    b. $df = 9$
    c. $t_{.05} = +1.83$
    d. $t = 2.5$
    e. $p < .05$
    f. Reject

15. **a.** $df = 27$
    b. $t_{.05} = \pm 2.052$ and $t_{.01} = \pm 2.771$
    c. $s_{\bar{x}_1 - \bar{x}_2} = 1.51$
    d. $C(-0.76 \leq (\mu_1 - \mu_2) \leq 5.42) = .95$
    e. $C(-1.85 \leq (\mu_1 - \mu_2) \leq 6.51) = .99$

Chapter 11

1.

SS	df	MS	F
141.3	3	47.10	3.54
1278	96	13.31	

Reject

3.

SS	df	MS	F
54.45	1	54.45	14.39
68.10	18	3.78	

Reject

5.

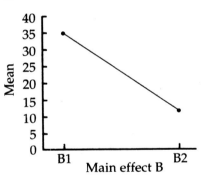

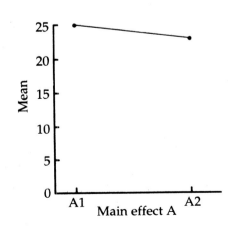

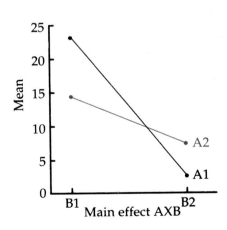

474 Answers to Selected Exercises

7. f.

Source	SS	df	MS	F	p
Between	56.00	2	28.00	5.92	$<\alpha$
Within	85.14	18	4.73		

9. g.

Source	SS	df	MS	F	p
A	16.67	1	16.67	0.11	>.05
B	8.17	1	8.17	0.05	>.05
AXB	383.99	1	383.99	2.58	>.05
WS	2981.00	20	149.05		
Total	3389.83	23			

h.

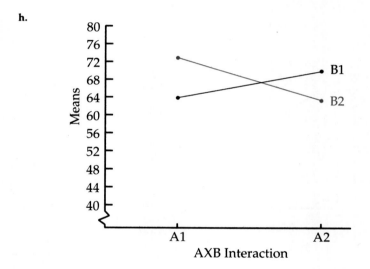

AXB Interaction

Chapter 12

1.
	Source	df
a.	Total	99
b.	Between subject	19
c.	Within subject	80
d.	Between treatment	4
e.	Subject by treatment	76

2.

Source	SS	df	MS	F	p
Between subjects	197.33	9			
Within subjects	1569.33	20			
Treatment	695.27	2	347.63	7.16	<.01
SXT	874.07	18	48.56		
Total	1766.67	29			

5.

Source	SS	df	MS	F	p
S	3559.81	15			
A	17.52	1	17.52	0.08	>.05
S(gps)	3542.29	14	221.39		
WS	1194.67	32			
B	401.79	2	200.90	18.18	<.01
AXB	439.35	2	219.68	19.88	<.01
S(gps)XB	353.52	28	11.05		
Total	4754.48	47			

7. j. F's are:
A = 2.24   B = 2.75   AXB = 2.05

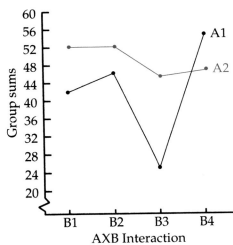

AXB Interaction

9.

Source	SS	df	MS	F
A	1602.47	2	801.23	7.66
S(gps)	2822.60	27	104.54	
B	2588.07	2	1294.03	15.17
AXB	205.47	4	51.37	0.60
S(gps)XB	4607.80	54	85.33	
Total	11826.4	89		

Chapter 13

1. $T_{crit} = \pm 2.083$
   Standard error = 7.05

Comparison	t
A_1B_1 vs. A_1B_2	−1.30
A_1B_1 vs. A_2B_2	−0.90
A_1B_1 vs. A_2B_2	0.07
A_1B_2 vs. A_2B_1	0.40
A_1B_2 vs. A_2B_2	1.37
A_2B_1 vs. A_2B_2	0.97

   There are no significant differences.

3. $F_s = 2.79$
   - **a.** $C = 1.6$
     $s_c = 1.33$
     $F' = 1.20$
     Fail to reject.
   - **b.** $C = 4.20$
     $s_c = 1.15$
     $F' = 3.65$
     Reject.
   - **c.** $C = 5.00$
     $s_c = 1.33$
     $F' = 3.76$
     Reject.

5.
	SS	df	MS	F
Between	28.40	2	14.20	9.26
Within	9.20	6	1.53	

	1 vs. 2	1 vs. 3	3 vs. 2	2&3 vs. 1	1&3 vs. 2	1&2 vs. 3
C	4.6	3.9	0.7	4.25	2.65	1.60
S_c	1.01	1.01	1.01	0.87	0.87	0.87
F'	4.55*	3.86*	0.69	4.89*	3.05	1.84

   *significant at $\alpha = .05$

   $F_s = 3.21$

7. **a.** HSD = 2.31
   b. NH–NL = 1.88   CH–NH = 1.50   CL–NH = 0.63   CH–NL = 3.38*
   CL–NL = 2.50*   CH–CL = 0.88

Chapter 14

1. **a.** df = 5 and $\chi^2_{.05} = 11.7$ **c.** df = 12 and $\chi^2_{.05} = 21.03$
   b. df = 1 and $\chi^2_{.01} = 6.64$ **d.** df = 1 and $\chi^2_{.01} = 6.64$

Answers to Selected Exercises 477

3. a. H_o: Strain and performance are independent
    H_a: Performance depends upon strain
    b. df = 1
    c. $\chi^2_{.05} = 3.84$
    d. $\chi^2 = 7.72$
    e. Reject
    f. Strain of rat and problem-solving success are dependent.

5. $\chi^2 = 4.3$ Fail to reject.

7. $\chi^2 = 8$ Reject.

9. $\chi^2 = 18.3$ Reject.

11. $\chi^2 = 4.19$ Fail to reject.

13. $\chi^2 = 35.88$ Reject.

15. $\chi^2 = 46.59$ Reject.

Chapter 15

1. $U_1 = 4$ $U_2 = 60$ $U_{crit} = 7$, for a two-tailed test at $\alpha = .01$
Reject because $4 < 7$
Conclusion: The populations from which the two groups come are not identical.

3. $H = 8.42$ Critical value of chi-square = 5.99   Reject.
Conclusion: The ratings of the three boats differ.

5.
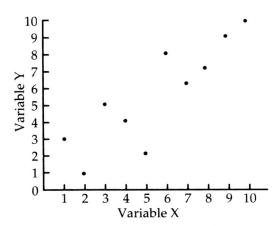

7. rho = -0.16

9. $H = 9.06$ $\chi^2_{crit} = 5.99$

Chapter 16

1.

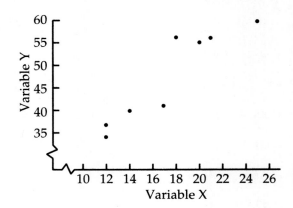

Positive correlation.

3. $\rho = 0.93$

5. $\rho = 0.88$

7. $\rho = -0.81$

9. rho $= 0.88$

Chapter 17

1. **a.** $b = 3.78$ $\mu_x = 5.53$ $\mu_y = 60$
b. $a = 39.11$
c.

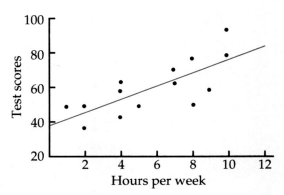

3. **a.** $Y' = 6.46$ **b.** $Y' = 11.50$ **c.** $Y' = 8.98$

5. **a.** $\rho = 0.81$ **b.** Coefficient of determination: $\rho^2 = 0.66$

7.   **a.** $\rho = 0.88$
    b. $b = 1.20$ $a = 41.35$
    c.

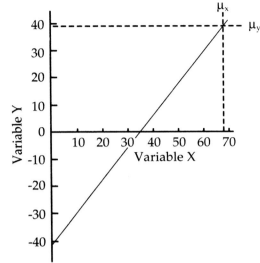

9. $MR = 0.58$

11. $R_p = 0.41$

Chapter 18

A-1. Two-way ANOVA.

A-3. One-way ANOVA.

A-5. t-test for independent means.

A-7. t-test for dependent means.

B-1. Kruskal-Wallis test.

B-3. Wilcoxon test for dependent groups.

B-5. Wilcoxon test.

C-1. Chi-square test for independence with 1 df.

C-3. Chi-square test for independence with 2 df.

C-5. Chi-square test for goodness of fit with 1 df or a Z-test for a proportion.

Index

A

A posteriori comparisons, 296-302
A posteriori hypothesis, 157
A priori comparisons, 294-296
A priori hypothesis, 157
Abscissa, 35
Absolute frequency, defined, 31
Acceptance region, 168
Alpha level, defined, 167
Alternative hypothesis
   defined, 165-166
   directional vs non-directional, 166
Analysis of variance, one-way, 218-232
   critical values. *See* Appendix B, Table B-3
   degrees of freedom, 228
   F-ratio, 229
   mean squares, 228
   null and alternative hypotheses, 221
   sums of squares, 224-226
Analysis of variance, one-way with repeated measures, 260-266
   critical values. *See* Appendix B, Table B-3
   degrees of freedom, 261
   F-ratio, 264
   mean squares, 263
   null and alternative hypotheses, 260
   sums of squares, 261-263
Analysis of variance, single factor. *See* Analysis of variance, one-way
Analysis of variance, summary table, 231, 245
Analysis of variance, two factor. *See* Analysis of variance, two-way
Analysis of variance, two-way, 232-248
   critical values. *See* Appendix B, Table B-3
   degrees of freedom, 242
   F-ratio, 242
   interaction in, 235
   logic of, 233
   main effects in, 233
   mean squares, 241
   null and alternative hypotheses, 248
   sums of squares, 238-241
Analysis of variance, two-way with repeated measures, 266-279
   critical values. *See* Appendix B, Table B-3
   degrees of freedom, 268
   F-ratio, 272
   interaction in, 278-279
   mean squares, 271-272
   null and alternative hypotheses, 267
   sums of squares, 269-271
ANOVA. *See* Analysis of variance
ANOVA summary table. *See* Analysis of variance, summary table
Arithmetic mean. *See* mean
Association, measures of, 317. *See also* Correlation
Attrition, 12
Average. *See* Mean; Median; Mode

B

Balance point, mean as, 65-67
Bar graph, 35
Beta, 177. *See also* Power
Between-subjects design, 200
Bias
   investigator, 12-13
   sampling, 13
Biased estimate of parameters, 187
Bimodal distributions, 58
Binomial
   expansion, 125-127
   probability, 125-127
Bivariate frequency distribution, 29, 39-41

C

Case study design, 15
Categorical data, 309
Causality, 9, 356
Central Limit Theorem, 138-139
Central tendency. *See* Mean; Median; Mode
Chi-square distribution, 310
Chi-square test
   for goodness of fit, 311-314
   for independence, 314-317
Coefficient of correlation. *See* Correlation
Coefficient of determination, 363, 383
Combinations, 124-125
Combined subgroups
   mean, 69-71
   standard deviation, 84-85
   variance, 84-85
Comparisons among means, *a posteriori* or *post hoc*

Index   481

with Scheffé test, 296-300
with Tukey test, 300-302
Comparisons among means, *a priori* or planned, 294-296
Compound probability, 119-122
Computer
   statistics packages, 18-19
   use in statistics, 16
Conceptual hypothesis, defined, 163
Conditional probability, 117-119
Confidence interval for the difference
   with normal curve, 161-162
   with t-distribution, 193-195
Confidence interval for the mean
   with normal curve, 158-161
   with t-distribution, 192-193
Confidence interval for the proportion, 162-163
Confidence limits. *See* Confidence interval;
   Interval estimation
Constant, 4
Continuous variable, 6
Contrast. *See* Comparisons among means
Control group, 14, 201
Correlated samples. *See* Dependent samples
Correlation, 9, 356
   chi-square, 317
   partial, 389-390
   Pearson, 357, 364
   Spearman, 342-345
Correlational design, 15
Correlational hypothesis, defined, 164
Correlational statistics, 4
Cramer's measure of association, 317
Critical region, 168
Critical values
   defined, 168
   for ANOVA. *See* Appendix B, Table B-3
   for chi-square. *See* Appendix B, Table B-4
   for Mann-Whitney U test. *See* Appendix B, Table B-6
   for Pearson correlation test. *See* Appendix B, Table B-9
   for Spearman rank-order correlation test. *See* Appendix B, Table B-8
   for t-test. *See* Appendix B, Table B-2
   for Tukey test. *See* Appendix B, Table B-5
   for Wilcoxon T test. *See* Appendix B, Table B-7
   for Z-test, 167-168
Cross-cultural design, 15
Cumulative frequency, 31
Curvilinear relationship, 361

D

Data collection procedures, 9
Degrees of freedom
   defined, 189-191
   for ANOVA, one-way, 228
   for ANOVA, one-way with repeated measures, 261
   for ANOVA, two-way, 242
   for ANOVA, two-way with repeated measures, 268
   for chi-square test of goodness of fit, 314
   for chi-square test for independence, 318
   for Kruskal-Wallis test, 342
   for Pearson correlation test, 364
   for Scheffé test, 298
   for t-test for a population mean, 197
   for t-test for the difference between dependent means, 205
   for t-test for the difference between independent means, 198
   for Tukey test, 300
Dependent event, 119
Dependent groups design, 200-203, 259-260, 334-339
Dependent samples
   in ANOVA with repeated measures, 259-260
   in t-test, 203-205
   in Wilcoxon test, 334-339
Dependent variable, 5
Derived score, defined, 92
Descriptive statistics, 2
Design
   between-subjects, 200
   case study, 15
   correlational, 15
   cross-cultural, 15
   dependent groups, 200-203, 259-260, 334-339
   evaluation research, 16
   experimental, 14
   factorial, 237
   matched-groups, 201
   repeated measures, 200-203
   within-groups, 200
Deviation score, defined, 65
Dichotomous variable, 125
Direct-difference method, in t-test, 204-205
Directional alternative hypotheses, 166
Discrete variable, 6
Dispersion, measures of. *See* Range; Standard Deviation; Variance
Distribution-free tests. *See* Non-parametric techniques

E

Empirical distributions, 103-104
Error term, defined, 201
Error variance, 223. *See also* Standard error
Errors of inference. *See* Inferential error
Estimate of parameter, defined, 185
Evaluation research design, 16
Exact limits, 36
Expected frequencies, in chi-square test, 316
Expected value
  of F statistic, 220
  of t for the difference, 204
  of Z for the difference, 172
Experiment-wise error rate
  in ANOVA, 249
  in multiple comparisons, 293-294
Experimental design, 14
Experimental hypothesis, defined, 163
Experimental mortality, 12
Experimental variable, 4
Experimenter bias, 12-13
External validity, 10

F

F-ratio, 229, 242, 264, 272
F' statistic, in Scheffé test, 298
Factorial, 123
Factorial design, 237
Field research, 9
Freedom, degrees of. *See* Degrees of freedom
Frequency
  absolute, 30
  cumulative, 31
  relative, 30
Frequency distributions
  bivariate, 29, 39-41
  graphing, 34-41
  grouped, 33-34
  simple, 30-33
  univariate, 29, 34-39, 41-43
Frequency polygon, 39

G

Goodness of fit test. *See* Chi-square test for goodness of fit
Graphing frequency distributions, 35-41
Grouped frequency distribution, 33-34

H

H statistic, in Kruskal-Wallis test, 340
Hawthorne effect, 13
Heteroscedasticity, in regression, 361-362
Histogram, 36
Homogeneity of variance
  assumptions of, in ANOVA, 248, 280-281
  assumptions of, in t-test for the difference, 199
  defined, 199
Homoscedasticity in regression, 361-362
Honestly significant difference (HSD), in Tukey test, 300
HSD. *See* Honestly significant difference
Hypotheses
  alternative, 165-166
  conceptual, 163
  correlational, 164
  directional alternative, 166
  experimental, 163
  non-directional alternative, 166
  null, 165-166
  research, 163
  statistical, 164-166
Hypothesis testing using the F-distribution. *See* Analysis of variance
Hypothesis testing using the normal curve
  for the difference, 172-174
  for the mean, 170-172
  for the proportion, 174-175
Hypothesis testing using the t-distribution
  for the difference between dependent means, 203-205
  for the difference between independent means, 197-199
  for the population mean, 196-197
Hypothesis testing, non-parametric. *See* Non-parametric techniques

I

Independent event, 119
Independent variable, 4
Inferential error
  in ANOVA, 249
  in multiple comparisons, 293-294
  Type I, defined, 176
  Type II, defined, 176
Inferential statistics, 3
Interaction, in ANOVA, 235, 278-279
Internal validity, 11-13
Interval estimation with the normal curve
  for the difference, 161-162
  for the mean, 158-161
  for the proportion, 162-163
Interval estimation with the t-distribution
  for the difference, 193-195
  for the mean, 192-193
Interval midpoint, 33

Interval variable, 6
Interval width (i), 33
Investigator bias, 12-13

K
Kruskal-Wallis test, 339-342
Kurtosis, 43

L
Laboratory research, 9
Least-squares criterion, in regression, 375-376
Leptokurtic distributions, 43
Limits, exact, 36
Linear regression. *See* Regression, linear
Lower exact limit, 36

M
Main effects, 233
Mann-Whitney U test, 330-335
  critical values. *See* Appendix B, Table B-6
  null and alternative hypotheses for, 330
  Z test for, 333
Matched-groups design, 201
Matched-pairs signed-ranks test. *See* Wilcoxon test
Mathematical variable, 6
Maturation, 12
Mean of population
  calculating, 63-64
  defined, 57
  interpreting, 65-67
  of combined subgroups, 69-71
Mean of sample, 137
Mean squares, 228, 241, 263, 271-272
Means, comparisons. *See* Comparisons among means
Median
  calculating, 59-62
  defined, 57
  interpreting, 65
Methods of measurement, 9
Mid-point of interval, 33
Mode
  calculating, 57-58
  defined, 57
  interpreting, 64-65
Multiple comparisons. *See* Comparisons among means
Multiple correlation coefficient, 385-386
Multiple regression. *See* Regression, multiple
Mutually exclusive interval, 33
Mutually exclusive events, 121

N
Negatively skewed distributions, 42
Nominal variable, 6
Non-directional alternative hypothesis, 166
Non-parametric techniques
  chi-square test for goodness of fit, 311-314
  chi-square test for independence, 314-317
  Kruskal-Wallis test, 339
  Mann-Whitney U test, 330-335
  Rank-order correlation test, 342
  Spearman rank-order correlation test, 342-345
  Wilcoxon test, 335-339
Normal curve
  defined, 104
  equation, 105
  properties, 105
Normality assumption, 179
Notation, statistical, 7
Null hypothesis, defined, 165-166

O
Observation, in measurement, 9
Ogive, 40
One-tailed test, described, 169
One-way ANOVA. *See* Analysis of variance, one-way
Open-ended distributions, 69
Operationalize, 163
Ordinal variable, 7
Ordinate, 35
Organismic variable, 5

P
Parameter
  biased estimate of, 187
  defined, 134
  estimate of, 185
Partial correlation, 389-390
Pearson correlation test
  coefficient, 357, 364
  degrees of freedom for, 364
  t-test for, 364
Percentile
  defined, 92
  calculations, 93-94
Percentile rank
  defined, 92
  calculations, 94-95
Permutations, 122-124
Planned comparisons, 294-296
Platykurtic distributions, 43
Pooled standard deviation, 84-85

Pooled variance, 84-85
Population
  defined, 3
  mean of, 57
  standard deviation of, 79
  variance of, 79
Positively skewed distributions, 42
Post-hoc, 157
Post-hoc comparisons, 296-302
Power
  defined, 177
  estimate of treatment effect, 206-207
Predictive statistics, 4
Proactive history, 11
Probability
  binomial, 125-127
  compound, 119-122
  conditional, 117-119
  dependent events in, 119
  independent events in, 119
  mutually exclusive events in, 121
  simple, 116-117

Q
Quartile, 92

R
Random sample, defined, 135
Random sampling distribution
  defined, 135-136
  of chi-square, 310
  of F, 220
  of H, 340
  of r, 363
  of T, 337
  of t, 188-189
  of the difference between means, 142-147
  of the mean, 136-142
  of the proportion, 148-150
  of U, 332
  of Z, 104-105, 189
Range, 77
Rank-order correlation test, 342
Ratio variable, 7
Real limits. *See* Exact limits
Region of acceptance, 168
Region of rejection, 168
Regression, multiple
  multiple correlation coefficient, 385-386
  multiple regression equation, 386
  partial correlation, 389
  slopes for line of, 387
  standard error of multiple estimate, 388
  Y-intercept for line of, 387

Regression, simple linear
  coefficient of determination, 363, 383
  equation for line of, 377
  homoscedasticity in, 361-362
  least squares criterion, 375-376
  line of, 374
  linearity of, 362
  on the mean, 384
  slope for line of, 377
  standard error of estimate, 381-382
  Y-intercept for line of, 378
Relative frequency, defined, 31
Repeated measures designs
  multi-group designs, 259-260
  non-parametric designs, 334-339
  two-group designs, 200-203
Research design. *See* Design
Research hypothesis, 163
Restriction of range, in correlation, 362
Retroactive history, 11
rho statistic, 343

S
Sample
  defined, 3
  mean of, 137
  notation, 8
  variance, 186
Sampling bias, 13
Sampling distribution. *See* Random sampling distribution
Scattergraph, 40-41
Scheffé test, 296-300
Self-report, in measurement, 9
Shape of frequency distributions, 41-43
Significance level, defined, 167
Simple frequency distribution, 30-33
Simples linear regression. *See* Regression, simple linear
Simple probability, 116-117
Skew, 42
Slope
  in multiple regression, 387
  in simple linear regression, 377
Spearman rank-order correlation test, 342-345
  critical values. *See* Appendix B, Table B-8
Spread sheet, 16
Standard deviation
  calculations, 77-82
  defined, 77
  interpretation, 83
  of combined subgroups, 84-85

of random sampling distribution. *See* Standard error
pooled, 84-85
Standard error
　defined, 137-138
　for planned comparisons, 294
　for the Mann-Whitney U test, 333
　for the r statistic in Pearson's correlation test, 364
　for the Scheffé test, 297
　for the Wilcoxon signed-ranks test, 337
　of estimate, 381
　of multiple estimate, 388
　of the difference, in normal distribution, 144
　of the difference, in t-test for dependent means, 204
　of the difference, in t-test for independent means, 194
　of the mean, in normal distribution, 138
　of the mean, in t-test, 196
　of the proportion, in normal distribution, 149
Standard normal distribution. *See* Normal distribution
Standard score, defined, 185
Standardized tests, in measurement, 10
Statistic, defined, 134
Statistical hypothesis, 164-166
Statistical significance, 171, 176
Stem and leaf diagrams, 38-39
Sums of squares, 224-226, 238-241, 261-263, 269-271
Symbols, statistical, 7-8
Symmetrical distributions, examples of, 41

T
t-distribution
　confidence intervals, 192-195
　defined, 186
　degrees of freedom for, 189
　hypothesis testing, 195-198
　properties of, 186-189
　unbiased estimates in, 186-187
t-score, 186
t-test
　for Pearson's correlation test, 364
　for planned comparisons, 292-295
　for the difference between dependent means, 203-205
　for the difference between independent means, 197-199
　for the population mean, 196-197
T statistic, 335-336. *See also* Wilcoxon signed-ranks test
Testing, effects on validity, 12

Theoretical distributions, 103-104
Treatment effect, 206-207
Tukey test, 300-302
　critical values. *See* Appendix B, Table B-5
Two-tailed test, 169
Two-way ANOVA. *See* Analysis of variance, two-way
Type I error, 176-178
Type II error, 176-178

U
U statistic, in Mann-Whitney test, 330
Unbiased estimates of parameters, 186-187
Univariate frequency distribution, 29, 34-39, 41-43
Upper exact limit, 36

V
Validity, 10
　external, 13-16
　internal, 11-13
Variability, measures of. *See* Range; Standard deviation; Variance
Variable
　continuous, 6
　defined, 4
　dependent, 5
　dichotomous, 125
　discrete, 6
　experimental, 4
　independent, 4
　interval, 6
　mathematical, 6
　nominal , 6
　ordinal, 7
　organismic, 5
　ratio, 7
Variance
　calculations, 77-82
　defined, 77
　interpretation, 82-83
　of combined subgroups, 84-85
　of sample, 186
　pooled, 84-85
　unbiased estimate, 187

W
Wilcoxon signed-ranks test, 335-336
　critical values. See Appendix B, Table B-7
Within-subjects design, 200

Y
Y-intercept
　in multiple regression, 387
　in simple linear regression, 378

Z
Z-distribution, 96-97. *See also* Normal curve
Z-score, 95, 186
Z-tests
    for the difference, 172-174
    for the Mann-Whitney U test, 333
    for the mean, 170-172
    for the proportion, 174-175
    for the Wilcoxon signed-ranks test, 337